Essentials of Anesthesiology

Essentials of Anesthesiology

Edited by Quentin Hardy

AMERICAN
MEDICAL PUBLISHERS
www.americanmedicalpublishers.com

American Medical Publishers,
41 Flatbush Avenue,
1st Floor, New York,
NY 11217, USA

Visit us on the World Wide Web at:
www.americanmedicalpublishers.com

ISBN: 978-1-63927-534-2

Cataloging-in-Publication Data

Essentials of anesthesiology / edited by Quentin Hardy.
p. cm.
Includes bibliographical references and index.
ISBN 978-1-63927-534-2
1. Anesthesiology. 2. Anesthesia. 3. Anesthesia services.
4. Anesthesia--Complications. I. Hardy, Quentin.

RD81 .E77 2022

617.96--dc23

Table of Contents

Preface

Anesthesiology is a medical branch which is concerned with the total perioperative care of patients required before, during and after the surgery. There are various sub-fields of anesthesiology including critical emergency medicine, intensive care medicine and pain medicine. It primarily makes use of anesthesia and anesthetics to support key functions of a patient's body during the perioperative period. Anesthesiology is a broader field that requires knowledge of various areas such as pharmacology, mechanical ventilation and other areas of medicine such as cardiology, pulmonology and obstetrics to evaluate the risk of anesthesia. It also includes the anatomical knowledge of the nervous system for nerve blocks. This book discusses the fundamentals as well as modern approaches to anesthesiology. From theories to research to practical applications, case studies related to all contemporary topics of relevance to this field have been included in this book. It is an essential guide for both academicians and those who wish to pursue this discipline further.

The information shared in this book is based on empirical researches made by veterans in this field of study. The elaborative information provided in this book will help the readers further their scope of knowledge leading to advancements in this field.

Finally, I would like to thank my fellow researchers who gave constructive feedback and my family members who supported me at every step of my research.

Editor

1

Sleep and anesthesia: can we use a physiologic model to decrease risks of a medical intervention

Samira Rajaei[1], **Ali Dabbagh**[2*]

Abstract

Anesthesiology is one of the most important creations of the modern science, basically based on the anesthetic drugs; however, there are a few concerns regarding the effects of the anesthetic drugs. Would there be any progress in the current trend of anesthesiology, both clinically and basically. There would be a possibility to use the physiologic mechanisms of sleep to be incorporated into clinical practice instead of pharmacologic agents in order to decrease their unwanted effects.

Keywords: Sleep, Anesthesia, Analgesia, Mechanism, Pain

1. Immunology Department, School of Medicine, Tehran University of Medical Sciences, Tehran, Iran
2. Cardiac Anesthesiology Department, Anesthesiology Research Center, Shahid Beheshti University of Medical Sciences, Tehran, Iran

Corresponding Author:
Ali Dabbagh, MD. Professor, Anesthesiology Research Center, Cardiac Anesthesiology Department, Shahid Beheshti University of Medical Sciences, Tehran, Iran.
E-mail: alidabbagh@yahoo.com

Introduction

Anesthesiology is a relatively new convention of medicine. Many surgeries are nowadays performed just because we can anesthetize patients; otherwise, there was no progress in the many fields of surgery. In the United States, nearly 60,000 patients are anesthetized each day, mainly for surgical operation.

The first time that anesthesia was "created", one of the greatest fears of mankind was overcome (1): since the first patient was anesthetized in October 16, 1846 by Dr William T. G. Morton at Massachusetts General Hospital, Boston, the science and practice of anesthesiology has made many great developments, increasing its efficacy and safety and at the same time, decreasing the anesthesia-related morbidity and mortality (2, 3).

In the current era of modern anesthesiology, the practice and science of anesthesia is composed of 4 basic elements; each being one of its permanent counterparts; without each of them, anesthesia is not complete. These 4 basic elements are (4, 5):

1) hypnosis (an iatrogenic pharmacologic-based coma)
2) amnesia (forgetting the unpleasant events during operation)
3) analgesia (painlessness)
4) akinesia (lack of movements in response to noxious stimuli, including the surgical incisions and manipulations).

Very interesting issue is that all of these basic elements of anesthesia are created after interaction of anesthetic drugs with different parts of the nervous system (including central, peripheral, and autonomic nervous systems). However, CNS remains the primary site of action for "anesthesia". In other words, anesthesia is an iatrogenic, reversible, pharmacologic-based coma; affecting CNS neuronal circuits at many levels including the molecular level; for example, the mechanism of anesthesia in some volatile agents (i.e. Isoflurane and Sevoflurane) is through inhibition of orexinergic neurons; also, ketamine acts through “pyramidal cells and also, seven different types of CA1 interneurons” (6-13) or amnesia is induced primarily through effects of anesthetics on hippocampus neurons (14-16). Also, the majority of CNS anesthetics act through N-methyl-D-aspartate (NMDA) receptor or gamma-amino butyric acid (GABA) receptor subunits (17-30).

Globally, some believe that anesthesia induction is due to “drug-induced global modulation of neuronal function”; meanwhile, termination of anesthesia is spontaneous and passive, occurring after termination of pharmacologic effects of anesthetics from “their sites in the central nervous system”; though this mechanism might be somewhat oversimplification and the neural inertia could have a role (31-36).

But are we doing anesthesia in a right way? Are the modern anesthetic drugs as safe and physiology-compatible as we want? To answer this questions, one could consider the many animal and human studies proving the very safe anesthetic agents and the very diminutive incidence of unwanted effects of anesthetic drugs. Despite the many available proofs for modern anesthesia safety, there are some considerations regarding the effects of anesthetics on organ functions described in the following paragraphs.

If we want to discuss more specifically, anesthesia is not so much physiologic. It is demonstrated in cerebral cortex and hippocampus neurons of rats that neuronal spikes from these sites are “very stable across physiologic states i.e. waking, slow-wave sleep and rapid-eye-movement sleep”; however, these neuronal spikes and avalanches “would collapse during anesthesia”. Also, waiting time distributions obey a single scaling function during all natural behavioral states, but not during anesthesia (34, 36-38).

From another viewpoint, anesthesia is an iatrogenic pharmacologic based coma; of course with a reversible nature. In fact, electroencephalographic studies performed in patients undergoing general anesthesia has demonstrated an EEG pattern similar to patients with coma; in other words, the EEG waves in "comatose patients" and "patients undergoing general anesthesia" both demonstrate high amplitude, low-frequency waves (4, 39, 40).

Now let's discuss the issue from a different viewpoint; i.e. the neurophysiologic point of view. During normal sleep, the arousal status is depressed and we would go unconscious. During the rapid eye movement (REM) phase of sleep, EEG waves have an active high-frequency, low-amplitude pattern; while in the non- rapid eye movement (Non-REM) phase of sleep the EEG waves are high amplitude, low frequency (33, 39-44). In contrast to this dual stage pattern of EEG in sleep, the EEG pattern in "general anesthesia" or "coma" has high amplitude, low-frequency waves. Although coma and general anesthesia have some similarities with the Non-REM phase of sleep, "coma and general anesthesia" are not the same as Non-REM (4, 32, 41, 45, 46). As we see, EEG assessments also suggest us that possibly; the current anesthetic pharmacologic agents are not as physiologic as we need.

Concerning the clinical point of view may be all above comments are not as worrying as the following lines of this paragraph; which addresses a sample of the many studies published mainly in the last decade. There are an increasing number of evidence demonstrating the unwanted effects of anesthetic agents on the synaptogenesis processes in the animal neonates receiving modern anesthetic agents; these animal and lab studies have demonstrated the clues to apoptotic effects of anesthetics; some even well demonstrating these effects on animal CNS; though human CNS studies are not so much available due to technical problems (12, 46-74); also, there are a number of studies raising the questions regarding the effects of some of the current anesthetic agents on the behavioral and learning aspects of the human neonates, though none of them still have not presented definite proof for this effect (75).

There are some new windows which could help us use the sleep mechanism as a “physiologic mechanism” instead of the current “pharmacologic mechanism” for anesthesia. In one direction, there is a concordance between interventions which disturb sleep and/or cause some types of somatic pain; in other words, these interventions have the “same direction effects” for pain and sleep; i.e. there is a concordance between them (76-79); so, possibly we could use the physiologic mechanisms maintaining normal sleep for suppressing those surgical stimuli which create pain. On the other hand, we could use some newer molecules like urethane which could induce anesthesia with mechanisms different from current anesthetics; it means that urethane induces anesthesia with a mechanism "closely mimicking natural sleep" (8, 80-83).

Conclusion

The above paragraphs are brief concerns regarding the importance of a new look at our current approach for a very common medical practice. In other words, in the current era of clinical and basic studies, the effects of anesthetic agents in creating the "pharmacological coma" is a very important concern with high priority, in medicine, in pharmaceutical studies and more importantly, in neuroscience. We anticipate a very important turning point, which would add another improvement to the safety of anesthesia and add another revolution to the previous "jump up's" of this field of medicine, as a number of relatively safe anesthetic agents have emerged and shown to be neuroprotective (5, 84-90); however, this time, the turning point would be at the cellular and subcellular levels.

Acknowledgment

The authors would like to acknowledge the kind help of Anesthesiology Research Center, Shahid Beheshti University of Medical Sciences, Tehran, Iran for their invaluable support.

Conflicts of Interest

The authors declare that there are no conflicts of interest.

References

1. Robinson DH, Toledo AH. Historical development of modern anesthesia. J Invest Surg. 2012;25(3):141-9.

2. LeVasseur R, Desai SP. Ebenezer Hopkins Frost (1824-1866): William T.G. Morton's first identified patient and why he was invited to the Ether demonstration of October 16, 1846. Anesthesiology. 2012;117(2):238-42.

3. Bause GS, Sim PP. C.T. Jackson's 15 October 1846 letter to J.-B.A.L. Elie de Beaumont: Jackson's thoughts on Ether Day's Eve? Bull Anesth Hist. 2011;29(1):12-4.

4. Brown EN, Lydic R, Schiff ND. General anesthesia, sleep, and coma. N Engl J Med. 2010;363(27):2638-50.

5. Sanders RD, Tononi G, Laureys S, Sleigh JW. Unresponsiveness not equal unconsciousness. Anesthesiology. 2012;116(4):946-59.

6. Kelz MB, Sun Y, Chen J, Cheng Meng Q, Moore JT, Veasey SC, et al. An essential role for orexins in emergence from general anesthesia. Proceedings of the National Academy of Sciences of the United States of America. 2008;105(4):1309-14.

7. Laorden ML, Ferenczi S, Pinter-Kubler B, Gonzalez-Martin LL, Lasheras MC, Kovacs KJ, et al. Hypothalamic orexin--a neurons are involved in the response of the brain stress system to morphine withdrawal. PLoS One. 2012;7(5):e36871.

8. Clement EA, Richard A, Thwaites M, Ailon J, Peters S, Dickson CT. Cyclic and sleep-like spontaneous alternations of brain state under urethane anaesthesia. PLoS One. 2008;3(4):e2004.

9. Seamari Y, Narvaez JA, Vico FJ, Lobo D, Sanchez-Vives MV. Robust off- and online separation of intracellularly recorded up and down cortical states. PLoS One. 2007;2(9):e888.

10. Reig R, Sanchez-Vives MV. Synaptic transmission and plasticity in an active cortical network. PLoS One. 2007;2(7):e670.

11. Kuang H, Lin L, Tsien JZ. Temporal dynamics of distinct CA1 cell populations during unconscious state induced by ketamine. PLoS One. 2010;5(12):e15209.

12. Chen G, Gong M, Yan M, Zhang X. Sevoflurane induces endoplasmic reticulum stress mediated apoptosis in hippocampal neurons of aging rats. PLoS One. 2013;8(2):e57870.

13. Forgacs PB, Frey HP, Velazquez A, Thompson S, Brodie D, Moitra V, et al. Dynamic regimes of neocortical activity linked to corticothalamic integrity correlate with outcomes in acute anoxic brain injury after cardiac arrest. Annals of clinical and translational neurology. 2017;4(2):119-29.

14. Perouansky M, Pearce RA. How we recall (or don't): the hippocampal memory machine and anesthetic amnesia. Can J Anaesth. 2011;58(2):157-66.

15. Wang DS, Orser BA. Inhibition of learning and memory by general anesthetics. Can J Anaesth. 2011;58(2):167-77.

16. Changeux JP. Conscious processing: implications for general anesthesia. Curr Opin Anaesthesiol. 2012;25(4):397-404.

17. Dong Y, Wu X, Zhang G, Xu Z, Zhang Y, Gautam V, et al. Isoflurane facilitates synaptic NMDA receptor endocytosis in mice primary neurons. Curr Mol Med. 2012.

18. Esencan E, Yuksel S, Tosun YB, Robinot A, Solaroglu I, Zhang JH. XENON in medical area: emphasis on neuroprotection in hypoxia and anesthesia. Med Gas Res. 2013;3(1):4.

19. Jin J, Gong K, Zou X, Wang R, Lin Q, Chen J. The blockade of NMDA receptor ion channels by ketamine is enhanced in developing rat cortical neurons. Neuroscience letters. 2013;539:11-5.

20. Kuhlmann L, Foster BL, Liley DT. Modulation of Functional EEG Networks by the NMDA Antagonist Nitrous Oxide. PLoS One. 2013;8(2):e56434.

21. Liu CL, Gao M, Jin GZ, Zhen X. GABA neurons in the ventral tegmental area responding to peripheral sensory input. PLoS One. 2012;7(12):e51507.

22. Liu F, Patterson TA, Sadovova N, Zhang X, Liu S, Zou X, et al. Ketamine-induced neuronal damage and altered N-methyl-D-aspartate receptor function in rat primary forebrain culture. Toxicol

Sci. 2013;131(2):548-57.
23. Wang S, Tian Y, Song L, Lim G, Tan Y, You Z, et al. Exacerbated mechanical hyperalgesia in rats with genetically predisposed depressive behavior: role of melatonin and NMDA receptors. Pain. 2012;153(12):2448-57.
24. Trudell JR, Bertaccini E, Maciver MB. Teaching an old GABA receptor new tricks. Anesth Analg. 2012;115(2):270-3.
25. Akk G, Steinbach JH. Structural studies of the actions of anesthetic drugs on the gamma-aminobutyric acid type A receptor. Anesthesiology. 2011;115(6):1338-48.
26. Forman SA. Clinical and molecular pharmacology of etomidate. Anesthesiology. 2011;114(3):695-707.
27. Saari TI, Uusi-Oukari M, Ahonen J, Olkkola KT. Enhancement of GABAergic activity: neuropharmacological effects of benzodiazepines and therapeutic use in anesthesiology. Pharmacological reviews. 2011;63(1):243-67.
28. Olsen RW, Li GD. GABA(A) receptors as molecular targets of general anesthetics: identification of binding sites provides clues to allosteric modulation. Can J Anaesth. 2011;58(2):206-15.
29. Drexler B, Antkowiak B, Engin E, Rudolph U. Identification and characterization of anesthetic targets by mouse molecular genetics approaches. Can J Anaesth. 2011;58(2):178-90.
30. Kafashan M, Ching S, Palanca BJ. Sevoflurane Alters Spatiotemporal Functional Connectivity Motifs That Link Resting-State Networks during Wakefulness. Frontiers in neural circuits. 2016;10:107.
31. Friedman EB, Sun Y, Moore JT, Hung HT, Meng QC, Perera P, et al. A conserved behavioral state barrier impedes transitions between anesthetic-induced unconsciousness and wakefulness: evidence for neural inertia. PLoS One. 2010;5(7):e11903.
32. Brown RE, Basheer R, McKenna JT, Strecker RE, McCarley RW. Control of sleep and wakefulness. Physiol Rev. 2012;92(3):1087-187.
33. Cannon J, McCarthy MM, Lee S, Lee J, Borgers C, Whittington MA, et al. Neurosystems: brain rhythms and cognitive processing. The European journal of neuroscience. 2014;39(5):705-19.
34. Kepecs A, Tan AY. Spatial diversity of spontaneous activity in the cortex. The Journal of neuroscience : the official journal of the Society for Neuroscience. 2015;9:48.
35. Vincent JL, Shehabi Y, Walsh TS, Pandharipande PP, Ball JA, Spronk P, et al. Comfort and patient-centred care without excessive sedation: the eCASH concept. Intensive Care Med. 2016;42(6):962-71.
36. Mitra A, Raichle ME. How networks communicate: propagation patterns in spontaneous brain activity. Philosophical transactions of the Royal Society of London Series B, Biological sciences. 2016;371(1705).
37. Ribeiro TL, Copelli M, Caixeta F, Belchior H, Chialvo DR, Nicolelis MA, et al. Spike avalanches exhibit universal dynamics across the sleep-wake cycle. PLoS One. 2010;5(11):e14129.
38. Lin SC, Brown RE. Optogenetic Dissection of the Basal Forebrain Neuromodulatory Control of Cortical Activation, Plasticity, and Cognition. 2015;35(41):13896-903.
39. Stamatakis EA, Adapa RM, Absalom AR, Menon DK. Changes in resting neural connectivity during propofol sedation. PLoS One. 2010;5(12):e14224.
40. Mitra A, Snyder AZ, Tagliazucchi E, Laufs H, Raichle ME. Propagated infra-slow intrinsic brain activity reorganizes across wake and slow wave sleep. eLife. 2015;4.
41. Lydic R, Baghdoyan HA. Sleep, anesthesiology, and the neurobiology of arousal state control. Anesthesiology. 2005;103(6):1268-95.
42. McCarthy MM, Ching S, Whittington MA, Kopell N. Dynamical changes in neurological diseases and anesthesia. Current opinion in neurobiology. 2012;22(4):693-703.
43. Picchioni D, Duyn JH, Horovitz SG. Sleep and the functional connectome. NeuroImage. 2013;80:387-96.
44. Purdon PL, Sampson A, Pavone KJ, Brown EN. Clinical Electroencephalography for Anesthesiologists: Part I: Background and Basic Signatures. Anesthesiology. 2015;123(4):937-60.
45. Brown EN, Purdon PL, Van Dort CJ. General anesthesia and altered states of arousal: a systems neuroscience analysis. Annu Rev Neurosci. 2011;34:601-28.
46. Sivadas N, Radhakrishnan A, Aswathy BS, Kumar VM, Gulia KK. Dynamic changes in sleep pattern during post-partum in normal pregnancy in rat model. Behavioural brain research. 2017;320:264-74.
47. Creeley CE, Olney JW. The young: neuroapoptosis induced by anesthetics and what to do about it. Anesth Analg. 2010;110(2):442-8.
48. Jevtovic-Todorovic V. Developmental synaptogenesis and general anesthesia: a kiss of death? Curr Pharm Des. 2012;18(38):6225-31.
49. Jevtovic-Todorovic V, Hartman RE, Izumi Y, Benshoff ND, Dikranian K, Zorumski CF, et al. Early exposure to common anesthetic agents causes widespread neurodegeneration in the developing rat brain and persistent learning deficits. The Journal of neuroscience : the official journal of the Society for Neuroscience. 2003;23(3):876-82.
50. Jevtovic-Todorovic V, Olney JW. PRO: Anesthesia-induced developmental neuroapoptosis: status of the evidence. Anesth Analg. 2008;106(6):1659-63.
51. McCann ME, Soriano SG. General anesthetics in pediatric anesthesia: influences on the developing brain. Current drug targets. 2012;13(7):944-51.
52. Mellon RD, Simone AF, Rappaport BA. Use of anesthetic agents in neonates and young children. Anesth Analg. 2007;104(3):509-20.
53. Persson J. Wherefore ketamine? Curr Opin Anaesthesiol. 2010;23(4):455-60.
54. Vutskits L. Anesthetic-related neurotoxicity and the developing brain: shall we change practice? Paediatr Drugs. 2012;14(1):13-21.
55. Allegaert K. The clinical pharmacology of short acting analgo-sedatives in neonates. Curr Clin Pharmacol. 2011;6(4):222-6.
56. Allegaert K, Tibboel D, van den Anker J. Pharmacological treatment of neonatal pain: In search of a new equipoise. Semin Fetal Neonatal Med. 2013;18(1):42-7.
57. Brambrink AM, Back SA, Riddle A, Gong X, Moravec MD, Dissen GA, et al. Isoflurane-induced apoptosis of oligodendrocytes in the neonatal primate brain. Annals of neurology. 2012;72(4):525-35.
58. Brambrink AM, Evers AS, Avidan MS, Farber NB, Smith DJ, Martin LD, et al. Ketamine-induced neuroapoptosis in the fetal and neonatal rhesus macaque brain. Anesthesiology. 2012;116(2):372-

84.
59. Brambrink AM, Evers AS, Avidan MS, Farber NB, Smith DJ, Zhang X, et al. Isoflurane-induced neuroapoptosis in the neonatal rhesus macaque brain. Anesthesiology. 2010;112(4):834-41.
60. Brambrink AM, Orfanakis A, Kirsch JR. Anesthetic neurotoxicity. Anesthesiol Clin. 2012;30(2):207-28.
61. Koerner IP, Brambrink AM. Brain protection by anesthetic agents. Curr Opin Anaesthesiol. 2006;19(5):481-6.
62. McCann ME, Soriano SG. Is anesthesia bad for the newborn brain? Anesthesiol Clin. 2009;27(2):269-84.
63. Reddy SV. Effect of general anesthetics on the developing brain. Journal of anaesthesiology, clinical pharmacology. 2012;28(1):6-10.
64. Schubert H, Eiselt M, Walter B, Fritz H, Brodhun M, Bauer R. Isoflurane/nitrous oxide anesthesia and stress-induced procedures enhance neuroapoptosis in intrauterine growth-restricted piglets. Intensive Care Med. 2012;38(7):1205-14.
65. Zhou ZW, Shu Y, Li M, Guo X, Pac-Soo C, Maze M, et al. The glutaminergic, GABAergic, dopaminergic but not cholinergic neurons are susceptible to anaesthesia-induced cell death in the rat developing brain. Neuroscience. 2011;174:64-70.
66. Bai X, Yan Y, Canfield S, Muravyeva MY, Kikuchi C, Zaja I, et al. Ketamine Enhances Human Neural Stem Cell Proliferation and Induces Neuronal Apoptosis via Reactive Oxygen Species-Mediated Mitochondrial Pathway. Anesth Analg. 2013;116(4):869-80.
67. Bajic D, Commons KG, Soriano SG. Morphine-enhanced apoptosis in selective brain regions of neonatal rats. Int J Dev Neurosci. 2013;31(4):258-66.
68. Boscolo A, Milanovic D, Starr JA, Sanchez V, Oklopcic A, Moy L, et al. Early Exposure to General Anesthesia Disturbs Mitochondrial Fission and Fusion in the Developing Rat Brain. Anesthesiology. 2013.
69. Jevtovic-Todorovic V, Boscolo A, Sanchez V, Lunardi N. Anesthesia-induced developmental neurodegeneration: the role of neuronal organelles. Frontiers in neurology. 2012;3:141.
70. Lei X, Guo Q, Zhang J. Mechanistic insights into neurotoxicity induced by anesthetics in the developing brain. International journal of molecular sciences. 2012;13(6):6772-99.
71. Liu JR, Liu Q, Li J, Baek C, Han XH, Athiraman U, et al. Noxious stimulation attenuates ketamine-induced neuroapoptosis in the developing rat brain. Anesthesiology. 2012;117(1):64-71.
72. Yu D, Jiang Y, Gao J, Liu B, Chen P. Repeated exposure to propofol potentiates neuroapoptosis and long-term behavioral deficits in neonatal rats. Neuroscience letters. 2013;534:41-6.
73. Mintz CD, Smith SC, Barrett KM, Benson DL. Anesthetics interfere with the polarization of developing cortical neurons. J Neurosurg Anesthesiol. 2012;24(4):368-75.
74. Lewis LD, Weiner VS, Mukamel EA, Donoghue JA, Eskandar EN, Madsen JR, et al. Rapid fragmentation of neuronal networks at the onset of propofol-induced unconsciousness. Proceedings of the National Academy of Sciences of the United States of America. 2012;109(49):E3377-86.
75. Davidson AJ. Anesthesia and neurotoxicity to the developing brain: the clinical relevance. Paediatr Anaesth. 2011;21(7):716-21.
76. Doufas AG, Panagiotou OA, Ioannidis JP. Concordance of sleep and pain outcomes of diverse interventions: an umbrella review. PLoS One. 2012;7(7):e40891.
77. Cascella M. Mechanisms underlying brain monitoring during anesthesia: limitations, possible improvements, and perspectives. Korean J Anesthesiol. 2016;69(2):113-20.
78. Ching S, Brown EN. Modeling the dynamical effects of anesthesia on brain circuits. Current opinion in neurobiology. 2014;25:116-22.
79. Horner RL, Hughes SW, Malhotra A. State-dependent and reflex drives to the upper airway: basic physiology with clinical implications. Journal of applied physiology (Bethesda, Md : 1985). 2014;116(3):325-36.
80. Pagliardini S, Greer JJ, Funk GD, Dickson CT. State-dependent modulation of breathing in urethane-anesthetized rats. The Journal of neuroscience : the official journal of the Society for Neuroscience. 2012;32(33):11259-70.
81. Whitten TA, Martz LJ, Guico A, Gervais N, Dickson CT. Heat synch: inter- and independence of body-temperature fluctuations and brain-state alternations in urethane-anesthetized rats. J Neurophysiol. 2009;102(3):1647-56.
82. Wolansky T, Clement EA, Peters SR, Palczak MA, Dickson CT. Hippocampal slow oscillation: a novel EEG state and its coordination with ongoing neocortical activity. The Journal of neuroscience : the official journal of the Society for Neuroscience. 2006;26(23):6213-29.
83. Sharma AV, Wolansky T, Dickson CT. A comparison of sleeplike slow oscillations in the hippocampus under ketamine and urethane anesthesia. J Neurophysiol. 2010;104(2):932-9.
84. Dabbagh A, Rajaei S. Xenon: a solution for anesthesia in liver disease? Hepat Mon. 2012;12(11):e8437.
85. Benggon M, Chen H, Applegate R, Martin R, Zhang JH. Effect of dexmedetomidine on brain edema and neurological outcomes in surgical brain injury in rats. Anesth Analg. 2012;115(1):154-9.
86. Blaudszun G, Lysakowski C, Elia N, Tramer MR. Effect of perioperative systemic alpha2 agonists on postoperative morphine consumption and pain intensity: systematic review and meta-analysis of randomized controlled trials. Anesthesiology. 2012;116(6):1312-22.
87. Hong JY, Kim WO, Yoon Y, Choi Y, Kim SH, Kil HK. Effects of intravenous dexmedetomidine on low-dose bupivacaine spinal anaesthesia in elderly patients. Acta Anaesthesiol Scand. 2012;56(3):382-7.
88. Lin Y, He B, Chen J, Wang Z. Can dexmedetomidine be a safe and efficacious sedative agent in post-cardiac surgery patients: a meta-analysis? Crit Care. 2012;16(5):R169.
89. Bantel C, Maze M, Trapp S. Neuronal preconditioning by inhalational anesthetics: evidence for the role of plasmalemmal adenosine triphosphate-sensitive potassium channels. Anesthesiology. 2009;110(5):986-95.
90. Bantel C, Maze M, Trapp S. Noble gas xenon is a novel adenosine triphosphate-sensitive potassium channel opener. Anesthesiology. 2010;112(3):623-30.

Anesthetic management of patients with Klippel-Feil syndrome

Kamran Mottaghi[1], Farhad Safari[1], Parisa Sezari[1], Naeime Gholizadeh[1], Masoud Nashibi[1]*

Abstract

Klippel-Feil syndrome (KFS) is a rare entity which is characterized by failure of normal segmentation of cervical vertebrae resulting in short neck with restricted movement and cervical instability. This anomaly increases the risk of neurological damage during airway instrumentation like laryngoscopy and positioning for surgery. We report three patients, a 42 years old man with KFS who scheduled for craniocervical fusion under general anesthesia, a 6 years old girl candidate for cleft palate repair and a 26 years old woman candidate for craniocervical fusion. All the patients were successfully managed using fiberoptic bronchoscope in first two cases and gum elastic bougie (GEB) in the last case.

Keywords: Klippel-Feil syndrome; Fiberoptic Bronchoscope; Gum Elastic Bougie

1. Anesthesiology Research Center, Shahid Beheshti University of Medical Sciences, Tehran, Iran

Corresponding Author:
Masoud Nashibi, MD, Assistant Professor, Anesthesiology Research Center, Shahid Beheshti University of Medical Sciences, Tehran, Iran, E-mail: masoudnashibi@sbmu.ac.ir

Introduction

Most of the rare genetic disorders are considered as great challenges for anesthesiologists (1-3). KFS is a rare congenital fusion of cervical vertebrae due to a failure in the segmentation process of the cervical vertebrae in the early weeks of gestation and also may have other associated anomalies. The clinical presentation is known as the classic triad of short neck, limited neck movements and a low posterior hairline (4, 5). There are three subtypes of the condition classified according to the extent of vertebral involvement. KFS appears to be an etiologically heterogeneous condition with sporadic occurrence, autosomal dominant and autosomal recessive modes of inheritance reported. Gunderson suggested that KFS is a genetic condition, whereas Gray found a low incidence of inheritance (6). Two small studies suggested that mutations of the MEOX1 gene, which codes for mesenchyme homeobox 1, may cause a recessive subtype of this syndrome (7, 8).

The incidence of KFS is 1:42,000 births and is one of the common congenital causes of difficult airway (4, 6).

The spinal deformities and increased risk of neurological damage during airway management is a challenge for anesthesiologist (9); hence, their anesthetic management should be carefully planned considering other comorbidities. We report successful anesthetic management in patients with KFS and associated anomalies and also review the literature regarding the various methods used for airway management in these cases.

Brief Report

Case 1

A 42 years old man was scheduled for craniocervical fixation. He was a known case of KFS with a short webbed neck. On examination the patient had a pulse rate of 86 beats/ min and a blood pressure of 125/82 mmHg. Examination of the airway showed that there was limited flexion and extension of the upper cervical spine, he had an adequate mouth opening and his Mallampati grade was 3. The systemic examination was normal. His other investigations were all within normal limits, except Magnetic Resonance Imaging (MRI) of the cervical spine which showed fusion of the upper cervical spines and brain stem compression (figure 1), scoliosis (figure 2) and sabre shaped tibial bone (figure 3).

Since anatomical landmarks in the neck were distorted and a difficult airway was anticipated, an awake fiberoptic intubation was planned.

The day before surgery, the procedure was explained to the patient. He was kept nil by mouth for 8 hours. On the day of surgery the patient was brought to the operating room where his ECG, SpO2 and BP were monitored and an intravenous access secured with an 18G cannula on his right hand. Atropine (0.25 mg/IV) injected to desiccate patient's saliva. After calculating the maximum safe dose of local anesthetic, the patient was given 2% lidocaine viscous gargles which he was asked to swallow so as to coat the posterior surface of the epiglottis. This was followed by aliquots of a 10% xylocaine spray which was installed into each nares, with the patient taking deep breaths. Minimal sedation with 1mg midazolam and 50μg fentanyl was given intravenously to keep the patient calm, while the reversal agents were at hand. Phenylephrine nasal drop applied to each nostril and 2% lidocaine gel sniffed by the patient. Fiberoptic bronchoscope advanced through the right nostril. After visualizing the vocal cords, two ml of 2% lidocaine was injected through the side port of the fiberoptic bronchoscope to anesthetize the airway and vocal cords. The fiberoptic bronchoscope was then introduced into the trachea, the tracheal rings and the carina identified, the endotracheal tube inserted and its position confirmed after removal of the fiberoptic

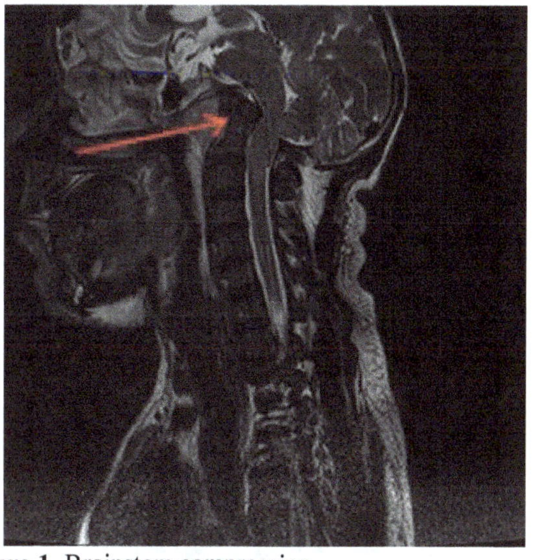

Figure 1. Brainstem compression.

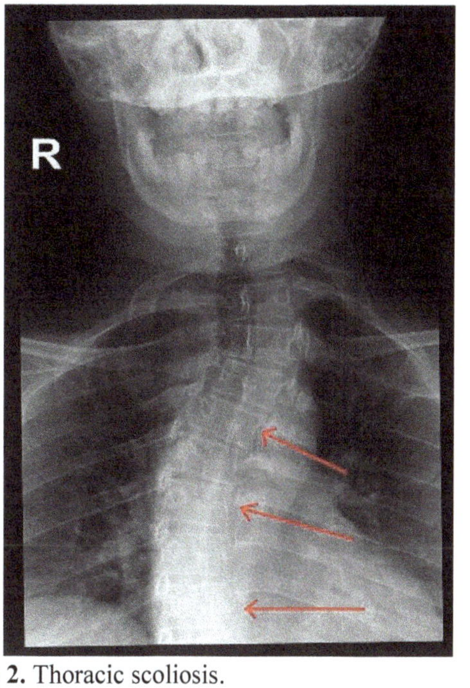

Figure 2. Thoracic scoliosis.

bronchoscope, by the chest movements as seen on inspection and bilateral symmetric air entry on auscultation. The EtCO2 further confirmed correct placement of the endotracheal tube which was then fixed properly. Then Propofol 100 mg was given intravenously, the patient was then paralyzed with a non-depolarizing neuromuscular blocker (Atracurium) and anesthesia was maintained with isoflurane, 50% nitrous oxide and 50% oxygen, and fentanyl 50μg/hour.

Surgery proceeded uneventfully and patient

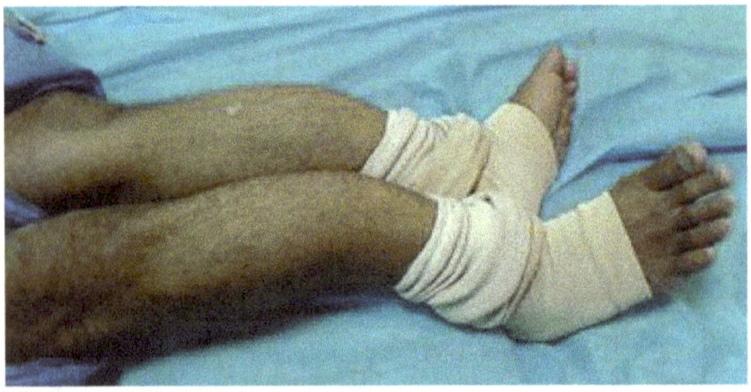

Figure 3. Sabre shaped tibia bone.

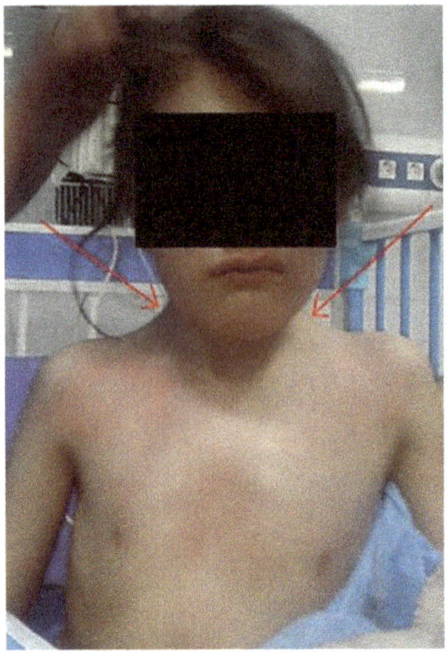

Figure 4. Webbed neck.

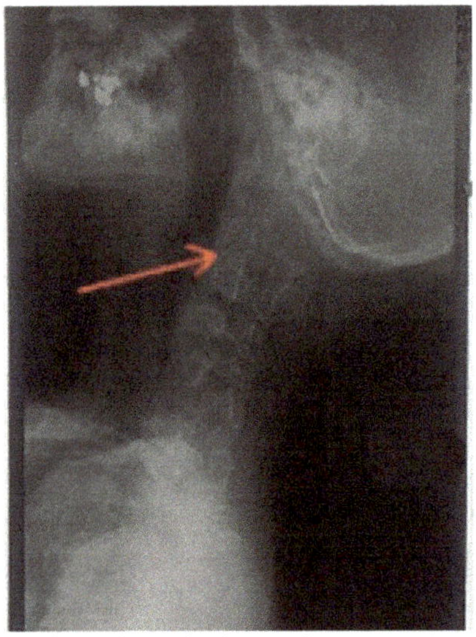

Figure 5. Fusion of cervical Vertebrae.

transferred to the Intensive Care Unit (ICU). On the next morning, he transferred to Operation theatre for extubation which was uneventful.

Case 2

A six years old girl, known case of KFS was a candidate for cleft palate repair. The patient had webbed neck (figure 4), cervical spine vertebrae fusion (figure 5), scoliosis, barrel chest (figure 6), dental deformities and severe limitation in head extension and rotation and mouth opening. The vital signs, lab data and respiration were normal. Since the patient was a six-year old girl, she was not cooperative enough to perform an awake fiberoptic tracheal intubation. On the other hand, we were concerned about airway management and probable difficulty in mask ventilation and tracheal intubation so we decided to intubate the patient using a fiberoptic bronchoscope after inhalational induction with sevoflurane. The incremental percentage of sevoflurane was used. After ten minutes patient's eyes were in central position, respiration had a regular pattern and Cerebral State Monitoring (CSM) showed the depth of anesthesia at 40. In the first attempt, we failed since the passage was obstructed by tongue. For the second attempt, jaw thrust performed which lifted the tongue and opened the passage and fiberoptic passed through the trachea and tracheal tube slit over. Surgery lasted about 2 hours. At the end the residual muscle relaxation reversed using neostigmine and atropine. The procedure completed uneventfully.

Case 3

A twenty-six years old woman complaining of mild weakness and paresthesia in all the four limbs was admitted for operative treatment of the cervical spine. The illness started one year back and had a progressive course necessitating her admission.

The patient had been diagnosed to have KFS several years previously and was a known case of hypothyroidism who was on levothyroxine treatment.

On examination the patient was a short, moderately built woman with a pulse rate of 85/ minute and a blood pressure of 130/80 mmHg. She had a short webbed neck and a low posterior hairline with a limited extension of the neck (figure 7). Flexion and rotation were however not limited. She had an adequate mouth opening and her Mallampati grade was 3. Thyromental span was 6 cm. No dental abnormality or occlusion was present.

Cervical spine x-rays showed fusions at C2 to

C3 levels and C5 to C7 (figure 8). Chest x-ray showed thoracic kypho-scoliosis (figure 9).

Induction was conducted using sevoflurane 8% and 50% mixture of N20 and O2. When sufficient depth of anesthesia was reached, head fixation was applied gently by an attending neurosurgeon, a check laryngoscopy (Macintosh blade 4) was done and there was difficulty in visualization of the vocal cords so we used GEB as the first alternative technique in case of difficult intubation. The endotracheal tube slit over GEB and its position confirmed by the chest movements as seen on inspection and bilateral equal air entry on auscultation. The EtCO2 further confirmed correct placement of the endotracheal tube.

After securing the orotracheal tube, the patient was rotated to the prone position with necessary precautions and maintenance of anesthesia managed with propofol infusion and non-depolarizing neuromuscular blocker.

After completion of the surgery, which lasted 300 min, the patient was returned back to the supine position and residual muscle paralysis reversed with neostigmine 4mg and atropine 1.2mg. Extubation of the trachea was accomplished after ensuring that the patient was awake and had adequate respiration. Post-operatively the patient was monitored in the recovery room after which she was sent to the ward.

Discussion

Rare congenital and genetic disorders are a great challenge for anesthesiologists. KFS occurs due to a failure of normal segmentation of the cervical spines in the 3rd to 8th week of gestation (10). Its etiology is unknown and clinical presentation is varied because of the different associated syndromes and anomalies that may occur. Other axial anomalies include cervical or fused ribs, cleft or hemi vertebrae, kyphosis, scoliosis, spina bifida occulta and sacral agenesis. Decreased range of movement of the neck with loss of rotation is the most consistent finding being more pronounced than the loss of flexion and extension. High cervical abnormalities can cause acute spinal cord compression following comparatively minor trauma. A Sprengel's anomaly occurs in 20-30% of patients. Renal anomalies are common in individuals with KFS. Laryngeal

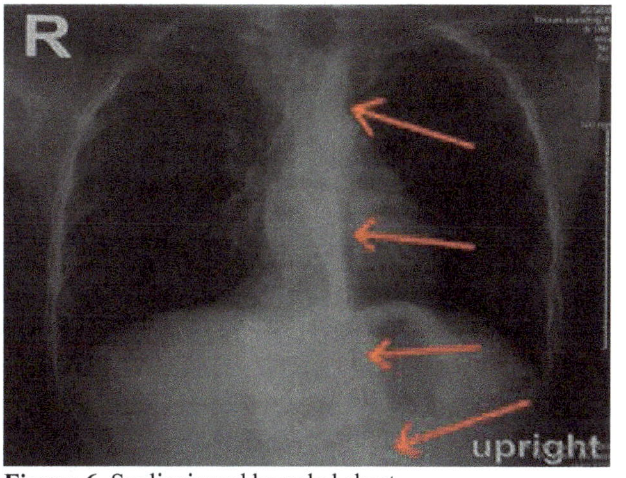

Figure 6. Scoliosis and barreled chest.

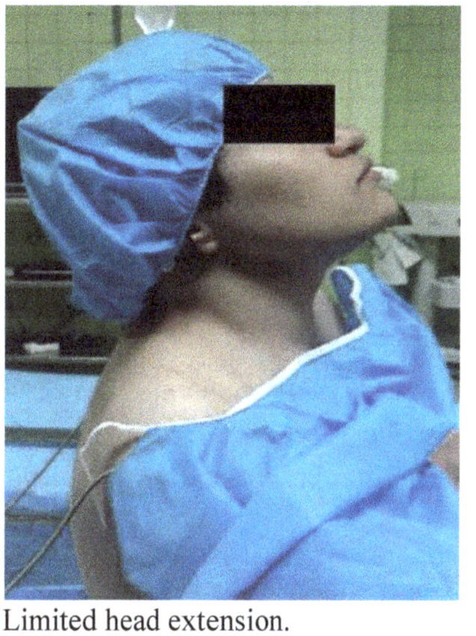

Figure 7. Limited head extension.

cartilages may be malformed, causing aphonia or other voice impairment. Cardiovascular anomalies occur in 14-29% of patients, the most common being Ventricular Septal Defect (11, 12). Other less common anomalies are congenital limb deficiencies, craniosynostosis, ear abnormalities and craniofacial abnormalities (13).

Out of three variants of KFS, Type I is an extensive abnormality in which several cervical and upper thoracic vertebrae are fused into a single block. In Type II variant, failure of complete segmentation occurs at one or two cervical interspaces. Associated anomalies were sprengel's deformity and deafness. Type III variant includes Type I or II deformities with coexisting segmentation defects in the lower thoracic or lumbar spine. Most common form is Type II and it

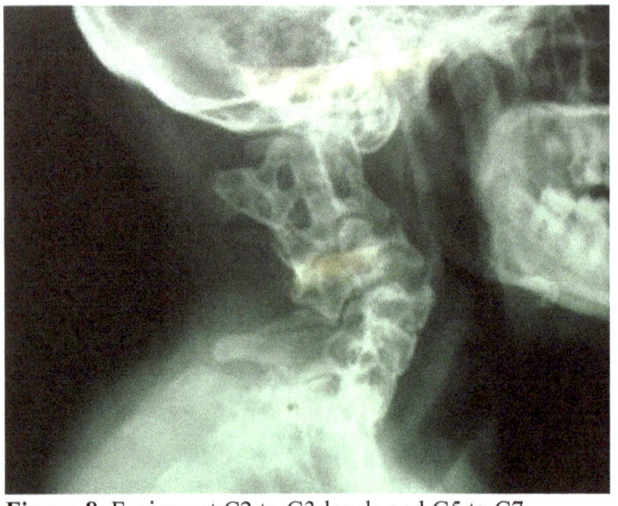

Figure 8. Fusions at C2 to C3 levels and C5 to C7.

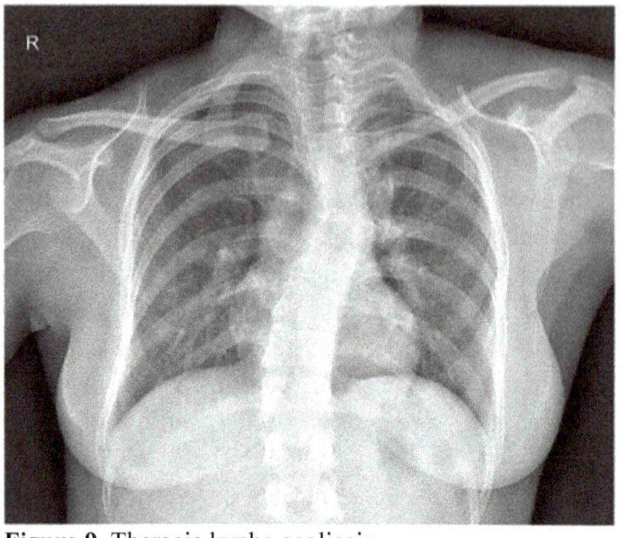

Figure 9. Thoracic kypho-scoliosis.

commonly involves C2-3 and C5-6 interspaces (13, 14).

In our first case, it is most likely type II variant with involvement of C2- C3 and C5 – C7 interspaces.

Patients with KFS may present for various surgical procedures at different ages. Commonly involved surgical procedures are cervical spine surgery, scoliosis correction, spinal canal stenosis surgery, renal surgery, cesarean section and eye or ear surgery.

The main anesthetic concern with these patients is the airway management during general anesthesia due to potential unstable cervical spine and abnormal atlanto-occipital junction, and an increased risk of neurological damage (15). Although several methods of having a secure airway have been reported in these patients, a specific standard recommendation on airway management does not exist. An awake fiberoptic intubation seems to be the most effective and safe method but sometimes difficult and time consuming as well (16).

Direct laryngoscopy with manual cervical stabilization has also been used successfully but even slight extension at atlanto-axial joint may cause damage to spinal cord (17). On the other hand, traction maneuver may limit the orolaryngeal alignment and make intubation more difficult. Neurological worsening following intubation under manual neck stabilization has not been reported (15). Cricothyrotomy is considered to be a good alternative, but an obstruction in the operative field remains a concern. Bullard laryngoscopy has been reported to be safe by some authors, but limited availability has made it less popular (18). The intubating LMA has also been used successfully for intubation without head and neck manipulation (19). But posterior displacement of the normal cervical spine due to cervical pressures generated by the laryngeal mask devices was also observed (20). O'Conner and Moysa reported that airway control could be temporarily lost after induction and an LMA might be required to secure the airway (21). Therefore, caution must be taken when dealing with an unstable cervical spine.

Due to earlier anticipation of difficult airway in these patients, it is indispensable to secure the airway before induction of general anesthesia especially in emergent patients. So we used awake fiberoptic intubation for airway management in our patients. This technique has some advantages, including but not limited to

- an awake, spontaneously breathing patient, who maintains own airway
- needs no spinal movement during intubation
- allows confirmation of tracheal tube placement
- a high success rate
- lower rate of complications
- better patient acceptance (19).

Despite the numerous advantages, failure of fiberoptic intubation with complications like massive subcutaneous emphysema or airway injury have also been reported (22, 23).

Conclusion

A thorough airway assessment and adequate preparation is a critical component for airway management in such cases. After considering all the modes of airway management, we advise awake fiberoptic intubation as one of the best and safest options for securing the airway in a patient with KFS, if it was not possible, inhalational induction and fiberoptic intubation would be a wise alternative.

Acknowledgment

The authors would like to thank the kind help of physicians and nurses, operating room and anesthesiology ward staffs, Loghman Hakim Hospital and Anesthesiology Research Center Shahid Beheshti University of Medical Sciences, Tehran, Iran for their kind help and support.

Conflicts of Interest

The authors declare that there are no conflicts of interest.

References

1. Nashibi M, Tajbakhsh A, MahdavipourVahdati S, Safari F, Mottaghi K. Didmoad (Wolfram) Syndrome: Case Report. Journal of Cellular & Molecular Anesthesia. 2016;1(3):126-8.

2. Nashibi M, Tajbakhsh A, Safari F, Mottaghi K. Anesthetic Consideration of Niemann-Pick Disease Type C. Journal of Cellular & Molecular Anesthesia. 2016;1(2):73-7.

3. Safari F, Mottaghi K, Fallahinejadghajari R, Nashibi M. Crouzon Syndrome: a fibroblast growth factor receptor 2 gene mutation. J Cell Mol Anesth. 2017;2(1):15-8.

4. Klippel M, Feil A. Un cas d'absence des vertébres cervicales cage thoracique remontant jusqu'a la base du crâne. Bulletins et Mémoires de la Société d'anthropologie de Paris. 1912:101-2.

5. Samartzis D, Lubicky JP, Herman J, Shen FH. Faces of Spine Care: From the Clinic and Imaging Suite. Klippel-Feil syndrome and associated abnormalities: the necessity for a multidisciplinary approach in patient management. The spine journal : official journal of the North American Spine Society. 2007;7(1):135-7.

6. Gunderson CH, Greenspan RH, Glaser GH, Lubs HA. The Klippel-Feil syndrome: genetic and clinical reevaluation of cervical fusion. Medicine. 1967;46(6):491-512.

7. Bayrakli F, Guclu B, Yakicier C, Balaban H, Kartal U, Erguner B, et al. Mutation in MEOX1 gene causes a recessive Klippel-Feil syndrome subtype. BMC Genet. 2013;14:95.

8. Mohamed JY, Faqeih E, Alsiddiky A, Alshammari MJ, Ibrahim NA, Alkuraya FS. Mutations in MEOX1, encoding mesenchyme homeobox 1, cause Klippel-Feil anomaly. Am J Hum Genet. 2013;92(1):157-61.

9. Khawaja OM, Reed JT, Shaefi S, Chitilian HV, Sandberg WS. Crisis resource management of the airway in a patient with Klippel-Feil syndrome, congenital deafness, and aortic dissection. Anesthesia and analgesia. 2009;108(4):1220-5.

10. Kaplan KM, Spivak JM, Bendo JA. Embryology of the spine and associated congenital abnormalities. The spine journal : official journal of the North American Spine Society. 2005;5(5):564-76.

11. Algom M, Schlesinger Z. Prolapse of the mitral valve in Klippel-Feil syndrome. Chest. 1981;79(1):127-8.

12. Falk RH, Mackinnon J. Klippel-Feil syndrome associated with aortic coarctation. Br Heart J. 1976;38(11):1220-1.

13. Chattopadhyay A, Shah AM, Kher A, Bharucha BA, Karapurkar AP. Craniosynostosis and Klippel-Feil syndrome: a rare association. Indian J Pediatr. 1996;63(6):819-22.

14. Nagib MG, Maxwell RE, Chou SN. Identification and management of high-risk patients with Klippel-Feil syndrome. J Neurosurg. 1984;61(3):523-30.

15. Whittle IR, Besser M. Congenital neural abnormalities presenting with mirror movements in a patient with Klippel-Feil syndrome. Case report. J Neurosurg. 1983;59(5):891-4.

16. Daum RE, Jones DJ. Fibreoptic intubation in Klippel-Feil syndrome. Anaesthesia. 1988;43(1):18-21.

17. Stallmer ML, Vanaharam V, Mashour GA. Congenital cervical spine fusion and airway management: a case series of Klippel-Feil syndrome. J Clin Anesth. 2008;20(6):447-51.

18. Baraka A, Muallem M, Sibai AN, Louis F. Bullard laryngoscopy for tracheal intubation of patients with cervical spine pathology. Can J Anaesth. 1992;39(5 Pt 1):513-4.

19. Al Zahrani T. Reverse LMA insertion in a neonate with Klippel-Feil syndrome--case report. Middle East J Anaesthesiol. 2007;19(3):625-9.

20. Keller C, Brimacombe J, Keller K. Pressures exerted against the cervical vertebrae by the standard and intubating laryngeal mask airways: a randomized, controlled, cross-over study in fresh cadavers. Anesthesia and analgesia. 1999;89(5):1296-300.

21. O'Connor PJ, Moysa GL, Finucane BT. Thoracic epidural anesthesia for bilateral reduction mammoplasty in a patient with Klippel-Feil syndrome. Anesthesia and analgesia. 2001;92(2):514-6.

22. Maktabi MA, Hoffman H, Funk G, From RP. Laryngeal trauma during awake fiberoptic intubation. Anesthesia and analgesia. 2002;95(4):1112-4, table of contents.

23. Richardson MG, Dooley JW. Acute facial, cervical, and thoracic subcutaneous emphysema: a complication of fiberoptic laryngoscopy. Anesthesia and analgesia. 1996;82(4):878-80.

Effect of intraarticular injection of ozone on inflammatory cytokines in knee osteoarthritis

Masoud Hashemi[1], Seyed Mehdi Hoseini Khameneh[2], Seyed Amir Mohajerani[1*], Peyman Dadkhah[1]

Abstract

Background: Knee Osteoarthrosis is one of the most debilitating diseases. Prolotherapy includes intra-articular injection of various drugs to decrease inflammation. Injection of intradiscal O_2-O_3 has reduced pain and disability in patients with low back pain due to prolapsed lumbar disk. To compare the effect of intraarticular injection of Ozone and steroids in improvement of clinical and cellular healing of knee osteoarthritis.

Materials and Methods: in a randomized clinical trial, 70 patients with knee osteoarthrosis were included in the study. In Ozone group, 5 ml (35 µg/ml) of Ozone and in steroid group 5ml (50 mg) Triamcinolone was injected intra-articular. In 1, 2, and 6 months, patients were followed for pain scale, disability index and IL-1β and TNF-α serum levels were measured.

Results: At 1 month after injection pain scale and disability index and IL-1β and TNF-α were decreased in both groups. However, at 2 and 6 month pain scale and disability index compared significantly lower in the Ozone group to steroid group ($p<0.05$). Besides, serum level of IL-1β and TNF-α compared also significantly lower at 2 and 6 months in the Ozone group in the steroid group ($p<0.05$).

Conclusion: Intraarticular Ozone induces significantly longer improvement of pain and disability in knee osteoarthrosis compare to steroid injection. In addition, serum inflammatory cytokines are also lower in Ozone group compared to the steroid group along with clinical improvements.

Keywords: Ozone, Inflammatory, Cytokines, Knee osteoarthritis

1- Anesthesiology Research Center, Department of Anesthesiology, Shahid Beheshti University of Medical Sciences, Tehran, Iran
2- Department of Orthopaedics Surgery, Shahid Beheshti University of Medical Sciences, Tehran, Iran

Corresponding Author: Seyed Amir Mohajerani, MD, Akhtar Hospital, Fereshteh St, Tehran, Iran.
E-mail: amirmhj@gmail.com

Introduction

Knee Osteoarthritis (OA) of the knee is a degenerative disease manifest as painful joint, articular stiffness and decreased function (1). Osteoarthritis affects the knee and it is currently leading cause of disability in adults (2). The number of adults with arthritis and its associated activity limitation will probably increase little by little; with the resulting great impact on the individual lifestyles, and of course, the health care system (3). The exact mechanism of pain and disability is not well known yet. Various parts have been named as the origin of pain such as articular capsule, ligaments, synovium, bone, lateral part of the meniscus, and involvement of extra-articular ligaments and tendons (4). The role of systemic inflammatory cytokines in the genesis and progression of osteoarthritis has been proposed by a considerable number of studies. In patients with painful knee, osteoarthritis after an intra-articular injection, alterations in serum cytokines are in good correlation with pain response (5, 6).

Total Knee replacement is the only surgical option but it is expensive. Prolotherapy is a novel technique to alleviate pain in chronic musculoskeletal pain and particularly in knee osteoarthritis (7). Intra-articular injection of various agents could lead to initiate proliferation and regeneration of damaged cartilage tissue. However, controversies over the type of drug injected, duration of action, the extent of pain relief, and retained function still persist. Several researches support the use of intra-articular knee injection as a valuable conservative intervention in the continuum of arthritis management (8). In other similar studies, various agents, including ozone have been tried for intra-articular injection (9-11).

Ozone is more active than oxygen in the universe. Prolotherapy by ozone uses the power of oxygen to regenerate damaged tissues, joints, ligaments, and tendons. This usually causes a partial or complete healing, and ends with pain. Mixture of ozone and oxygen. Injected into cartilaginous tissue could inhibit inflammation and start the regeneration of tissue (12, 13). Ozone affects nucleus pulposus macromolecular structures (proteoglycans and collagens) and has a longer duration of action compared to steroid injection in previous reports (14). The objective of this study is to compare the effect of intra-articular injection of ozone and steroids in improvement of clinical and cellular healing of knee osteoarthritis.

Methods

The study was reviewed and approved by the Shahid Beheshti University of Medical Sciences Ethics Committee. All procedures that performed in this study, were in accordance with the ethical standards of the institution and/or national research committee. Information about the study was given comprehensively both orally and in written form to all patients or their accompanying adult. They gave their informed written consent prior to their inclusion in the study.

In a randomized clinical trial, 70 patients with chronic osteoarthritis were enrolled in this randomized clinical trial. Patients were randomly assigned to a computer based accidental number by which patient group was determined. Physician administering drug and evaluating patients were blind to each other and patient group. All demographic variables, including age, sex, and BMI were measured and recorded on a specified data sheet for each patient.

The inclusion criteria were patients with chronic osteoarthritis aged between 35 to 75 years and knee osteoarthritis. Exclusion criteria were severe underlying disease, any contraindication to steroids and ozone, and indication for surgical arthroplasty.

Intra-articular ozone and steroid injection

Intraarticular injection of 5 ml (35μg/ml) of ozone was injected using regular size syringes. In steroid group 5ml of Triamcinolone (10mg/ml) was injected into the intra-articular space.

Pain and disability measurement

After injection patients were scheduled for follow up visits at 1, 3, and 6 months. At each visits pain scale was measured using numeric rating score (NRS). Disability was measured using an Oswestry Disability Index (ODI) at each visit. Evaluation of pain and disability was performed by a physician blinded to the patient group and were recorded in a specified data sheet.

Blood samples (2ml) were collected at each visit and were stored at -80°C freezer until sent to the laboratory for measurement of IL-1b and TNF-alpha at 37°C.

Il-1b and TNF-α ELISA measurement

Samples were thawed on 4°C on ice bucket and centrifuged at 2000 rpm for 3 minutes. Then 100μl of aqueous phase were transferred on prepared 96 well-plates. For 96 well plates preparation, plates were washed twice the night before and primary antibody for IL-1beta (IL-1β Antibody (H-153), rabbit polyclonal IgG, Santa Cruz, CA, USA) and TNF-alpha (TNF-α antibody (sc-133192), mouse IgG2a, Santa Cruz, CA, USA) were loaded and incubated at 37°C until the next morning. Next morning after proper washing of plates, samples were loaded on the plate. Then secondary antibodies (goat anti-rabbit IgG-HRP, and goat anti-mouse IgG-HRP (sc-2005), Santa Cruz, CA, USA) were added to the samples. IL-1b and TNF-a were measured using an ELISA plate reader by a standard curve.

Statistical Analysis

Statistical calculations were conducted using SPSS 20 (Chicago, IL, USA). The variables were presented as mean ± standard deviation and were analyzed by the student t-test; parametric texts were used. Other variables were analyzed by Chi-Square, Mann-Whitney U-test or non-parametric tests. P<0.05 was considered as statistically significant. The sample size was estimated using sample size calculator software with 95% confidence interval, p=0.05 and power of 80% and difference between two groups of 30% in primary outcome based on the pilot study.

Results

In this randomized clinical trial, 75 patients with knee osteoarthritis were enrolled and randomly assigned to one of steroid or ozone groups. Five patients in ozone group and 9 patients in the steroid group were lost to follow-up, and 30 patients with ozone and 31 patients in the steroid group finished the study. There were no significant differences in age, sex or BMI, of patients (p>0.05). Mode of osteoarthritis grade at the time of inclusion in the study was 2 in both groups. Mean of osteoarthritis grade were not significantly different in two groups of patients (p=0.33) (Table1). Duration of pain before injection (NRS>4) was 14.5±5.7 months in ozone and 14.9±7.3 months in steroid group which was not significantly different. The mean pain score before injection (NRS score) was 6.8±1.7 in ozone and 6.9±1.5 in steroid group which was not significantly different (p=0.1) (Table 1).

Comparison of pain scale (Numerical rating scale) before and after injection during follow-up time is depicted in figure1. Pain scale was not significantly different at 1 month (p=0.35) after injection, but was different at 2 and 6 month post injection (p=0.011, 0.025; respectively) (Figure 1).

Disability index

Function of joints after injection were measured by the Oswestry disability index (ODI) % (Figure 2). At the beginning of the study before intra-articular injection ODI score was not significantly different between two groups (p=0.44). ODI score was not significantly different between two groups at 1 month after intraarticular injection (p=0.28).

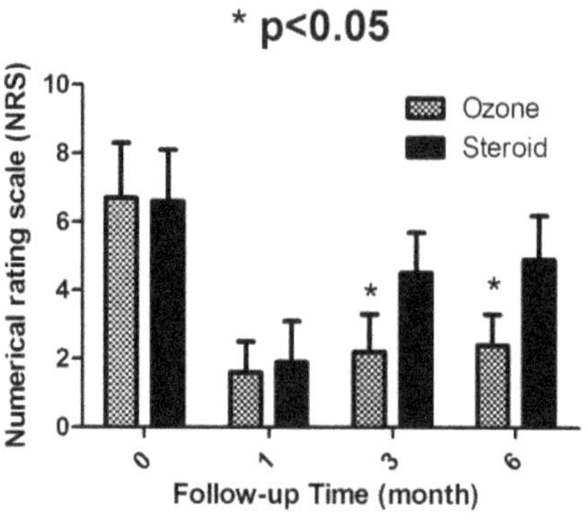

Figure 1. Comparison of pain scale (Numerical rating scale) between patients with knee osteoarthritis after intraarticular injection of ozone and steroid injection (*Mann-Whitney test).

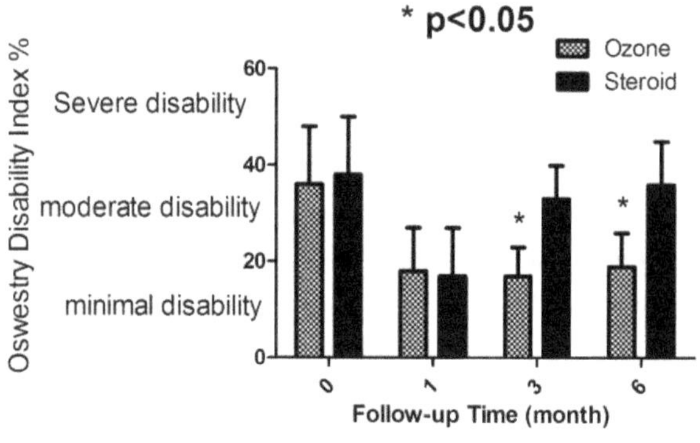

Figure 2. Comparison of functional disability (Oswestry Disability Index) between patients with knee osteoarthritis after intraarticular injection of ozone and steroid injection.

However, ODI score was significantly different at 2 and 6 month post injection (p=0.02, 0.03; respectively).

Inflammatory cytokines

IL-1b and TNF-α were measured and compared in two groups of patients. At baseline samples before intra-articular injection, there were no significant differences in in IL-1b and TNF- α between ozone and steroid groups. At 1 month samples also, there were no significant differences in IL-1b and TNF- α between ozone and steroid groups. However, at 3 and 6 month follow up samples, Il-1b and TNF- α were significantly lower in ozone group compared to steroid groups (Figure 3).

Discussion

In the study, we compared intra-articular

Table 1: Demographic characteristics of patients with intraarticular injection of ozone and steroid.

	Ozone (n=30)	Steroid (n=31)	p-value
Age	56.7±16.9	54.8±19.5	0.19†
Sex (male/female)	11/19	11/20	0.26‡
BMI	22.6±4.3	21.4±3.8	0.35*
Grade of osteoarthritis (Mode/Mean ± SD)	2 /2.2±0.8	2/2.3±0.9	0.33*
Duration of pain before injection (NRS>4) (m)	14.5±5.7	14.9±7.3	0.74‡
Pain score before injection (NRS score)	6.8±1.7	6.9±1.5	0.10‡

Mann-Whitney test ‡ † Wilcoxon-signed rank test *t-test

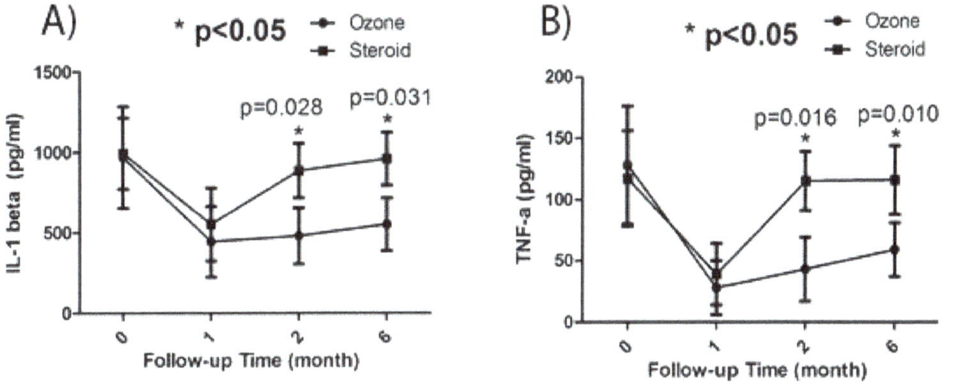

Figure 3. Comparison of serum IL-1 and TNF-α between patients with knee osteoarthritis after intraarticular injection of ozone and steroid injection.

injection of ozone and steroid in decreasing pain and disability and inflammatory response in patients with knee osteoarthritis. Patients who were injected with ozone had less pain and disability after 6 months follow up compare to steroid group.

Ozone effects in decreasing pain were longer compared to steroid. Steroid has been the mainstay of minimally invasive therapies for osteoarthritis. However, there is much debate about the duration of effect in these patients. It is important to note that ozone has invariably showed a longer duration of action in decreasing pain and disability in joint pain. On the other hand, a comprehensive systematic review showed that intra-articular corticosteroid injection results in clinically and statistically significant reduction in osteoarthritis knee pain and the beneficial effect could last for 3 to 4 weeks, but is unlikely to continue beyond that (15).

Specific inflammatory cytokines, IL-1b and TNF-α decreased significantly in ozone group compare to steroid group. Chemical factors include systemic and local inflammatory responses along with mechanical factors could affect cartilage tissue and its destruction (16). The Intracartilaginous ozone injection was first introduced by Muto et al. (17) with positive results in clinical and inflammatory responses. Ozone decreases inflammation and joint injury, providing reduction of pro-inflammatory cytokines, TNF-α and IL-1β transcripts and re-establishment of cellular redox balance (18, 19). Intraarticular glucocorticoid (GC) therapy diminishes synovial cell infiltration, vascularity, expression of pro-inflammatory cytokines (TNF, IL-1beta), and adhesion molecule levels (ICAM-1, VEGF) in patients with chronic arthritis (20). Although steroid has robust anti-inflammatory action against inflammatory cytokines, however, this effect in cartilaginous tissue was shorter compared to ozone in our study coherently with others (21). Actually, their trend reflects a similar pattern in pain and disability, decrease in these patients. These two cytokines showed to be the mainstay of initiation and propagation of chondrocyte destruction. Ozone has probably more stable anti-inflammatory effect, compared to steroid. Besides, ozone, anti-oxidant action could also help to diminish the inflammatory response. Ozone injection has shown to significantly decrease intradiscal inflammation and the inflammatory response (22).

We did not observe any adverse effects in ozone injected patients. It is an important aspect of our study. On the other hand, intra-articular steroid therapy has not side effects. In a recent paper, researchers showed that the outcome of combination of O_2O_3 and hyaluronic acid demonstrated improved results compared with hyaluronic acid in patients affected by knee OA (23). Meanwhile, a combination of ozone with platelet-rich plasma (PRP) or dextrose could be effective (24, 25).

Conclusion

Patients with chronic knee osteoarthritis could respond better and longer to intra-articular ozone injection compared to intraarticular steroid injection. In addition, serum inflammatory cytokines are also lower in Ozone group compared to the steroid group along with clinical improvements.

Acknowledgment

None.

Conflicts of Interest

The authors declare that they have no conflict of interest.

References

1. Lee J, Song J, Hootman JM, Semanik PA, Chang RW, Sharma L, et al. Obesity and other modifiable factors for physical inactivity measured by accelerometer in adults with knee osteoarthritis. Arthritis Care Res (Hoboken). 2013;65(1):53-61.
2. Lawrence RC, Felson DT, Helmick CG, Arnold LM, Choi H, Deyo RA, et al. National Arthritis Data Workgroup.Estimates of the prevalence of arthritis and other rheumatic conditions in the United States. Part II. Arthritis Rheum. 2008;58(1):26-35.
3. Yelin E. Cost of musculoskeletal diseases: impact of work disability and functional decline. J Rheumatol Suppl. 2003;68:8-11.
4. Felson DT. The sources of pain in knee osteoarthritis. Curr Opin Rheumatol. 2005;17(5):624-8.
5. Singh JA, Noorbaloochi S, Knutson KL. Cytokine and neuropeptide levels are associated with pain relief in patients with chronically painful total knee arthroplasty: a pilot study. BMC Musculoskelet Disord. 2017;18(1):17.
6. King W, Bendele A, Marohl T, Woodell-May J. A human blood-based anti-inflammatory solution inhibits osteoarthritis progression in a meniscal-tear rat study. J Orthop Res. 2017.
7. Rabago D, Slattengren A, Zgierska A. Prolotherapy in primary care practice. Prim Care. 2010;37(1):65-80.
8. Cheng OT, Souzdalnitski D, Vrooman B, Cheng J. Evidence-based knee injections for the management of arthritis. Pain Med. 2012;13(6):740-53.
9. Dhillon MS, Patel S, Marwaha N. Platelet-rich plasma for knee osteoarthritis--authors' response. Am J Sports Med. 2013 Sep;41(9):NP43-4
10. Stein A, Yassouridis A, Szopko C, Helmke K, Stein C. Intraarticular morphine versus dexamethasone in chronic arthritis. Pain. 1999;83:525–32.
11. Elvis AM, Ekta JS. Ozone therapy: A clinical review. J Nat Sci Biol Med. 2011;2(1):66-70.
12. Gautam S, Rastogi V, Jain A, Singh AP. Comparative evaluation of oxygen-ozone therapy and combined use of oxygen-ozone therapy with percutaneous intradiscal radiofrequency thermocoagulation for the treatment of lumbar disc herniation. Pain Pract. 2011;11(2):160-6.
13. Hashemi M, Poorfarokh M, Mohajerani SA, Jalili P, Akhyani V, Barikani A, Farivar F. Injection of intradiscal o2-o3 to reduce pain and disability of patients with low back pain due to prolapsed lumbar disk. Anesth Pain Med. 2014;4(5):e19206.
14. Masini M, Calaça A. Minimally invasive treatment for refractory low back pain, targeted by epidural endoscopy with O2/O3 and steroid therapy. Acta Neurochir Suppl. 2011;108:33-7.
15. Godwin M, Dawes M. Intra-articular steroid injections for painful knees. Systematic review with meta-analysis. Can Fam Physician. 2004;50:241-8
16. Magalhaes FN, Dotta L, Sasse A, Teixera MJ, Fonoff ET. Ozone therapy as treatment for low back pain secondary to herniated disc: a systematic review and meta-analysis of randomized controlled trials. Pain Physician. 2012 Mar-Apr;15(2):E115-29.
17. Muto M, Avella F. Percutaneous treatment of herniated lumbar disc by intradiscal oxygen-ozone injection. Interv Neuroradiol. 1998;4(4):279-86.
18. Vaillant JD, Fraga A, Díaz MT, Mallok A, Viebahn-Hänsler R, Fahmy Z, Barberá A, Delgado L, Menéndez S, Fernández OS.Ozone oxidative postconditioning ameliorates joint damage and decreases pro-inflammatory cytokine levels and oxidative stress in PG/PS-induced arthritis in rats. Eur J Pharmacol. 2013;714(1-3):318-24.
19. Chen H, Yu B, Lu C, Lin Q. The effect of intra-articular injection of different concentrations of ozone on the level of TNF-α, TNF-R1, and TNF-R2 in rats with rheumatoid arthritis. Rheumatol Int. 2013;33(5):1223-7.
20. Klint E, Grundtman C, Engström M, Catrina AI, Makrygiannakis D, Klareskog L, Andersson U, Ulfgren AK. Intraarticular glucocorticoid treatment reduces inflammation in synovial cell infiltrations more efficiently than in synovial blood vessels. Arthritis Rheum. 2005;52(12):3880-9.
21. Kullenberg B, Runesson R, Tuvhag R, Olsson C, Resch S. Intraarticular corticosteroid injection: pain relief in osteoarthritis of the hip? J Rheumatol. 2004;31(11):2265-8.
22. Chang JD, Lu HS, Chang YF, Wang D. Ameliorative effect of ozone on cytokine production in mice injected with human rheumatoid arthritis synovial fibroblast cells. 2005;26(2):142-51.
23. Giombini A, Menotti F, Di Cesare A, Giovannangeli F, Rizzo M, Moffa S, Martinelli F. Comparison between intrarticular injection of hyaluronic acid, oxygen ozone, and the combination of both in the treatment of knee osteoarthrosis. J Biol Regul Homeost Agents.

2016;30(2):621-5.
24. Duymus TM, Mutlu S, Dernek B, Komur B, Aydogmus S, Kesiktas FN. Choice of intra-articular injection in treatment of knee osteoarthritis: platelet-rich plasma, hyaluronic acid or ozone options. Knee Surg Sports Traumatol Arthrosc. 2016 Apr 7.
25. Hashemi M, Jalili P, Mennati S, Koosha A, Rohanifar R, Madadi F, et al. The Effects of Prolotherapy with Hypertonic Dextrose Versus Prolozone (Intraarticular Ozone) in Patients With Knee Osteoarthritis. Anesth Pain Med. 2015;5(5):e27585.

4

Effect of Intravenous Infusion of Lidocaine on Pain Reduction after Cesarean Section under General Anesthesia

Anahita Hirmanpour[1], Reihanak Talakoub[1], Hamed Mansouri[1]

1. Anesthesia and Critical Care Research Center, Alzahra Hospital, Department of Anesthesiology, School of Medicine, Isfahan University of Medical Sciences, Isfahan, Iran

Corresponding Author: Reihanak Talakoub, MD, Associate Professor, Anesthesiology and Critical Care Research Center, Isfahan University of Medical Science, Isfahan, Iran;
Email: reihanak.talakoub@gmail.com

Abstract

Background: The present study was conducted to evaluate the effect of Lidocaine on pain reduction during and ileus and the need for opioids after caesarean section.

Materials and Methods: This study was randomized double-blind controlled clinical trial. 40 ASA I, II pregnant women were candidates for caesarean section with general anesthesia. They were randomly allocated into two groups of Lidocaine receivers and placebo using randomized block design; the Lidocaine group received 1.5 mg/kg of Lidocaine right before the surgery and then its infusion with a dose of 2 mg/Kg/h until the end of the surgery and the placebo group received normal saline with the same volume and application. Patients' pain intensity was measured using numerical rating scale (NRS), 0 (entering the recovery), 0.5, 1, 4, 12 and 24 hours after the surgery.

Results: Lidocaine decreased the systolic and diastolic pressures of the patients only during the first minute after intubation. There was decrease in mean of arterial blood pressure at the 10th minute after intubation and 40th minute after surgery. In addition, decreased the mean of patients' pain intensity, Diclofenac and Pethidine consumption, side effects (nausea and vomiting), and reduced the time interval before the first time of tolerating oral liquids; but it had effect on infants' Apgar score 1 and 5 minutes after delivery.

Conclusion: Lidocaine was definitely effective on reducing the intensity of pain, opioid and non-steroidal anti-inflammatory drugs consumption and ileus after surgery with the least occurrence of side effects for mothers and infants.

Keywords: Caesarean Section, Postoperative Pain, Lidocaine, General Anesthesia

Introduction

One of the most common complications of caesarean section is postoperative pain (1). Also the most common and important cause of dissatisfaction among mothers who has been under caesarean section at health centers is postoperative pain (1). Pain, during the first days after delivery, is an important obstacle for taking care of the infant and breastfeeding; therefore specialists' attention for controlling postoperative pain is necessary (1, 2).

Proper management of postoperative pain has been of great importance during the recent years. The intensity of postoperative pain depends on various factors like patient's perception of pain and threshold, the type and duration of surgery, the type of anesthesia and used anesthetics and patient's mental and psychological condition (example: differences in mental condition in laparotomy for caesarean section against laparotomy for uterus cancer) (1, 3).

The important matter in controlling postoperative pain after caesarean section is reducing morbidity and mother's faster recovery for returning home (4). There are different methods for getting mothers back to the desirable condition for taking care of their infant, breastfeeding, and pain management after caesarean. Like systemic analgesia methods and regional analgesia methods (constant infusion or injecting a dose of analgesic drug to the site of surgery), which would be used after evaluating their complications and advantages and patient's condition (1, 2).

In many Iranian health centers, which is a developing country, the rate of caesarean section is higher than the standard rate (30% of all the deliveries) and this would make it impossible to provide pain control strategies for all the patients (4).

Using non-steroidal anti-inflammatory drugs and opioids is the traditional and most common method for controlling post-operative pain. However there are also some regional analgesic methods which are more powerful than opioid drugs. Also, using narcotic injections compared to regional methods is associated with side effects such as nausea, vomiting, respiratory distress, constipation and dizziness (1, 2). Modern methods such as constant epidural infusion or patient controlled analgesia (PCA), besides needing trained personnel and special facilities, are expensive and associated with some side effects (spinal hematoma). On the other hand, due to low cultural and educational level of the patients who refer to most of the health centers, it is not possible to use advanced pain management devices patient controlled analgesia pumps or PCA (1, 2, 4, 5). Another study has evaluated the effect of using oral painkillers like Dipyrone and Morphine right after delivery (1, 2, 5, 6).

One of the commonly used analgesic drug in this field is Lidocaine which is used as an antiarrhythmic IB class drug for treating ventricular tachycardia and sometimes myocardial ischemia. This drug has analgesic and anti-hyperalgesia effects (7). Lidocaine is not teratogenic and it is a safe drug in its therapeutic doses and, except for neonatal inter-scalp injections that could cause neonatal toxicity, it has few side effects. Lidocaine has a low excretion into breast milk and its half-life is 90 to 120 minutes. Using Lidocaine during early pregnancy would not increase the risk for embryonic defects but it would decrease the blood supply for the placenta and increase the uterine myometrium tone. In high dose injections, it would temporarily and transiently decrease the Apgar score of infants (1, 5, 6). Furthermore, Lidocaine is an inexpensive, easily injectable and relatively safe drug (7).

The mechanisms of anesthetic drugs are numerous. The anesthetic effect of drugs, when prescribed before trauma to the tissue, is based on the preventive theory of central pain sensitization. Prescribing anesthetics before trauma would linger the pharmacokinetic effects of the anesthetic method (1).

Therefore the anesthetic drug would be administered through different methods of intramuscular, intravenous, epidural, regional peripheral nerve block, slowly intraperitoneal injection or subcutaneous injection (8, 9). The effect of Lidocaine on pain reduction in surgeries has previously been studied. In a study, local injection of Lidocaine before making the incision in caesarean section led to pain reduction during the early hours after the surgery in mothers without any side effects; it also reduced the need for opioids. Also injecting IM injection, SC injection or both of Lidocaine after making the incision in caesarean section into rectus abdominus muscle would reduce post-operative pain and the duration of hospitalization (6).

Therefore, considering the importance of pain control after caesarean section, preventive use of analgesic agents during surgery could be reasonable for reducing post-operative pain (7). Considering the advantages of local injection methods and the appropriateness of lidocaine for this matter, this study evaluated the effect of intravenous injection of

Lidocaine during caesarean section with general anesthesia on pain, ileus and the need for opioids after surgery.

Methods

This study was a randomized controlled double-blind clinical trial which was conducted from winter 2015 to autumn 2015 at Al-Zahra and Beheshti hospitals after taking permission from ethics committee of Isfahan University of Medical Sciences. ASA I and II term pregnant women (more than 37 weeks), who were candidates for caesarean section with general anesthesia were enrolled in the study.

The exclusion criteria were: receiving antiarrhythmic drugs, having any previous diagnosed allergy to Lidocaine, having diabetes, having neurologic problems, being an addict, chronic use of opioids or analgesics, having any type of heart blocks, having any type of arrhythmia, having a history of myopathy, having renal or hepatic problem or a GFR < 40% and having a heart problem or EF<45%. Surgeries that lasted more than 2 hours, were associated with complications such as bladder injury which required urology intervention, hysterectomy, blood transfusion (due to major bleeding) which led to acid-base disorders and diagnosed or pregnancy-related treatment-resistant hypotension, were also led to patient's exclusion. Participants were allocated into two groups of Lidocaine receivers and placebo (normal saline) through block random allocation

The drug and the placebo were prepared and coded in similar syringes by an anesthesia technician. The person who injected the syringes was different from the one who prepared them. The Lidocaine group received 1.5 mg/kg of Lidocaine right before the surgery and its infusion with a dose of 2 mg/kg.h lasted from clamping the umbilical cord and taking out the neonate until the end of the surgery and putting the bandages.

Patients of the placebo group received similar doses of normal saline. Then necessary measures for general anesthesia and then transfer to the recovery room were performed. Patients were monitored for ECG, SPO2 and NIBP from the beginning and all of the vital signs of the patients were measured and recorded before the induction, before intubation, 1, 5 and 10 minutes after intubation and then every half an hour until the end of the surgery. Also, after the surgery and the infusion ended, patients' vital signs were recorded every 15 minutes at the recovery room.

Patients' pain intensity at 0, 0.5, 1, 4, 12 and 24 hours after the surgery were measured and recorded.

Pain's scoring was based on numerical rating scale (NRS) and the scales were no pain (0), mild (1-4), moderate (5-7) and severe (8-10); an NRS of 4 or more required intervention and treatment. Treatment was first started by prescribing Diclofenac 100 mg suppository and in case the pain did not stop, 50 mg of Pethidine was injected intravenously.

After being transferred to the ward, patients who received standard treatment with Diclofenac and Pethidine, based on their own request and NSR of 4 or more, received another suppository of Diclofenac and if needed, 50 mg of IM Pethidine. The time of entering the recovery room and the time for the first request for pain killers at the recovery room and the ward were recorded. The extra doses of Diclofenac and Pethidine were also measured and recorded. Regarding sedation, patients were categorized into 4 groups of 0 = alert, I = sleepy but arousable, II = stupor and III = coma.

Side effects after surgery including lightheadedness, numbness and tingling in the extremities, nausea, vomiting and severe drowsiness were recorded. The duration of anesthesia, from the time of induction of anesthesia until transferring to the recovery room was calculated and recorded.

The duration of extubation, from the time of cutting the anesthetic until removing the tracheal tube was calculated and recorded. If the patient had hypotension of SBP < 90 mmHg or less than 20% of the baseline pressure drop, 5 mg of Ephedrine was injected intravenously. In case of Bradycardia (HR < 50), 0.5 mg Atropine was prescribed.

The duration of staying in the recovery room was measured and recorded from the time of entering until the time of being discharged from the recovery room based on modified aldreet score. Infant's Apgar score was measured and recorded 1 and 5 minutes after birth. The sample size was estimated to be 20 for each group with a confidence interval of 95%, test power of 0.84 and accuracy of 0.5. Data were analyzed using SPSS 21 (Chicago, Illinois, USA). A p value of less 0.05 was considered significant. For analyzing qualitative data, t test and chi-square were used. Mann-Whitney test was used for analyzing categorical variables. Variance analysis with repeated measures, Newman-Kelus test and post hoc student tests were used for analyzing hemodynamic variables at different times in both groups.

Results

Forty pregnant women were enrolled as the participants for this study. Demographic characteristics and the duration of surgery and recovery are respectively presented in tables 1 and 2.

The mean changes of systolic and diastolic blood pressure had a significant difference between both groups only one minute after intubation ($p< 0.05$) (Figure 1, 2).

The mean of changes in the arterial blood pressure of patients, at the same time intervals, had a significant difference between both groups 10 and 40 minutes after the surgery ($p< 0.05$) (Figure 3).

The mean of changes in the patients' heart rate, at the same time intervals, had a significant difference between both groups 1 minute after intubation ($p< 0.05$) (Figure 4).

The mean of changes in patients' oxygen saturation, at the same time intervals, had a significant difference between both groups 40 minutes after the surgery ($p< 0.05$) (Figure 5).

The mean of changes in patients' blood pressure, heart rate and oxygen saturation are shown in diagrams 1 to 5.

Measurement times on the horizontal axis of diagrams 1 to 5

Measurement time on the basis of intubation	1	2	3	4	5	6	7	8	9	10	11	12
	Right before	1 minutes after	5 minutes after	10 minutes after	40 minutes after	70 minutes after	100 minutes after	130 minutes after	160 minutes after	190 minutes after	220 minutes after	250 minutes after

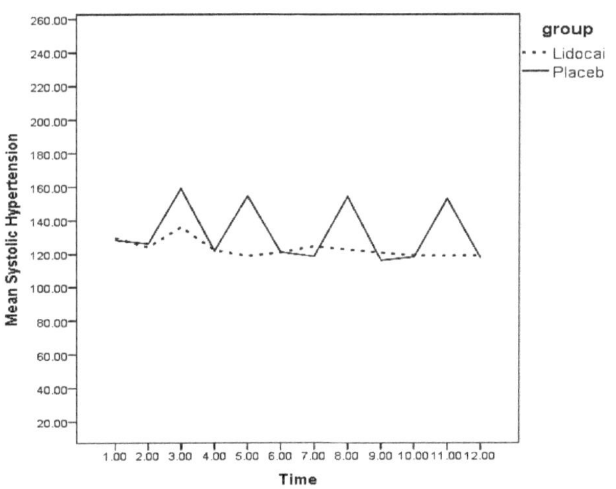

Figure 1. The linear diagram of the mean of systolic blood pressure for each studied group separately (mmHg).

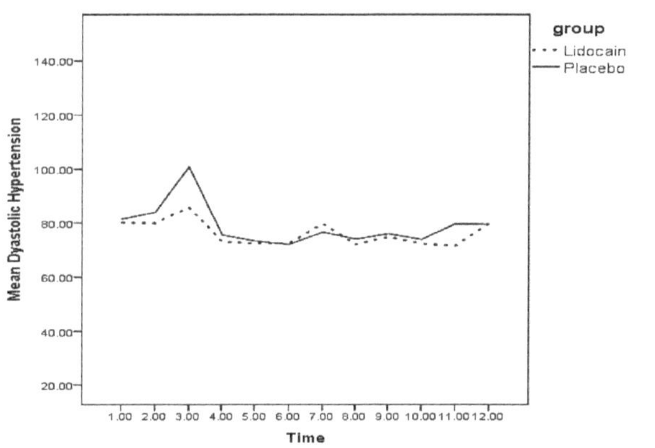

Figure 2. The linear diagram of the mean of diastolic blood pressure for each studied group separately (mmHg).

The mean of patients' intensity of pain based on NRS at the time of entering the recovery room, 15 minutes into the recovery room and then 4, 12, and 24 hours after the surgery had a significant difference between both groups ($p < 0.05$). No significant difference was observed between both groups at any other measurement time ($p > 0.05$) (Figure 6).

The mean of consuming extra doses of Diclofenac suppository, at the moment of entering the recovery room, 15 and 60 minutes into the recovery

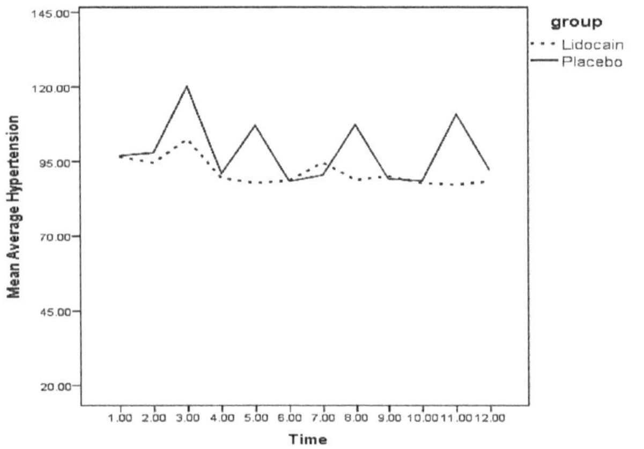

Figure 3. The linear diagram of the mean of arterial blood pressure for each studied group separately (mmHg).

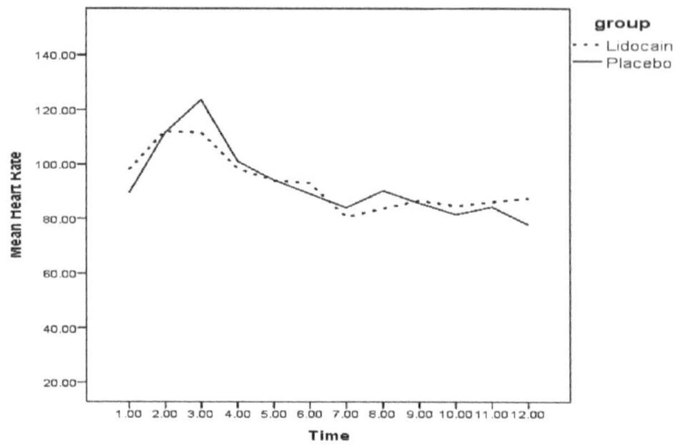

Figure 4. The linear diagram of patients' heart rate for each studied group separately.

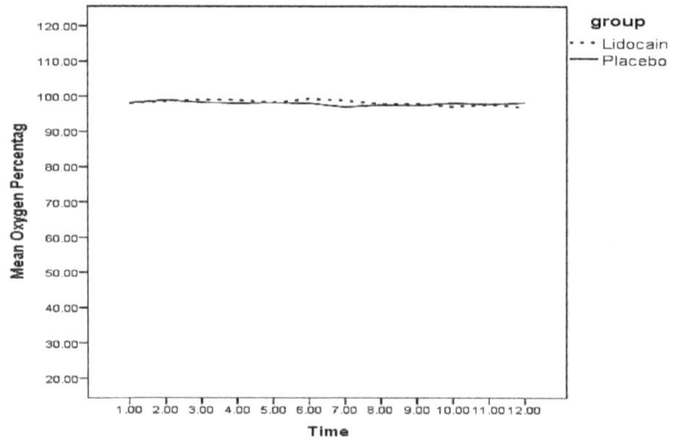

Figure 5. The linear diagram of patients' oxygen saturation for each studied group separately.

and 4 and 12 hours after the surgery was significantly lower in the Lidocaine receiving group compared to the placebo group; their difference was significant ($p < 0.05$). Considering the injection of extra doses of Pethidine, at the moment of entering the recovery room and 15 minutes into the recovery room and also 4 hours after the surgery, it was lower in the Lidocaine receiving group compared to the placebo group and their difference was significant ($p < 0.05$) (Figures 7 and 8).

The level of drowsiness at all the measurement times had no significant difference between both groups ($p > 0.05$) (Figures 9, 10, 11).

The frequency of the incidence of nausea and vomiting had a significant difference between both groups ($p < 0.05$) (Figure 12).

The frequency of the incidence of side effects had no significant difference between both groups ($p > 0.05$) (Figure 13).

The mean of Apgar score of infants one and five minutes after birth showed no significant difference between both studied groups ($p > 0.05$).

Discussion

The present study revealed that intravenous bolus injection of Lidocaine during surgery would decrease systolic and diastolic blood pressure and heart rate during the first minute after laryngoscopy and endotracheal intubation. However, according to previous studies, which had not used (10-12) this drug, could be effective on hemodynamic stability of pregnant women during laryngoscopy and endotracheal intubation. Furthermore, pain intensity and consumption of extra doses of analgesic drugs were lower in the Lidocaine receiving group compared to the placebo group.

The effect of local application of Lidocaine for pain reduction during surgeries has been previous studied. In one study, local injection of Lidocaine before making the incision in caesarean section, with no side effects for the mother, decreased the pain during the first hours after surgery and also decreased the need for opioids. Also subcutaneous injection of Lidocaine or intramuscular injection into rectus abdominis or both after making the incision in caesarean section would decrease post-operative pain intensity and duration of hospitalization (1, 6, 13). Intravenous injection during and after abdominal surgeries in different studies (14), would decrease the duration of hospitalization and would also decrease ileus, as the most important factor in lingered hospitalizations. Also patients would experience less

Table 1: Frequency distribution and dispersion of demographic characteristics for each group.

Variable	Lidocaine receiving group	Placebo group	P value
Age (years)	29.3 ± 3.3	29.3 ± 4.6	0.938
Gestational age (weeks)	39.9 ± 0.5	38.4 ± 1.1	0.066
Height (cm)	160 ± 4.8	161.5 ± 6.4	0.408
Weight (kg)	80.9 ± 12	79.75 ± 10.4	0.749
Body Mass Index (BMI)	31.59 ± 4.4	30.49 ± 2.8	0.345

- Variables are presented as mean ± SD
- P values less than 0.05 indicate statistically significant difference

Table 2: Comparing the mean duration of surgery and recovery between both groups.

Variable	Lidocaine receiving group	Placebo group	P value
Duration of surgery (minutes)	59.75 ± 18.3	51.5 ± 10.2	P ≥ 0.05
Duration of recovery	60 ± 0.0	60 ± 0.0	P > 0.05

- P values less than 0.05 indicate statistically significant difference

Measurement times on the horizontal axis of diagram 6

Measurement time on the basis of intubation	1	2	3	4	5	6	7	8
	At the time of entering the recovery room	15 minutes into the recovery room	30 minutes into the recovery room	45 minutes into the recovery room	60 minutes into the recovery room	4 hours after the surgery	12 hours after the surgery	24 hours after the surgery

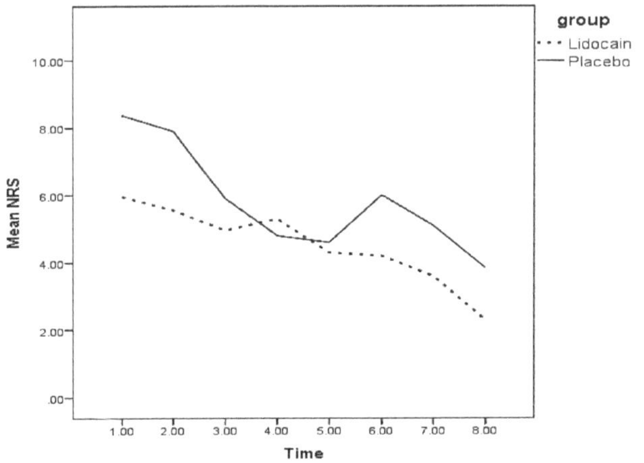

Figure 6. The linear diagram of patients' intensity of pain based on intensity.

nausea and vomiting during the first 24 hours after surgery and would need less Morphine (15, 16). The present study also approved the reduction of nausea and vomiting and less consumption of opioids. Intravenous injection of Lidocaine in radical prostatectomy, along with similar effects, was also effective in return of bowel functions (17). Intravenous injection of Lidocaine would decrease the intensity of permanent pain in women after breast surgeries (18).

Lidocaine had similar analgesic effects after cholecystectomy surgeries and laparoscopic cholecystectomy; it led to a decrease in the need for opioids, faster resolve of ileus and sooner discharges of the patient from the hospital (7, 19, 20). The present study also approved the safe and uncomplicated analgesic and hyper analgesic effect of Lidocaine 21) in pregnant women who were candidates for caesarean section. One of the limitations of this study was not measuring the serum level of Lidocaine, but considering all the conducted monitoring and patients' vital signs, no toxicity was

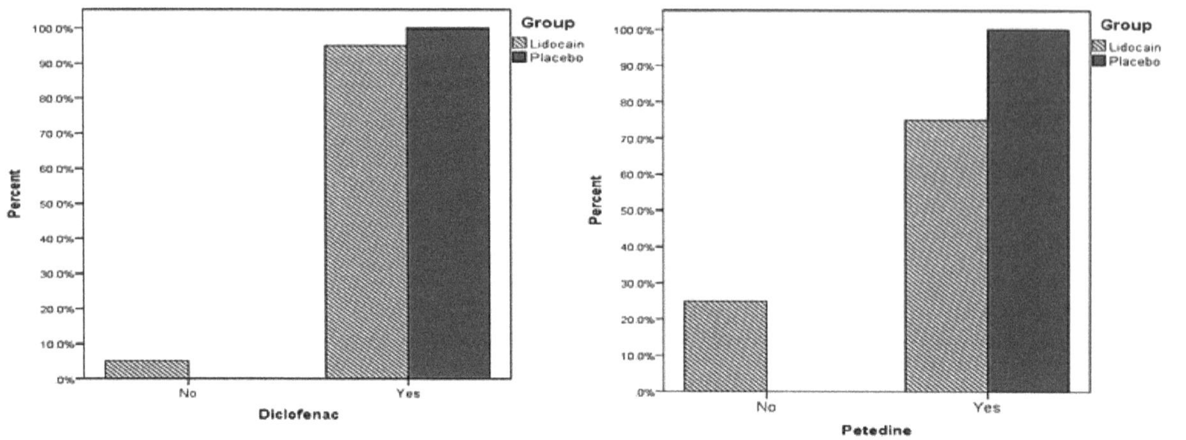

Figures 7 & 8. The frequency histogram for consuming Diclofenac suppository & Pethidine in each group separately.

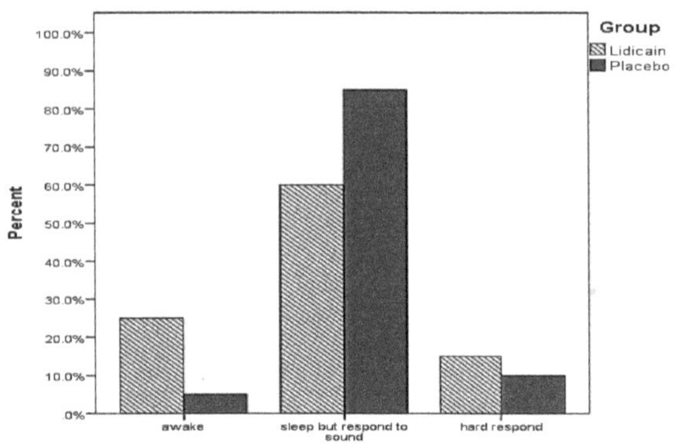

Figure 9. The frequency histogram for the level of drowsiness in both groups at the time of entering the recovery room.

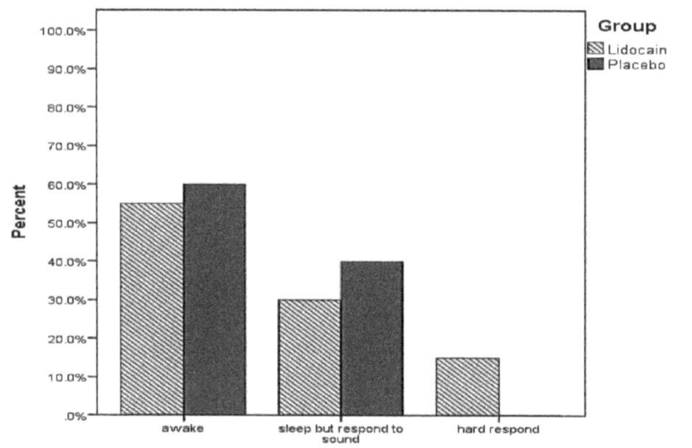

Figure 10. The frequency histogram for the level of drowsiness in both groups 30 minutes into the recovery room.

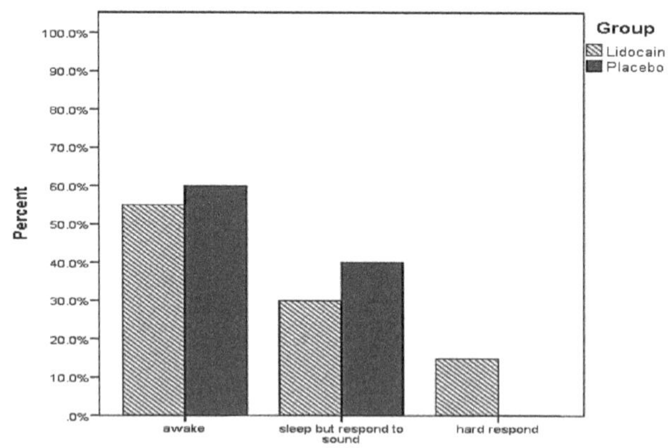

Figure 11. The frequency histogram for the level of drowsiness in both groups 60 minutes into the recovery room.

observed with this drug and the applied dosage. But conducting further studies with larger sample size and measurement of the serum level of Lidocaine is recommended. Another limitation of this study was not measuring the chronic pain of the patients after caesarean section. Since, the helpful effect of Lidocaine in controlling chronic pain after surgeries (18, 22, 23) has been approved, future studies could assess this matter; because in the present study patients could only be observed for 24 hours after the surgery. Therefore prescribing Lidocaine during the induction and also during the caesarean section, with no adverse effect on mothers' hemodynamics during the surgery or infants' Apgar score, could decrease the intensity of pain and also nausea and vomiting after surgery. It could also lead to a significant reduction in the use of opioids and pain killers after surgery and ileus (in case of any). Since this drug has a suitable price and could be applied easily, it could be afforded for being used during caesarean sections.

Table 3: Determining and comparing the mean of Apgar score of infants in both the studied groups.

Variable	Lidocaine receiving group	Placebo group	P value
The mean of Apgar score 1 minute after birth	8.55	8.70	0.701
The mean of Apgar score 5 minutes after birth	9.95	10.95	0.395

. P values less than 0.05 indicate statistically significant difference

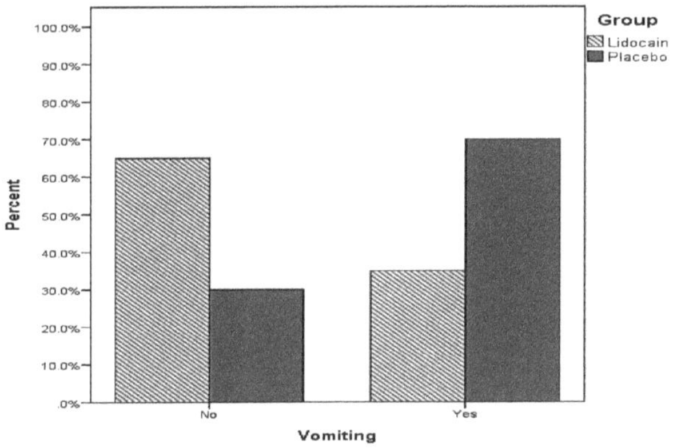

Figure 12. The frequency histogram for nausea and vomiting in both groups.

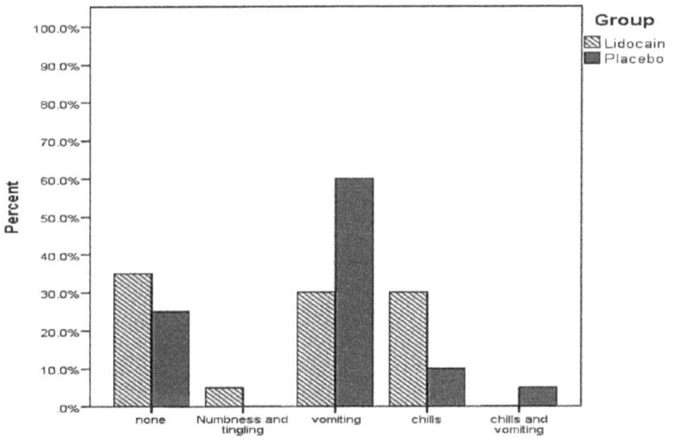

Figure 13. The frequency histogram for the incidence of side effects after surgery for both groups.

Conclusion

Using systemic Lidocaine during surgery with a bolus dose of 1.5 mg/kg and infusion dose of 2 mg/kg/h during caesarean section with general anesthesia, along with the hemodynamic stability of the mother after laryngoscopy and endotracheal intubation, could significantly decrease the intensity of post-operative pain, consumption of opioids and non-steroidal anti-inflammatory drugs and also ileus after the surgery.

Acknowledgment

The authors would like to thank the personnel of the operating room and maternity ward of Shahid Beheshti hospital for their cooperation during data collection and Ms. Asadi for her help in conducting data analysis. I would also like to thank my dear family who has always supported me.

Conflicts of Interest

The authors declare that they have no conflict of interest.

References

1. Sekhavat L, Behdad S. Preoperative analgesia with local lidocaine for cesarean delivery pain relief. J Matern Fetal Neonatal Med. 2011;24(7):891-3.

2. Choquette A, Troncy E, Guillot M, Varin F, Del Castillo JR. Pharmacokinetics of Lidocaine Hydrochloride Administered with or without Adrenaline for the Paravertebral Brachial Plexus Block in Dogs. PLoS One. 2017;12(1):e0169745.

3. Pan PH, Coghill R, Houle TT, Seid MH, Lindel WM, Parker RL, Washburn SA, Harris L, Eisenach JC.. Multifactorial Preoperative Predictors for Postcesarean Section Pain and Analgesic Requirement. Anesthesiology. 2006;104(3):417-25.

4. Shahin AY, Osman AM. Intraperitoneal lidocaine instillation and postcesarean pain after parietal peritoneal closure: a randomized double blind placebo-controlled trial. Clin J Pain. 2010;26(2):121-7.

5. Tan HL, Lie KI. Treatment of tachyarrhythmias during pregnancy and lactation. Eur Heart J. 2001;22(6):458-64.

6. Chow T, Galvin J, McGovern B. Antiarrhythmic drug therapy in pregnancy and lactation. Am J Cardiol. 1998 20;82(4A):58I-62I.

7. Kaba A, Laurent SR, Detroz BJ, Sessler DI, Durieux ME, Lamy ML, et al. Intravenous lidocaine infusion facilitates acute rehabilitation after laparoscopic colectomy. Anesthesiology. 2007;106(1):11-8.

8. Moiniche S, Kehlet H, Dahl JB. A qualitative and quantitative

systematic review of preemptive analgesia for postoperative pain relief: the role of timing of analgesia. Anesthesiology. 2002;96(3):725-41.

9. Kaufman E, Epstein JB, Gorsky M, Jackson DL, Kadari A. Preemptive analgesia and local anesthesia as a supplement to general anesthesia: a review. Anesth Prog. 2005;52(1):29-38.

10. El-Tahan MR, Warda OM, Diab DG, Ramzy EA, Matter MK. A randomized study of the effects of perioperative i.v. lidocaine on hemodynamic and hormonal responses for cesarean section. J Anesth. 2009;23(2):215-21.

11. Kord Valeshabad A, Nabavian O, Nourijelyani K, Kord H, Vafainejad H, Kord Valeshabad R, et al. Attenuation of Hemodynamic Responses to Laryngoscopy and Tracheal Intubation: Propacetamol versus Lidocaine-A Randomized Clinical Trial. Anesthesiol Res Pract. 2014;2014:170247.

12. Qi DY, Wang K, Zhang H, Du BX, Xu FY, Wang L, et al. Efficacy of intravenous lidocaine versus placebo on attenuating cardiovascular response to laryngoscopy and tracheal intubation: a systematic review of randomized controlled trials. Minerva Anestesiol. 2013;79(12):1423-35.

13. Barreveld A, Witte J, Chahal H, Durieux ME, Strichartz G. Preventive analgesia by local anesthetics: the reduction of postoperative pain by peripheral nerve blocks and intravenous drugs. Anesth Analg. 2013;116(5):1141-61.

14. De Oliveira GS Jr, Duncan K, Fitzgerald P, Nader A, Gould RW, McCarthy RJ. Systemic lidocaine to improve quality of recovery after laparoscopic bariatric surgery: a randomized double-blinded placebo-controlled trial. Obes Surg. 2014;24(2):212-8.

15. Marret E, Rolin M, Beaussier M, Bonnet F. Meta- analysis of intravenous lidocaine and postoperative recovery after abdominal surgery. Anesth Analg. 2004;98(4):1050-5.

16. Koppert W, Weigand M, Neumann F, Sittl R, Schuettler J, Schmelz M, et al. Perioperative intravenous lidocaine has preventive effects on postoperative pain and morphine consumption after major abdominal surgery. Anesthesia & Analgesia. 2004;98(4):1050-5.

17. Groudine SB, Fisher HA, Kaufman RP, Patel MK, Wilkins LJ, Mehta SA, et al. Intravenous lidocaine speeds the return of bowel function, decreases postoperative pain, and shortens hospital stay in patients undergoing radical retropubic prostatectomy. Anesth Analg. 1998;86(2):235-9..

18. Grigoras A, Lee P, Sattar F, Shorten G. Perioperative intravenous lidocaine decreases the incidence of persistent pain after breast surgery. Clin J Pain. 2012;28(7):567-72.

19. Saadawy I, Kaki A, Abd El Latif A, Abd- Elmaksoud A, Tolba O. Lidocaine vs. magnesium: effect on analgesia after a laparoscopic cholecystectomy. Acta Anaesthesiol Scand. 2010;54(5):549-56.

20. Tikuišis R, Miliauskas P, Samalavičius N, Žurauskas A, Samalavičius R, Zabulis V. Intravenous lidocaine for post-operative pain relief after hand-assisted laparoscopic colon surgery: a randomized, placebo-controlled clinical trial. Tech Coloproctol. 2014;18(4):373-80.

21. McCarthy GC, Megalla SA. Impact of intravenous lidocaine infusion on postoperative analgesia and recovery from surgery. Drugs. 2010;70(9):1149-63.

22. Vigneault L, Turgeon AF, Côté D, Lauzier F, Zarychanski R, Moore L, et al. Perioperative intravenous lidocaine infusion for postoperative pain control: a meta-analysis of randomized controlled trials. Can J Anaesth. 2011;58(1):22-37.

23. Reddi D, Curran N. Chronic pain after surgery: pathophysiology, risk factors and prevention. Postgrad Med J. 2014: 90(1062):222-7.

5

Preoperative Oral Valiflore Reduces Anxiety in Laparoscopic Cholecystectomy

Nazanin Babaei[1], Alireza Saliminia[2], Omid Azimaraghi[2], Yasaman Aghajani[1], Noushin Khazaei[1], Ali Movafegh*

Abstract

Background: Many patients undergoing surgical procedures experience preoperative anxiety. Therefore; develop a drug as a premedication with strong anxiolytic effect and minimal psychomotor impairment is desirable.
Materials and Methods: Under ethics committee approval, eighty patients, who met the inclusion criteria, were randomly assigned to two groups to receive either oral Valiflore (600 mg, Niak) or placebo as a premedication, 90 minutes before surgery. A numerical rating scale (NRS) for anxiety and the Ramsay sedation scale were measured at baseline, and 15, 30, 60, 90 minutes after premedication. Psychomotor function recovery was assessed using the Digit Symbol Substitution Test and the Trieger Dot Test on arrival in the operating room, 30 and 90 minutes after tracheal extubation. The duration of anesthesia, surgery and recovery time were recorded for each patient.
Results: There were no significant differences in the patients' demographic characteristics, ASA physical status, basal NRS score, the sedation level at different time intervals, duration of anesthesia, surgery and recovery time in the two groups ($p>0.05$). The NRS anxiety scores were significantly lower in the Valiflore group in comparison with the control group ($p<0.001$). There was no significant difference in psychomotor function test in both groups.
Conclusion: Oral administration of Valiflore as a premedication reduces anxiety before surgery without inducing sedation.
Keywords: Anxiety, Herbal medicine, Premedication, Preoperative anxiety, Valiflore

1. Research Development Center, Dr. Ali Shariati Hospital, Tehran University of Medical Sciences, Tehran, Iran
2. Department of Anesthesiology and Critical Care, Dr. Ali Shariati Hospital, Tehran University of Medical Sciences, Tehran, Iran

*Corresponding Author:
Ali Movafegh, M.D, Professor of Anesthesiology, Department of Anesthesiology and Critical Care, Dr. Ali Shariati Hospital, North Kargar Ave. Tehran University of Medical Sciences.Tehran, Iram

Email: movafegh@sina.tums.ac.ir

Introduction

Patients undergoing surgical procedures often experience high levels of anxiety (1, 2). This anxiety may induce adverse effects resulting in unfavorable physiological changes, including elevated blood cortisol levels and sympathetic hyperactivity leading to slower wound healing, decrease immune response and increase risk of infection. High anxiety may also adversely impact patients' experience of the surgery and intrude treatment process (2-4).

To reduce patient anxiety, anxiolytic premedications are highly recommended (2). Benzodiazepines are the most commonly used anxiolytic in reducing preoperative anxiety. These drugs are frequently accompanied by side effects, such as drowsiness, respiratory suppression and may interact with anesthetic agents to prolonged recovery and discharge of the patient (3, 5). Therefore, safe alternative treatments are considered.

Phytotherapeutic products have been administered increasingly to control anxiety (6, 7). Valiflore is an herbal medication containing combined extracts of *Passiflora incarnata Linneaus* and *Valeriana* officinalis.

Passiflora incarnata L. (Passion Flower) is a plant in the family of *Passifloraceae* that has traditionally been used as an anxiolytic and sedative worldwide since ancient times (8, 9). *Valeriana officinalis* (Valerian root) is a traditional herbal supplement from the *Valerianaceae* family, which has been widely used to reduce anxiety, restlessness, somatic arousal, as well as improve sleep disorders (10-13).

The therapeutic efficacy of valerian has been confirmed by the European Medicines Evaluation Agency in an actual monograph (Committee on Herbal Medicinal Products (HMPC/ EMEA) (11).

To our knowledge, the use of Valiflore on anxiety before inducing anesthesia has never been evaluated. In this double-blinded, placebo-controlled clinical trial, we hypothesized that the use of Valiflore as a premedication alleviates preoperative anxiety with limited impact on anesthesia and recovery. The primary outcome of the present study was to investigate the efficacy of preoperative oral administration of Valiflore on anxiety levels of patients during the preoperative period. The sedative effects, psychomotor function, anesthesia duration, surgery duration and the recovery period were assessed as secondary outcomes.

Methods

The study protocol was approved by the Tehran University of Medical Sciences Ethics Committee and written informed consent was obtained from all patients. The trial is registered at the Iranian Registry of Clinical Trials (IRCT.ir) with the registration number IRCT201404115175N13.

Eighty patients aged 20–55 years, classified as American Society of Anesthesiologists (ASA) physical status I and II, who were undergoing elective surgical laparoscopic cholecystectomy were enrolled in this randomized, double-blinded, placebo-controlled study. Patients with a history of chronic diseases, anxiety and other mental and psychological disorders, those consuming any medication chronically, including anti-depressant, sedative, analgesic and antiepileptic drugs, patients with pre-operative numerical rating scale for anxiety less than one were excluded from the study.

At the preoperative visit, all patients received an explanation of the study plan and the different scales used in the study by a trained investigator. An anesthesiologist who was not involved in anesthesia administration or in patient allocation prepared all drugs; thus, patients and investigators were blinded to group assignment. Patients were randomly allocated into two groups, control (group C, n=40) and intervention (group V, n=40) using a computer generated randomization list.

Approximately 2 hours before surgery, patients were transferred to a quiet room in the operating suite. All patients were assessed by monitoring with an electrocardiogram, noninvasive arterial blood pressure, and pulse oximetry on arrival to the operating room.

The patients' level of anxiety was evaluated using a Numeric Rating Scale (NRS); a 0–10 scale, where 0= no anxiety and 10=the worst possible anxiety. Patients' level of sedation was assessed using the Ramsay sedation scale where 1=agitated, anxious or restless; 2=cooperative, oriented and tranquil; 3=responds to commands only, 4=asleep, brisk response to light glabellar tap or auditory stimulus; 5=asleep, sluggish response to light glabellar tap or auditory stimulus; 6=asleep, no response (14).

Instantly prior to receiving the premedication or placebo, each patient was assessed for their baseline anxiety score using a Numeric Rating Scale and their baseline sedation level using the Ramsay sedation scale.

Patients in the control group received a placebo tablet and patients in the intervention group received a Valiflore tablet orally 90 minutes before surgery. The placebo and the active forms of drugs were identical in appearance.

The NRS score and Ramsay sedation score were repeated at 15, 30, 60 and 90 (immediately before induction of anesthesia) minutes after drug taken.

Psychomotor function was assessed using Trieger Dot Test (TDT) and Digit-Symbol Substitution Test (DSST) at preoperative baseline, 30 and 90 minutes after tracheal extubation. The TDT is a variation of the Bender-Gestalt test in which the patients were required to arrange a series of dots connected in a specific pattern. Points are subtracted for missing a dot. TDT deviation represents the cumulative distance (in millimeters) between the drawn line and missed dots. The DSST is a subtest of the Wechsler Adult Intelligence Scale. It is a timed paper and pencil test in which patients are asked to appropriately match numbers and symbols. The number of correct symbols matches during 90 seconds is the score (6).

In the operating room, a standard general anesthesia method was used in all patients. Anesthesia was induced with Alfentanil 15 μg/kg and Propofol 2.5mg/kg. Cisatracurium 0.2 mg/kg was administrated to facilitate orotracheal intubation. Anesthesia was maintained with Propofol 60-100μg/kg/min and 1 μg/kg/min Alfentanil.

Mechanical ventilation was adjusted to maintain end-tidal carbon dioxide (ETCO2) pressure at 35-40mmHg level. Patients were actively warmed to maintain body core temperature (esophageal normothermic). At the end of the surgery, neuromuscular block was resolved by the administration of neostigmine 2.5mg and atropine 1mg. The duration of anesthesia, surgery and recovery were assessed and recorded for all patients.

At the post-anesthesia care unit (PACU), patients received supplemental oxygen via a nasal cannula at 4 liters/minute-1. Postoperative pain was treated with 3mg/kg-1 Tramadol during 10 minutes infusion. Postoperative nausea and vomiting were treated with 4mg Ondansetron intravenously.

Patients were discharged from the PACU when they were awake and oriented, and were able to breathe deeply and cough freely, their arterial blood pressure was within 20% of preoperative values, their body temperature>36°C, and there was no shivering, minimal pain, and minimal nausea (15).

Based on the pilot study of 10 patients, 63% of patients experienced moderate to severe anxiety (score 4 to 10) before surgery (at 90 minutes). For a predicted 50% reduction in the percentages of patients experienced anxiety and bringing it to 32 was calculated that a sample size of 40 patients in each group would be sufficient to detect a three score difference in the mean of anxiety score between the two groups considering a power of 80%, and a significance level of $\alpha=0.05$.

Statistical analyses were performed using SPSS software (SPSS Inc., Chicago, IL, USA), version 20. To compare demographic data, ASA physical status, the basal NRS anxiety score, the duration of anesthesia, surgery and recovery time between the two groups, independent sample t-test was performed.

The repeated measures analysis of variance (ANOVA) was utilized to assess the changes in NRS for anxiety between groups and the changes over time in each group.

To compare the sedation scores between groups at each measurement time, the Fisher's exact test was used and to compare the sedation scores in groups within time, the Friedman test was used.

Data are presented as mean ± standard deviation (SD), median (range), or number (incidence) as appropriate. Statistical significance was considered significant when P value<0.05.

Results

We randomized 80 patients. No patients dropped out and all patients were included in the data analysis. A flow diagram of conduct of the trial is presented in figure 1.

Patients' characteristics, ASA physical status, the duration of anesthesia, surgery and recovery time were similar in the two groups (Table 1).

The basal NRS anxiety scores were similar in the Valiflore group (5.62±0.89) and in the control group (5.87±1.06) ($p>0.05$). A significant difference in the mean NRS anxiety scores from the baseline was found in the Valiflore group over time ($p<0.001$) (Figure 2).

Based on Ramsay sedation scores, the sedation levels of the patients were similar over time within and between groups (Fisher's exact test, $p>0.05$; Friedman test, $p>0.05$) (Table 2).

Psychomotor function scores were similar in both groups. The psychomotor function scores were

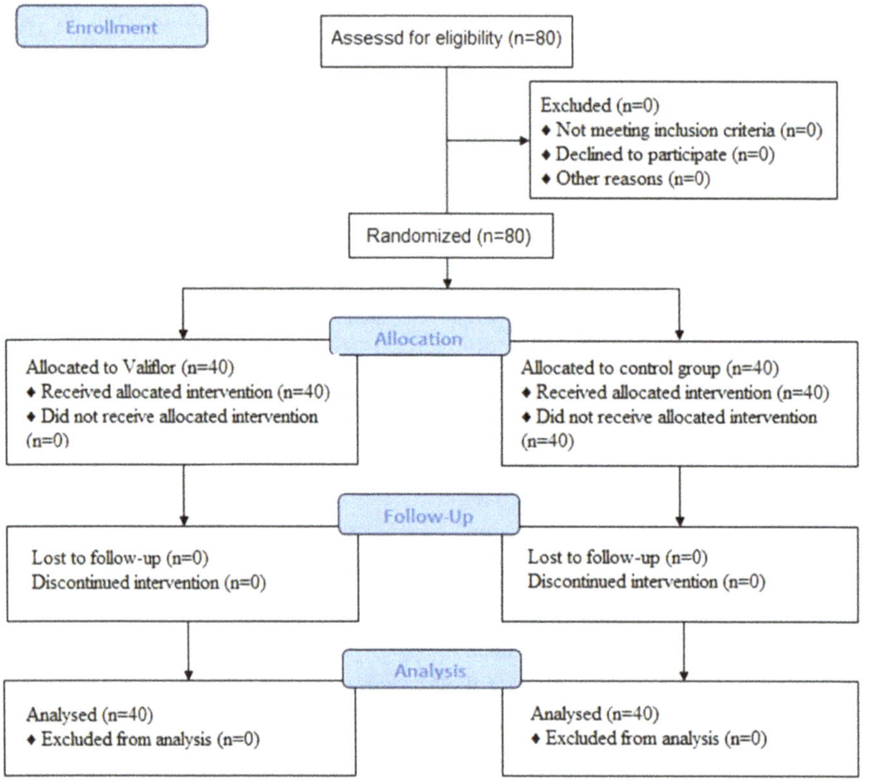

Figure 1. Flow diagram according to CONSORT statement.

Table 1: Patient Characteristics. There was no significant difference between groups.

	Valiflore group (n=40)	**Control group (n=40)**
Age (years)	37.1±8.7	39.5±6.3
Weight (kg)	64.4±9.4	67.0±10.0
ASA I/II	21/19	19/21
Anesthesia duration (min)	118.6±5.9	118.0±7.6
Surgery duration (min)	86.4±6.0	87.0±7.1
Recovery duration (min)	29.3±4.9	28.8±5.7

significantly reduced 30 minutes after tracheal

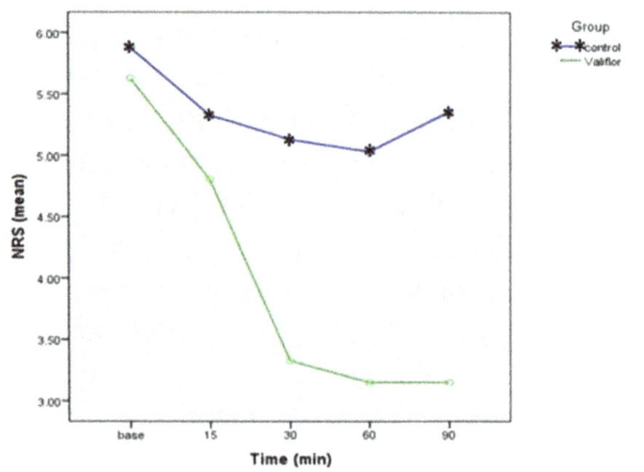

Figure 2. Numeric Rating Scale (NRS) of anxiety at different time intervals.

extubation in both groups; however, within 90 minutes after extubation they reached baseline values (Table 3).

Discussion

This study demonstrates that patients who received oral premedication with Valiflore experienced lower preoperative anxiety compared with patients who received placebo.

Table 2: Sedation in Groups. There was no significant difference.

	Valiflore group (n=40)	**Control group (n=40)**
Before premedication		
Agitated, anxious or restless	0	0
Cooperative, oriented and tranquil	40 (100%)	40 (100%)
Responds to commands only	0	0
Brisk response to light glabellar tap or auditory stimulus	0	0
Sluggish response to light glabellar tap or auditory stimulus	0	0
No response	0	0
15 min after premedication		
Agitated, anxious or restless	0	0
Cooperative, oriented and tranquil	40 (100%)	40 (100%)
Responds to commands only	0	0
Brisk response to light glabellar tap or auditory stimulus	0	0
Sluggish response to light glabellar tap or auditory stimulus	0	0
No response	0	0
30 min after premedication		
Agitated, anxious or restless	0	0
Cooperative, oriented and tranquil	40 (100%)	40 (100%)
Responds to commands only	0	0
Brisk response to light glabellar tap or auditory stimulus	0	0
Sluggish response to light glabellar tap or auditory stimulus	0	0
No response	0	0
60 min after premedication		
Agitated, anxious or restless	0	1 (2.5%)
Cooperative, oriented and tranquil	40 (100%)	39 (97.5%)

Responds to commands only	0	0
Brisk response to light glabellar tap or auditory stimulus	0	0
Sluggish response to light glabellar tap or auditory stimulus	0	0
No response	0	0
90 min after premedication		
Agitated, anxious or restless	0	0
Cooperative, oriented and tranquil	40 (100%)	40 (100%)
Responds to commands only	0	0
Brisk response to light glabellar tap or auditory stimulus	0	0
Sluggish response to light glabellar tap or auditory stimulus	0	0
No response	0	0

The onset and the peak effects of Valiflore's anxiolytic activity were observed at 15 and 60 minutes following oral administration. It was notable that the single dose of the Valiflore tablet led to 43% decrease in the level of anxiety.

In both groups, psychomotor impairment occurred 30 minutes after surgery; although, they returned to the basic levels after 90 minutes.

Also, the recovery time was similar in both groups which present that the administration of Valiflore as a premedication does not affect psychomotor function or discharge time to home. Preoperative Anxiety has been reported in 11–80% of adult patients, which can lead to unfavorable health outcomes result in longer recovery time and hospital stays. Prevention of preoperative anxiety, improves surgical outcome and decreases inpatient stay (3, 16).

Passiflora incarnata and Valerian root are popular medicinal plants for the treatment of anxiety with a long history of usage in the world (10, 17, 18). In Iran, compound drug has been introduced to the market with the trade name ''Valiflore'' (Niak R). In the present study, the effect of this almost new herbal combination on preoperative anxiety was evaluated.

Passiflora incarnata's anxiolytic effects have been supported in many well-documented studies, though; the active phytoconstituents and the exact mechanism of action responsible for the therapeutic properties have not been identified yet (19).

The anxiolytic activity of *Passiflora incarnata* has been attributed to mediate via benzodiazepine and γ-aminobutyric acid receptors (6, 17). Flavonoids are considered for the most probable active ingredient; they have anxiolytic properties similar to benzodiazepines, and modulate or inhibit GABAA and GABAC receptor currents. Chrysin has been shown to act as a partial agonist of benzodiazepine receptors and GABA was found to be a prominent ingredient of Passiflora extract (20, 21).

The evidences also support the *Valeriana officinalis*'s efficacy and clinical safety in the treatment of anxiety with no effect on psychomotor performance, alertness or concentration (7, 22). *Valeriana officinalis* was the most reported product (19.4%) among herbal products which is used in preoperative patients (23). The main active constituents of *Valeriana officinalis* are valerenic acid and valepotriates (24). The presence of the anxiolytic flavone 6-methylapigenin (MA) in *Valeriana officinalis* also has been reported (13). The exact mechanism of action of *Valeriana officinalis* has remained unknown. Neurobiological studies showed that valerenic acid interacts within the GABAA-ergic system, similarly to a mechanism of action of the benzodiazepine drugs, by binding to specific subunits of the GABAA receptor complex, result in opening of chloride channels and producing neural inhibition. Valerenic acid also has been attributed to work via

Table 3: Psychomotor Function tests.

	Valiflore group (n=40)	Control group (n=40)
TDTmm Preoperative baseline	0.8 ± 0.5	0.8 ± 0.3
TDTmm 30 min after extubation [a]	1.8 ± 1.0	2.0 ± 1.0
TDTmm 90 min after extubation	0.6 ± 0.2	0.7 ± 0.2
TDTnr Preoperative baseline	0.8 ± 0.3	0.8 ± 0.2
TDTnr 30 min after extubation [a]	1.9 ± 1.1	1.8 ± 0.8
TDTnr 90 min after extubation	2.8 ± 0.3	0.9 ± 0.5
DSST Preoperative baseline	25.1 ± 7.2	24.0 ± 6.3
DSST 30 min after extubation [a]	18.1 ± 7.2	18.2 ± 6.6
DSST 90 min after extubation	21.4 ± 6.2	22.1 ± 6.6

a There was a significant difference

modulation of the serotonergic system, adenosine receptors or melatonergic effects (10, 25).

In a double-blinded, randomized, controlled trial (RCT) 60 patients who were scheduled for spinal anesthesia were randomly allocated into two groups to receive oral *Passiflora incarnata* aqueous extract 700 mg 5 ml-1 or placebo. The result of this study showed that preoperative oral administration of *Passiflora incarnata* extract suppresses the increase in anxiety levels of patients before spinal anesthesia without changing in sedation level, psychomotor function test results, or hemodynamics (17).

In another study *Passiflora incarnata* extract was administered as a premedication to control presurgical anxiety in patients undergoing elective surgery under general anesthesia. A total of 60 patients was randomized into two groups to receive a *Passiflora incarnata* or a placebo tablet as a premedication, 90 minutes before surgery (n=30 for each group). The results revealed a significant reduction of preoperative anxiety in Passiflora group compared with placebo without inducing sedation or changing psychomotor function (6).

Contrary to all these reports, the study by Elsas and colleagues; in 2010 showed that Passiflora extracts have anxiogenic effects instead of the expected anxiolytic effects. The unexpected anxiogenic activity of Passiflora extracts may attributed to some conditions, such as dosage changes in flavonoids, which act as weak agonists to weak antagonists at specific GABAA receptor subtypes (20).

There are a few reports of adverse effects associated with *Passiflora incarnata* consumption (26), there are no such reports about *Valeriana officinalis*. Nausea, vomiting, prolonged QT, and ventricular arrhythmias developed following self-administration of *Passiflora incarnata* in a 34 year-old female patient (27). Hypersensitivity with cutaneous vasculitis, urticaria, asthma, and rhinitis after ingestion of tablets containing Passiflora extract has also been reported (6). Furthermore, Passiflora has been attributed to induce uterine contraction so its use is contraindicated during pregnancy (6, 17, 27). Altered consciousness has been reported after taking an herbal compound containing *Passiflora incarnata.* It was recommended not to take *Passiflora incarnata* with CNS depressants or stimulants to minimize possible adverse effects on CNS (27) although; these side effects are sporadic, and only occurred after chronic usage.

In the study, we used the 600 mg Valiflore tablet introduced by Niak pharmaceutical company-Iran, which may differ from other products in constituents or efficacy. It consists of dry extracts from Passion flower (30mg) and Valerian (100mg).

Valeriana officinalis extract ratio of 33% and *Passiflora incarnata* extract ratio of 9.9% is prepared.

The therapeutic dose of Valiflore for anxiety is 1-2 tablet/s once or twice a day. As Oral administration of Valiflore to reduce preoperative anxiety has not been evaluated, we used the minimum effective dose, a single dose of tablet (600 mg) to minimize few possible side effects. At the end of surgery, Valiflore presented a better effect than placebo. In this study, the patients were not required to complete side effect questionnaires, but they were asked to verbally report if they experienced any side effects both during and at the end of the day and no evidence of side effects were reported.

One limitation of this study was that we evaluated the psychological stress with subjective assessment tools which are not reliable parameters to assess anxiety as they are patient dependent. Therefore more physiological parameters such as stress biomarkers may have been able to assess subtle effects of the medication on the patients' level of anxiety. This would be an interesting consideration for future studies.

Conclusion

In conclusion, preoperative oral administration of Valiflore tablet was effective in reducing anxiety without changing in the sedation level or impairing psychomotor function compared with placebo. As this trial was the first study on the issue, more trials are required.

Acknowledgment

This study received no external funding. The authors declare no conflict of interest.

Conflicts of Interest

The authors declare that they have no conflict of interest.

References

1. Fortier MA, Martin SR, MacLaren Chorney J, Mayes LC, Kain ZN. Preoperative anxiety in adolescents undergoing surgery: a pilot study. Pediatric Anesthesia. 2011;21:969-73.

2. Bradt J, Dileo C, Shim M. Music interventions for preoperative anxiety. The Cochrane Library; 2013.

3. Arai Y-C, Kawanishi J, Sakakima Y, et al. The Effect of the Kampo Medicine Yokukansan on Preoperative Anxiety and Sedation Levels. Evidence-Based Complementary and Alternative Medicine. 2014;2014.

4. Ravitskiy L, Phillips PK, Roenigk RK, et al. The use of oral midazolam for perioperative anxiolysis of healthy patients undergoing Mohs surgery: Conclusions from randomized controlled and prospective studies. Journal of the American Academy of Dermatology. 2011;64:310-22

5. White PF, Tufanogullari B, Taylor J, Klein K. The effect of pregabalin on preoperative anxiety and sedation levels: a dose-ranging study. Anesthesia & Analgesia. 2009;108:1140-5.

6. Movafegh A, Alizadeh R, Hajimohamadi F, Esfehani F, Nejatfar M. Preoperative oral Passiflora incarnata reduces anxiety in ambulatory surgery patients: a double-blind, placebo-controlled study. Anesthesia & Analgesia. 2008;106:1728-32.

7. Pinheiro MLP, Alcântara CEP, de Moraes M, de Andrade ED. Valeriana officinalis L. For conscious sedation of patients submitted to impacted lower third molar surgery: A randomized, double-blind, placebo-controlled split-mouth study. Journal of pharmacy & bioallied sciences. 2014;6:109.

8. Dhawan K, Kumar S, Sharma A. Comparative anxiolytic activity profile of various preparations of Passiflora incarnata linneaus: a comment on medicinal plants' standardization. The Journal of Alternative & Complementary Medicine. 2002;8:283-91.

9. Sampath C, Holbik M, Krenn L, Butterweck V. Anxiolytic effects of fractions obtained from Passiflora incarnata L. In the elevated plus maze in mice. Phytotherapy Research. 2011;25:789-95.

10. Murphy K, Kubin Z, Shepherd J, Ettinger R. Valeriana officinalis root extracts have potent anxiolytic effects in laboratory rats. Phytomedicine 2010; 17: 674-8.

11. Hattesohl M, Feistel B, Sievers H, Lehnfeld R, Hegger M, Winterhoff H. Extracts of Valeriana officinalis L. Sl show anxiolytic and antidepressant effects but neither sedative nor myorelaxant properties. Phytomedicine. 2008;15:2-15.

12. Weeks BS. Formulations of dietary supplements and herbal extracts for relaxation and anxiolytic action: Relarian. Annals of Transplantation. 2009;15: RA256-RA62.

13. Fernández S, Wasowski C, Paladini AC, Marder M. Sedative and sleep-enhancing properties of linarin, a flavonoid-isolated from Valeriana officinalis. Pharmacology Biochemistry and Behavior. 2004;77: 399-404.

14. Ramsay M, Savege T, Simpson B, Goodwin R. Controlled sedation with alphaxalone-alphadolone. British medical Journal. 1974;2:656.

15. Marshall SI, Chung F. Discharge criteria and complications after ambulatory surgery. Anesthesia & Analgesia. 1999;88:508-17.

16. Yilmaz M, Sezer H, Gürler H, Bekar M. Predictors of preoperative anxiety in surgical inpatients. Journal of clinical nursing. 2012;21:956-64.

17. Aslanargun P, Cuvas O, Dikmen B, Aslan E, Yuksel MU. Passiflora incarnata Linneaus as an anxiolytic before spinal anesthesia. Journal of anesthesia. 2012;26:39-44.

18. Pakseresht S, Boostani H, Sayyah M. Extract of valerian root

(Valeriana officinalis L.) vs. placebo in treatment of obsessive-compulsive disorder: a randomized double-blind study. Journal of Complementary and Integrative Medicine. 2011;8.
19. Miyasaka LS, Atallah ÁN, Soares B. Passiflora for anxiety disorder. The Cochrane Library; 2007.
20. Elsas S-M, Rossi D, Raber J, et al. Passiflora incarnata L. (Passion flower) extracts elicit GABA currents in hippocampal neurons in vitro, and show anxiogenic and anticonvulsant effects in vivo, varying with extraction method. Phytomedicine. 2010;17:940-9.
21. Fiebich BL, Knörle R, Appel K, Kammler T, Weiss G. Pharmacological studies in an herbal drug combination of St. John's Wort (Hypericum perforatum) and passion flower (Passiflora incarnata): in vitro and in vivo evidence of synergy between Hypericum and Passiflora in antidepressant pharmacological models. Fitoterapia. 2011;82:474-80.
22. Kennedy DO, Little W, Haskell CF, Scholey AB. Anxiolytic effects of a combination of Melissa ofcinalis and Valeriana ofcinalis during laboratory induced stress. Phytotherapy research. 2006;20:96-102.
23. Lucenteforte E, Gallo E, Pugi A, et al. Complementary and alternative drugs use among preoperative patients: a cross-sectional study in Italy. Evidence-Based Complementary and Alternative Medicine. 2011;2012.
24. Sarris J, McIntyre E, Camfield DA. Plant-based medicines for anxiety disorders, part 2: a review of clinical studies with supporting preclinical evidence. CNS drugs. 2013;27:301-19.
25. Sarris J, Panossian A, Schweitzer I, Stough C, Scholey A. Herbal medicine for depression, anxiety and insomnia: a review of psychopharmacology and clinical evidence. European Neuropsychopharmacology. 2011;21:841-60.
26. Nunes A, Sousa M. Use of valerian in anxiety and sleep disorders: what is the best evidence? Acta Médica Portuguesa. 2011;24:961-6.
27. Dhawan K, Dhawan S, Sharma A. Passiflora: a review update. Journal of Ethnopharmacology. 2004;94:1-23.

Distribution of Bupivacaine in Epidural Space

Hamid Haji Gholam Saryazdi[1], Gholamreza khalili[1], Reihanak Talakoub[1*], Masoud Shahbazi[1], Saeed Abbasi[1]

Abstract

Background: There is no consensus regarding the spread of local anesthesia in thoracic epidural space to obtain regional analgesia or anesthesia. We aimed to determine the distribution of Bupivacaine injected into the thoracic epidural space to evaluate its cranial or caudal spread in patients undergoing epidural anesthesia.

Materials and Methods: In a prospective clinical trial, thirty adults patients (12 males and 18 females) with ASA class I and II, scheduled for elective cholecystectomy under thoracic epidural anesthesia with 0.5% Isobaric Bupivacaine were studied. Clinical and radiological outcomes were evaluated to assess the correlation between the volume of the local anesthetic injected to the thoracic epidural space and the extension of its spread within the epidural space. Immediately after insertion and fixation of epidural catheter, patients were transferred to MRI unit to receive 8 mL of 5% Bupivacaine plus 1 mL Magnevist through the epidural catheter. Then, the patterns of spread were evaluated. Data were obtained prospectively during the procedure.

Results: Mean distribution of bupivacaine in thoracic epidural space was 0.64 level/ml of local anesthetics and the average of spread was 5.21 levels. The mean spread of bupivacaine was more in females (5.5 ± 1.1) than males (4.8 ± 1.1); but the difference was not significant. Unlike Patients' age and weight, the height and body mass index had a significant negative correlation with the distribution of Bupivacaine.

Conclusion: Distribution of Bupivacaine in epidural space in female patients is more than male ones and the tendency of spread is more toward the cephalad direction than caudal.

Keywords: Bupivacaine distribution, Epidural anesthesia, Local Anesthesia, Bupivacaine, Magnevist

1. Anesthesia and Critical Care Research Center, Alzahra Hospital, Department of Anesthesiology, School of Medicine, Isfahan University of Medical sciences, Isfahan, Iran.

*Corresponding Author: Reihanak Talakoub, MD, Associate Professor, Anesthesiology and Critical Care Research Center, Isfahan University of Medical Science, Isfahan, Iran;

Email: reihanak.talakoub@gmail.com

Introduction

Epidural anesthesia is one of the common methods employed to control pain and is indicated for surgical procedures such as thoracic, upper and lower abdominal, cervical, gynecological, urological and lower extremity operations (1, 2). One of the favorable advantages of epidural anesthesia is providing better condition of pain control for several days post operatively (3, 4) by using patient controlled analgesia (PCA). In addition to patient's satisfaction, this method of pain control can prevent the dangerous and intense complications of uncontrolled pain that usually threat patients within the first couple of days after operation. Myocardial infarction causes uncontrolled pain and atelectasis induced by inappropriate ventilation due to postoperative pain is two of the most important complications (5, 6).

During epidural anesthesia, local anesthetic drug acts on the sodium channels on spinal nerves. The sensory and motor blockade is attributed to the direct contact of local anesthetics with the superficial layers of the nerve roots in the spinal cord (7, 8). The distribution of drugs within the epidural space can be influenced by different factors, including the injection volume, rate of infusion, intervertebral foramina status, body position, epidural fat, vascular absorption and the anatomy of a particular species (9–11).

The cranial spread of Methylene blue (MB) into the epidural space studied *in vivo*, and a correlation between the volume administered and the cranial distribution of the dye was observed. Moll and his colleagues studied the distribution of different volumes of MB solution injected into the epidural space in anaesthetized pregnant and non-pregnant sheep. The results showed that the volume of MB injected epidurally into pregnant and non-pregnant sheep correlated directly with its cephalic distribution into the epidural space; and a volume of 0.1 mL/kg or 0.2 mL/kg stained up to the first lumbar segment in pregnant and non-pregnant sheep, respectively. In addition, the results suggested that the volume of drugs administered into the epidural space of the pregnant sheep should be half than in the non-pregnant one (12).

In another study, the spread of labeled blood in epidural space of patients who suffered from severe uncontrollable post spinal postural headaches was detected. In this study, the labeled red blood cells were injected into the patients' epidural space, and in evaluation by imaging techniques using a gamma camera with a parallel-hole collimator, it was found that the blood injected into the epidural space tended to travel more easily upward in a cranial direction. The mean spread of blood was six spinal segments upward and three spinal segments downward (13).

Our study was aimed to evaluate the spread of Bupivacaine in patients who have not any deformity, manipulation or operation in their spinal column. In this study we used the combination of Bupivacaine and the radio-opaque marker Magnevist (gadopentetate dimeglumine) injected in the thoracic epidural space in candidates of cholecystectomy to evaluate the spread of local anesthetic detected by magnetic resonance imaging.

Methods

This prospective clinical trial was conducted in Alzahra University Hospital in Isfahan, Iran. The study protocol was approved by Anesthesiology Department and Ethic Committee of Isfahan Medical University and written informed consent was obtained from each patient.

We studied thirty, ASA I and II adult patients candidates of elective cholecystectomy who had no history of acute or chronic kidney disease, deformity or history of operation in the spinal area and severe hypersensitivity reactions to Magnevist.

Participants were selected by non-probable simple sampling method. The patients were prepared for epidural anesthesia on a side railed table in the room adjacent to the magnetic resonance imaging (MRI) section under full standard monitoring. To achieve appropriate sedation, 50 mg Fentanyl plus 1mg Midazolam was injected intravenously. After sterilizing the patient's thoracic area and determining the space of T7 based on the scapula tip marker, 5cc Lidocaine 1% was injected under the skin area of T7-T8 space.

By using a Tuohy 18G epidural needle and a midline approach through the T7-T8 space, by using one of the techniques of loss of resistance or hanging drop and being certain of the place of needle in the epidural space, 3cc test dose of Lidocaine 2% and Epinephrine 1/200000 was injected in the epidural space and the patient was monitored for two to three minutes. After complete assurance of intact dura and the placement of the needle (by checking patient's heart rate (HR) and lack of motor-sensory block in the lower extremities), the epidural catheter (Gauge 20) was inserted and advanced 3 – 5 cm in epidural space. Then the epidural needle was slowly pulled away from the epidural catheter while care was taken for the catheter not to displace.

After fixing the catheter on the patient's back, patient was quickly transferred to the MRI room and 8cc Bupivacaine 5% isobaric plus 1cc Magnevist (gadopentetate dimeglumine) was injected through the epidural catheter with a rate of 1ml/sec by an anesthesiologist's assistant and then the MRI was done. The MRI was set at 1.5 Tesla. During MRI procedure, the patient was under blood Oxygen saturation (SPO2) monitoring and under direct supervision of the anesthesiologist's assistant.

The extent of contrast spread was determined by calculating numbers of the intervertebral foramina completely covered by contrast medium. The radiologist performed the interpretations of the epidurograms and the spread of contrast medium to the upper and lower segments regarding to the seventh thoracic segment.

Upon completion of MRI, while the patient was under full supervision and cardiovascular and pulmonary monitoring, the patient was transferred to the operating room (OR) within 10 min maximally. HR, systolic and diastolic blood pressor (BP) and mean arterial BP were recorded at 0, 5 and 10 minutes after epidural anesthesia. Then, the MRI cliché was reviewed by the same radiologist and its report recorded.

We also determined patient characteristics such as gender, age, weight, height and body mass index (BMI) to determine differences in spread of local anesthetic in thoracic epidural anesthesia.

Our data was analyzed by using repeated measured design analysis of variance (ANOVA), Pearson correlation coefficient and t-paired test by applying SPSS version 22, Chicago IL, for Windows statistical programs. P values of <0.05 were considered statistically significant.

Results

A total of 24 patients including 18 females (60%) and 12 males (40%) were studied and all of the patients completed the study and were evaluable. The mean of HR at 5 and 10 minutes after thoracic epidural block was significantly lower when compared with the values at the time of 0 (P<0.001), but there was no significant difference between mean HR at 5 and 10 minutes after epidural block (p<0.14). The mean changes of systolic, diastolic and mean arterial blood pressure at 5 and 10 minutes after thoracic epidural block were also reduced significantly when compared with the values at the time 0.(p<0.001).

The mean distribution of Bupivacaine in thoracic epidural space was 0.64 level/ml of local anesthetics and the average of spread was 5.21 levels. The mean spread of Bupivacaine was more in females (5.5 ± 1.1) than males (4.8 ± 1.1), but this difference was not significant. The spread of Bupivacaine in the thoracic epidural space in men was 2.2 levels higher and 1.56 levels lower than the injection site (T7 space) and in females these measures were 2.8 levels higher and 1.7 levels lower. A comparison of the spread of local anesthetic in female and male patients is given in Table 1.

It showed that, Bupivacaine was spread in a wider range in females than males; although it was not statistically significant. Moreover, the spread of Bupivacaine in the thoracic epidural space has been more toward cephalad rather than caudal. Table 2 shows the Pearson correlation coefficient between the variables of spread of Bupivacaine in thoracic epidural space and the patients' age, weight, height and BMI. The Pearson correlation test showed a correlation coefficient between age and thoracic epidural local anesthetic spread of -0.03.

Table 1: Distribution of Bupivacaine according to Gender in Epidural Space.

	Females (Mean± SD)	Males (Mean± SD)	P- value
The mean spread of Bupivacaine in the thoracic space	5.5±1.1	4.8± 1.1	0.08
Number of distribution levels higher than the injection site	2.8±1.15	2.2± 0.83	0.1
Number of distribution levels lower than the injection site	1.7± 0.82	1.56± 0.53	0.36

Variables are presented as mean ± SD
P values less than 0.05 indicate statistically significant difference

Table 2: Distribution of Bupivacaine according to Age, Weight, Height and BMI in Epidural Space.

	Pearson Correlation Coefficient	**P- value**
Age (Years)	0.03	0.445
Weight (Kg)	0.2	0.17
Height (Cm)	0.71	<0.001*
BMI (Kg/m2)	0.34	0.05*

*significant difference

We also found a significant inverse relationship between height and Bupivacaine spread in thoracic epidural space (r=-0.71, P<0.001). The average height of our patients was 1.68cm. In the case of BMI, we found a significant positive relationship (r=0.34, P=0.05) between BMI and thoracic spread of Bupivacaine. The spread of Bupivacaine had weak relationship with Patient's weight with a correlation coefficient of -0.2 and this correlation was not significant.

Discussion

The aim of this study was to identify a relationship between the injection volume of Bupivacaine and the degree of its migration during thoracic epidural anesthesia. There are several factors, mentioned in the introduction, that influence the spread of drugs injecting in the epidural space. Our results showed that the mean distribution of Bupivacaine in thoracic epidural space was 0.64 level/ml of local anesthetics and the average of spread was 5.21 levels. We found that the mean spread of Bupivacaine level was more in females (5.5 ± 1.1) than males (4.8 ± 1.1), although this difference was not significant.

According to our findings in order to block one intervertebral level in males 1.88 cc and in females 1.63cc 0.5% isobaric Bupivacaine was required. A number of variables determine how far a local anesthetic will spread after injection into the epidural space. Some variables are regarding the patient and some are extrinsic, depending on variations in technique and the drugs given (14).

Burn et al. reported that it is impossible to predict accurately the level attained after epidural injection of contrast medium. The unpredictable pattern of spread is likely due to anatomical variation of the epidural space (15). Recent reports have indicated that the structure of the epidural space is more complex and variable than ever thought and this intrinsic factor makes the spread of solution in the epidural space unpredictable (16).

Szeinfeld et al, in a study, evaluated the volume and spread of blood injected to the epidural space in patients experienced postural headaches after spinal anesthesia. They injected an average volume of 14.8 cc labeled blood in lumbar epidural space and reported that the mean number of segments of blood spread was nine and the average volume of blood spread per spinal segment was 1.6 cc (13). In our study as well, this value was calculated as 1.88 cc and 1.63cc of 0.5% Isobaric Bupivacaine for males and females, respectively and was almost similar to the former study.

Coombs et al, also injected 18cc blood with 2cc tracer Maglumine (total 20cc) in lumbar epidural space for epidural blood patching and showed that this substance can spread in 5 intervertebral levels; i.e. 4cc blood was needed for each level. This difference might have been due to the fact that, in this study the subjects were women who had been recently given birth. Those, whose spinal column curve, body physiology, absorption and excretion of medicines are affected by pregnancy up to 40 days after childbirth. In addition, the mentioned study was carried out on the lumbar epidural space whereas our study was done on the thoracic epidural space (17). Moreover, in our study we used 0.5% isobaric Bupivacaine while in the previous studies, blood was injected in epidural space. It is obvious that the absorption of 0.5% isobaric Bupivacaine in epidural space is different from blood absorption in this region. On the other hand, in our study, for every one level drop in local anesthetic, 1.6 level rises in the thoracic epidural blood absorption space was seen, but in the study carried out on women after childbirth in lumbar epidural space, 2.5 levels blood absorption was raised for every blood fall level. This difference may be attributed to the difference of the epidural space in studied groups and studied solutions (blood vs. 0.5% isobaric Bupivacaine). In addition, in mentioned studies, there were no reports of differentiation of distribution of any injected solutions in epidural space according to the gender. Moreover, most studies in this regard performed on pregnant or post-childbirth women.

In contrast to the conflicting reports on lumbar epidural anesthesia, the few studies investigating the effects of age on thoracic epidural spread. It suggested that there is a positive correlation between age and spread of blockade, but recently Wink et al, reported that after injection of a fixed loading dose of Ropivacaine at the T3–T4 level, they were unable to demonstrate an effect of age on the maximal number of spinal segments blocked after thoracic epidural anesthesia (18). Similarly, in our study, we demonstrated almost no effect of age on thoracic epidural spread of local anesthetic.

It seems that taller patients require more local anesthetics to establish a certain level of blockade than shorter subjects, but clinical trials evaluating the relationship between height and spread of blockade after epidural administration of local anesthetics are lacking in thoracic epidural anesthesia. In thoracic epidural anesthesia, correlation coefficients from -0.25 (14) to -0.37 (19) have been found between the spread of epidural injected contrast medium and patient height. We also found a significant negative relationship (correlation coefficient of -0.71) between Bupivacaine spread in thoracic epidural space and the height of patients, which is almost similar to the findings of other studies.

Few studies report on the correlation between weight and spread of local anesthetics in thoracic epidural space. Yokoyama, et al, reported that weight was not correlated with epidural spread of contrast in thoracic epidural anesthesia. We also found that spread of Bupivacaine had weak relationship with Patient's weight (14).

Since a total of 8cc local anesthetic was injected, it could be concluded that to block each level of epidural space 1.6 and 1.88cc 0.5% isobaric Bupivacaine is required in female and male patients respectively. Moreover, the local anesthetic in thoracic epidural space raised 1.38 levels in males and 1.65 levels in females toward cephalic for each one level moving caudally. In the present study, Bupivacaine injection rate was 1cc/sec. which was similar to many other studies; however, in one study where analgesic injection was infused at the rate of 1cc per 3 seconds, the spread of the injected solution for each intervertebral level was reported as 1.96cc. This difference with our results may be due to the injection rate.

Conclusion

In conclusion, our study indicated that the distribution of Bupivacaine in epidural space is more in females than males and the tendency of spread is more toward the cephalad direction than caudal.

Acknowledgment

None.

Conflicts of Interest

The authors declare that they have no conflict of interest.

References

1. Miller RD. Miller`s Anesthesia. In: Cray RS, Chales BB, eds. Anesthesia for Obstetrics. Philadelphia: Elsevier. 2010:2224.
2. Djurhuus H, Rasmussen M, Jensen EH. Epidural blood Patch illustrated by CT-Epidurography. Acta Anaestheisol Scand. 1995;39(5):613-7.
3. Philip JH, Brown WU. Total Spinal Anesthesia late in the course of Obstetric Bupivacaine Epidural Block. Anesthesiology. 1976;44(4):340-1.
4. Gaiser R. Postdural Puncture Headache. Curr Opin Anaesthesiol. 2006;19(3):249-53.
5. Hall LW, Clarke KW, Trim CM. General principles of local analgesia. Hall LW, Clarke KW, Trim CM, eds. Veterinary Anesthesia. 2001:225–45.
6. Eisenach JC. Combined Spinal-Epidural Analgesia in Obstetrics. Anesthesiology. 1999;91(1):299-302.
7. Bernards CM. Sophistry in Medicine: Lessons from the Epidural Space. Reg Anesth Pain Med. 2005;30(1):56-66.
8. Valverde A. Epidural analgesia and anesthesia in dogs and cats. Vet Clin North Am Small Anim Pract. 2008;38:1205–30.
9. Lee I, Yamagishi N, Oboshi K. Distribution of new methylene blue injected into the lumbosacral epidural space in cats. Vet Anaesth Analg. 2004;31:190–4.
10. Lee I, Yamagishi N, Oboshi K, et al. Eliminating the effect of epidural fat during dorsolumbar epidural analgesia in cattle. Vet Anaesth Analg. 2004;31:86–9.
11. Gorgi AA, Hofmeister EH, Higginbotham MJ, et al. Effect of body position on cranial migration of epidurally injected methylene blue in recumbent dogs. Am J Vet Res. 2006;67:219–21.
12. Moll X, García F, Ferrer RI. Distribution of Methylene Blue after Injection into the Epidural Space of Anaesthetized Pregnant and Non-Pregnant Sheep. Plos One. 2014;9(4):e92860
13. Szeinfeld M, Ihmeidan IH, Moser MM, et al. Epidural blood Patch: Evaluation of the Volume and Spread of Blood injected into the Epidural Space. Anesthesiology. 1986;64(6):820-2.
14. Yokoyama M, Hanazaki M, Fujii H,et al. Correlation between the distribution of contrast medium and the extent of blockade during epidural anesthesia. Anesthesiology. 2004;100:1504–10.
15. Burn JM, Guyer PB, Langdon L: The spread of solutions injected into the epidural space: A study using epidurograms in patients with the lumbosciaticsyndrome. Br J Anaesth. 1973;45:338–45.
16. Savolaine ER, Pandya JB, Greenblatt SH, et al: Anatomy of the human lumbar epidural space: New insights using CT-epidurography. Anesthesiology. 1988;68:217–20.
17. Coombs DW, Dennis W, Hooper D. Subarachnoid Pressure with Epidural Blood Patch. Regional Anesthesia & Pain Medicine. 1979;4(3):3-6.
18. Wink J, Wolterbeek R, Aarts LP. Upper thoracic epidural anaesthesia: effects of age on neural blockade and cardiovascular parameters. Acta Anaesthesiol Scand. 2013;57(6):767–75.
19. Saitoh K, Hirabayashi Y, Shimizu R. Extensive extradural spread in the elderly may not relate to decreased leakage through intervertebral foramina. Br J Anaesth. 1995;75:688–91.

Preventive Effect of Paracetamol and Dexamethasone on Nausea, Vomiting, and Pain after Laparoscopic Cholecystectomy

Reihanak Talakoub[1*], Gholam Reza Khalili[1], Babak Haghanifar[1]

1-Anesthesiology and Critical Care Research Center, Isfahan University of Medical Sciences, Isfahan, Iran.

Corresponding Author: Reihanak Talakoub Associate Professor, Anesthesiology Department, Alzahra Hospital, Soffeh Blvd, Isfahan, Iran.
Email:
Reihanak.Talakoub@gmail.com

Abstract

Background: The currently used antiemetic drugs are not effective in all post-operative patients due to multifactorial origin of nausea and vomiting. Therefore, the present study was designed to evaluate the preventive effect of paracetamol on postoperative nausea and vomiting (PONV) in comparison with dexamethasone in patients undergoing elective laparoscopic cholecystectomy.
Materials and Methods: in this double-blinded clinical trial 105 patients were selected using a random sampling method; they were American standards association (ASA) class I and II, 18-75 years and candidate for laparoscopic cholecystectomy; randomly assigned into three groups: Paracetamol, Dexamethasone, and control. They were anesthetized using the same method, using sodium thiopental, Fentanyl, Atracurium, and Lidocaine. Anesthesia was maintained with oxygen, Isoflurane and Morphine. They also received 6 mL/kg/h ringer lactate. Patients data were recorded and analyzed.
Results: The mean severity of nausea and vomiting in the recovery room at minutes 30, 45, and 60 had a significant difference between the groups ($p<0.05$). The satisfaction score at minutes 45 and 60 had a significant difference between the groups ($p<0.05$). However, the mean scores of satisfaction of patients at 15 and 30 minutes were almost the same and no significant difference between the three groups was reported ($p>0.05$).
Conclusion: The severity of nausea and vomiting was low in the Paracetamol group and Paracetamol was more effective than Dexamethasone in terms of reducing the rate of nausea and vomiting.
Keywords: Paracetamol, Dexamethasone, laparoscopic cholecystectomy

Introduction

Laparoscopic cholecystectomy (LC) is a gold standard surgical procedure for cholelithiasis and some cases of cholecystitis and gallbladder stone. Although the surgical techniques are improved and have satisfied outcomes, postoperative nausea and vomiting (PONV) is a common and disturbing effect arisen from operation and anesthesia and is often more irritating than surgical pain. The prevalence of PONV depends on many factors including anesthesia type, length and type of operation, and patient gender since women develop PONV more than men do. Patients with motion sickness are more affected by

PONV. Routine use of antiemetic drugs is not required in all surgeries because according to statistics, 30% of patients develop this effect after surgery.

Patients undergoing laparoscopic cholecystectomy (LC) are more prone to PONV with a reported occurrence of 53-72%, and this increases the length of recovery, the delay in patient discharge, patient dissatisfaction, and hospital costs. The reason for LC-induced PONV is not clear yet, however, some factors are involved such as using isoflurane and fentanyl during operation, peritoneum stretching, increased blood pressure in the peritoneal cavity, and narcotics injection after operation.

Different efforts have been done to reduce the occurrence of PONV, and many antiemetic drugs have been studied. However, given the multifactorial origin of PONV, these medicines are not completely effective in all patients. Meanwhile, Dexamethasone is used as an effective antiemetic drug, which mechanism has not been understood, but it may act through central inhibition of prostaglandin synthesis, serotonin inhibition in intestine, inhibition of endorphin release, and change in permeability of blood brain barrier to serum proteins (1-3). Various studies have investigated the impact of Dexamethasone alone or in combination with other medicines on PONV.

In a double-blinded randomized clinical trial in 2009, Fuji *et al.* studied the effect of Dexamethasone in reducing nausea, vomiting, and the need for analgesics after operation. In this study, 90 patients who were candidate for LC were divided into three groups of Dexamethasone 8 mg, Dexamethasone 4 mg, and placebo, and were evaluated in terms of nausea, vomiting, and the need for analgesics after operation. Finally, it was concluded that dexamethasone 8 mg is effective in reducing nausea, vomiting, and the need for analgesics after operation in patients undergoing LC (4).

Sanchez-Rodriguez *et al.* (2010) investigated the preventive effect of Dexamethasone on PONV in a double-blinded randomized clinical trial. They divided 210 patients elected for LC into two groups of 8 mg dexamethasone and placebo. The results showed that the pharmaceutical regimen used was safe with no specific adverse effect and significantly reduced PONV in patients undergoing LC (5). Intravenous paracetamol or acetaminophen is other drug studied for reducing nausea and vomiting.

Intravenous Paracetamol or Acetaminophen is widely used as an analgesic and despite its known little anti-inflammatory and anti-pyretic effects; it has sufficient impact on peripheral and central pain systems (12). It acts through inhibitory mechanism of bradykinin in the peripheral system and through mediators such as NMDA, substance P, and nitric oxide pathway in the central system (6, 7).

In 2011, Cok *et al.* studied the effect of Paracetamol on PONV. A total of 90 patients of 2 to 14 years old undergoing strabismus surgery were divided into two groups of Paracetamol (15 mg/kg) and normal saline and were evaluated in terms of postoperative nausea and vomiting and the need for analgesics. The results showed that Paracetamol significantly reduced postoperative nausea and vomiting and the need for analgesics in the first 24 hours (8).

The objective in the present study was to prevent this condition, and most studies address this issue rather than treatment. Review of the literature showed that previous studies have investigated the effects of Paracetamol and Dexamethasone on PONV individually in comparison with placebo, however, no study was found regarding the comparison of Paracetamol and Dexamethasone. Therefore, this study was designed to compare the effect of Paracetamol and Dexamethasone on PONV in patients electively undergoing laparoscopic cholecystectomy.

Methods

This double-blinded clinical trial was performed in Al-Zahra Medical Center of Isfahan in 2014-2015, after obtaining permits from the ethics committee of the university and informed consent of patients. A total of 105 men and women ASA (I, II) aging from 18 to 75 years who were candidate for laparoscopic cholecystectomy under general anesthesia were randomly divided into three groups.

Exclusion criteria: history of drug addiction and long-term use of oral sedatives or analgesics, history of motion sickness, pregnancy, previous heart or lung disease, liver, kidney, or thyroid dysfunction, investigational drug intake within 30 days before surgery, nausea and vomiting or the use of antiemetic or H2 blockers within 48 hours before surgery, history of sensitivity to dexamethasone and paracetamol (in the case of drug sensitivity, severe hemodynamic impairment more than 30% of the baseline lasting more than 15 minutes), patients requiring transfusion, changing laparoscopic surgery to open surgery, and changing anesthesia method or the anesthetic drugs.

All patients were nil per os (NPO) for at least 8 hours and received 1/3-2/3 serum according to "1-2-4 rule of thumb". Patients were anesthetized with a completely similar method. To induce anesthesia, they received Thiopental sodium (6 mg/kg), Fentanyl (2 μg/kg), Atracurium (0.6 mg/kg), and Lidocaine (1.5 mg/kg). Anesthesia was continued with oxygen (6 L/min), Isoflurane (1.2-1.8%), and Morphine (0.15 mg/kg). They also received 6 mL/kg/h ringer lactate.

The patients selected through the simple randomized sampling method were divided into three groups.

Paracetamol group received 15 mg/kg intravenous Paracetamol in 15 minutes before closing the wound within a micro-set with 100 mL normal saline through infusion and 2 mL normal saline through intravenous injection. Dexamethasone group received 100 mL normal saline within 15 minutes before closing the wound through infusion and 8 mg dexamethasone (2 mL) through intravenous injection. Placebo group received 100 mL normal saline within 15 minutes before closing the wound through infusion and 2 mL normal saline through intravenous injection.

During anesthesia, mean arterial pressure, mean end-expiratory CO_2/SpO_2, and heart rate were monitored. All information including age, gender, weight, length of anesthesia and surgery, length of stay in the recovery room, length of extubating, nausea severity, vomiting frequency, and satisfaction scores were recorded. Mean arterial pressure and heart rate were measured before anesthesia and every 30 minutes during the operation. Bradycardia (heart rate <50 per min) was treated with 1 mg IV atropine.

At the end of operation, occurrence of nausea and vomiting, frequency of vomiting and severity of nausea were recorded and scored based on VAS; then, ranked from 0 to 10: zero for no nausea and 10 standing for unbearable vomiting. Also, vomiting scored from 0 to 3 (0 = no vomiting, 1 = 1 time vomiting, 2 = 2 times vomiting, and 3 = 3 or more times vomiting); retching equivalent to vomiting.

If the nausea score was 4 or higher and vomiting score was 3 or higher, 4 mg Ondansetron was slowly injected intravenously. The first time for receiving Ondansetron and the total received of that in 24 hours were recorded. The incidence of nausea and vomiting and the vomiting frequency were also recorded up to 24 hours. Pain intensity was scored using VAS from 0 to 10. If the pain score was 4 or greater, fentanyl (0.5 mg/kg) was administered.

The time of pethidine painkiller request, *i.e.* the time between surgery and the first dose of analgesic given at the request (VAS >4) and the total dose of consumed analgesic after 24 h were calculated and recorded. Postoperative VAS was recorded at minutes 15, 30, 45, and 60 in the recovery and at hours 6, 12, 24. Satisfaction was scored from 1 to 4 (1 = mild, 2 = moderate, 3 = good, 4 = excellent). Sedation level in the recovery room was evaluated and recorded at minutes 15, 30, 45, and 60 through Kulka method.

The Kulka method for evaluation of sedation: 0=Awake, 1=Drowsy or calm waking up easily, 2=Drowsy responding quick to verbal stimulation, 3=Drowsy responding late to verbal stimulation, 4=Unconsciousness, Criteria for discharging from recovery room was based on the modified Aldrete score (1). After collecting and completing, the data were analyzed using SPSS® software version 18 (SPSS Inc., Chicago, Ill., USA).

Results

Similar letters indicated no significant differences between the means according to Duncan's post hoc test (table 1). The mean severity of nausea at 6 hours after surgery had a significant difference between the three groups ($p<0.05$). However, the mean severity of nausea at 12 and 24 hours were almost identical between the three groups and had no significant difference ($p >0.05$). Using Duncan's post hoc test, the mean severity of nausea was also compared between the three groups two by two. Based of Duncan's test, the highest and the lowest mean of nausea severity at 6 hours were seen in the control group and in the paracetamol group, respectively.

Similar letters indicate no significant differences between the means according to Duncan's post hoc test (table 2). The mean patient satisfaction score at 6, 12 and 24 hours after surgery had significant differences between the three groups ($p<0.05$). Using Duncan's post hoc test, the mean severity of nausea was also compared between the three groups two by two. Based of Duncan's test, the highest and the lowest mean of patients satisfaction score were seen in the dexamethasone group and in the control group, respectively.

In table 3, the frequency of vomiting was compared between the three groups using Chi-square test at every step of measuring. The significance level of this test for 6 hours after surgery was calculated less than 0.05. Therefore, the vomiting rate at 6 hours after surgery had a significant difference between the three groups, but no significant difference existed at 12 and 24 hours after surgery. It can be seen that the vomiting rate at 6 hours after surgery was higher in the control group than other groups (the severity percent of vomiting 0 was higher in other groups than the controls). The vomiting rate at 6 hours after surgery was higher in the dexamethasone group than the paracetamol group (the severity percent of vomiting 0 in the Paracetamol group was higher than the Dexamethasone).

Similar letters indicate no significant differences between the means according to Duncan's post hoc test (table 4). The mean time of the first narcotic request had significant differences between the three groups ($p<0.05$). In the control group, the narcotic was requested approximately 2 hours earlier than the Dexamethasone group and in the Dexamethasone group almost 1 hour earlier than Paracetamol group.

The frequency of sedation level was compared between the three groups using Chi-square test at every step of measuring. The significance level of this test for different minutes was calculated less than 0.05. Therefore, the sedation level at these minutes had a significant difference between the three groups. It was observed that the sedation levels at minutes 15, 30, 45 and 60 in the recovery room were higher in the control and Dexamethasone groups than the Paracetamol group. In other words, the rate of sedation levels 3 and 4 in the control and Dexamethasone groups was higher than the Paracetamol group and the rate of sedation levels 0 and 1 in the Paracetamol group was higher than the control and Dexamethasone groups.

Similar letters indicate no significant differences between the means according to Duncan's post hoc test (table 5). The pain scores at 6 and 12 hours after surgery had significant differences between the three groups ($p<0.05$). The mean pain intensity at 24 hours after surgery was nearly identical between the groups and had no significant difference ($p>0.05$). Using Duncan's post hoc test, the mean pain intensity was also compared between the three groups two by two. Based of Duncan's test, the highest and the lowest mean of pain intensity at 6 and 12 hours after operation were seen in the control group and in the Paracetamol group, respectively. In other words, postoperative pain was lower in Paracetamol group than other groups.

Results showed that the mean arterial blood pressure during surgery was nearly identical between the three groups and had no significant difference ($p>0.05$). The mean arterial blood pressure measured every 30 minutes in the recovery room was almost identical between the three groups and there was no significant difference ($p>0.05$). Although the lowest mean arterial blood pressure at different times was seen in the dexamethasone group, this decline was not statistically significant.

The mean heart rate during surgery were significantly different between the three groups ($p<0.05$). According to Duncan's test, the maximum heart rate during surgery was seen in the paracetamol group and lowest in the dexamethasone group. The mean heart rate measured every 30 minutes in the recovery room was almost identical in the three groups and there was no significant difference ($p>0.05$). The lowest mean heart rate at different times was seen in the dexamethasone group, but this reduction was not statistically significant.

Discussion

Difference in pain intensity among the groups was a result obtained in this study. The results indicated that pain intensity was lower in the paracetamol group, while the findings of Waldron *et al.* in 2013 were in contrast with ours. They stated that pain was lower in the dexamethasone group (9). However, Karnak *et al.* reported findings similar to ours. Pain intensity was lower in the paracetamol group (10). This difference may be attributed to this fact that Waldron *et al.* performed a systematic review and meta-analysis including 5796 patients.

Patient satisfaction and sedation level, both higher in the dexamethasone group than in other groups, were other results obtained by this study. In this regard, a number of similar findings have been reported. For example, Chan *et al.* (2014) stated the higher satisfaction of patients in the dexamethasone group (11). In 2016, Jessen *et al.* reported a higher level of sedation and satisfaction in the dexamethasone group (12).

In this study, the groups were also compared in terms of heart rate during surgery, and it was observed that the maximum heart rate during surgery was seen in the paracetamol and the lowest in the dexamethasone group. In this case, Powell *et al.* (2016) reported findings similar to ours. They stated that the lowest heart rate during operation had a significant relationship with dexamethasone injection (13).

Difference in nausea severity and vomiting rate among groups was another result in this study. According to our findings, both cases were lower in the paracetamol group. While Guay *et al.* (2016) reported contrary findings (14). However, in 2016, Zou *et al.* provided findings similar to ours. They also confirmed low level and severity of nausea in the paracetamol group (15). According to differences in the results in one year and different sample size, it is recommended to perform the future studies with higher sample size to could make decisions that are more confident.

Conclusion

In this study, the effect of paracetamol on post-operative nausea and vomiting (PONV) and pain was compared with dexamethasone in patients who underwent elective laparoscopic cholecystectomy, and it was found that the severity of nausea and vomiting was lower in the paracetamol group, and paracetamol was more effective in reducing the rate of nausea and vomiting. In contrast, patient satisfaction and sedation level between the studied groups was higher in the dexamethasone group than other groups.

Acknowledgment

The authors appreciate the kind help of all physicians and nurse, Al-Zahra Medical Center Isfahan, Iran.

Conflicts of Interest

The authors declare that they have no conflict of interest.

References

1. Aapro ms,Albert Ds. Dexamethasone as an antiemetic in patients treated with ciplatin. N Engl J Med. 1981;305:520.
2. Rich WM, Abdulhayoglu G, DiSaia PJ.Methylprednisolone as an antiemetic during cancer chemotherapy – a pilot study. Gynecol Oncol. 1980;9:193–8.
3. Fredrikson M, Hursti T, Furst CJ. Nausea in cancer chemotherapy is inversely related to urinary cortisol excretion. Br J Cancer. 1992;65:779 80.
4. Harris AL. Cytotoxic-therapy-induced vomiting is mediated via enkephalin pathways. Lancet. 1982;1:714–6.
5. Elhakim M, Ali NM, Rashed I, Riad MK, Refat M. Dexamethasone reduces postoperative vomiting and pain after pediatric tonsillectomy. Can J Anaesth. 2003;50 (4):392-7.
6. Bianchin A, De Luca A, Caminiti A. Postoperative vomiting reduction after laparoscopic cholecystectomy with single dose of dexamethasone. Minerva Anestesiol. 2007;73(6):343-6.
7. Fujii Y, Itakura M. Reduction of postoperative nausea, vomiting, and analgesic requirement with dexamethasone for patients undergoing laparoscopic cholecystectomy. Surg Endosc. 2010;24(3):692-6.
8. Fukami Y, Terasaki M, Okamoto Y, Sakaguchi K, Murata T, Ohkubo M, Nishimae K. Efficacy of preoperative dexamethasone in patients with laparoscopic cholecystectomy. J Hepatobiliary Pancreat Surg. 2009;16(3):367-71.
9. Waldron NH1, Jones CA, Gan TJ, Allen TK, Habib AS. Impact of perioperative dexamethasone on postoperative analgesia and side-effects: systematic review and meta-analysis. Br J Anaesth. 2013;110(2):191-200.
10.Kranke P1, Jokinen J, Pace NL, Schnabel A, Hollmann MW, Hahnenkamp K, Eberhart LH, Poepping DM, Weibel S. Continuous intravenous perioperative lidocaine infusion for postoperative pain and recovery. Cochrane Database Syst Rev. 2015;(7):CD009642.
11.Chan EY1, Fransen M, Parker DA, Assam PN, Chua N. Femoral nerve blocks for acute postoperative pain after knee replacement surgery. Cochrane Database Syst Rev. 2014;(5):CD009941.
12. Jessen Lundorf L1, Korvenius Nedergaard H, Møller AM. Perioperative dexmedetomidine for acute pain after abdominal surgery in adults. Cochrane Database Syst Rev. 2016; 2:CD010358.
13.Powell R1, Scott NW, Manyande A, Bruce J, Vögele C, Byrne-Davis LM, Unsworth M, Osmer C, Johnston M. Psychological preparation and postoperative outcomes for adults undergoing surgery under general anaesthesia. Cochrane Database Syst Rev. 2016 ;(5):CD008646.
14.Guay J1, Nishimori M, Kopp S. Epidural local anaesthetics

versus opioid-based analgesic regimens for postoperative gastrointestinal paralysis, vomiting and pain after abdominal surgery. Cochrane Database Syst Rev. 2016;7:CD001893.

15.Zou Z1, An MM, Xie Q, Chen XY, Zhang H, Liu GJ, Shi XY. Single dose intra-articular morphine for pain control after knee arthroscopy. Cochrane Database Syst Rev. 2016;(5):CD008918.

Table 1: Comparison of the mean severity of nausea in three groups at 6, 12, and 24 hours postoperatively

Severity of Nausea	Groups	Mean	Standard deviation	*p*-value
at 6 hours after operation	Control	0.8890a	0.51400	
	Paracetamol	0.0010c	0.61400	0.037
	Dexamethasone	0.1814b	1.01400	
at 12 hours after operation	Control	0.4929a	1.30094	
	Paracetamol	0.1120a	0.01400	0.094
	Dexamethasone	0.4857a	1.62956	
at 24 hours after operation	Control	1.5714a	1.44070	
	Paracetamol	1.1714a	1.01419	0.736
	Dexamethasone	1.3429a	1.57074	

Table 2: Comparison of the mean patient satisfaction score at 6, 12 and 24 hours after surgery in three groups

		Mean	Standard deviation	*p*-value
Satisfaction at 6 hours after operation	Control	1.9333c	1.00491	
	Paracetamol	2.8286b	1.0008	0.044
	Dexamethasone	3.5455a	1.67801	
Satisfaction at 12 hours after operation	Control	1.0000c	1.20015	
	Paracetamol	2.7143b	1.90867	0.035
	Dexamethasone	3.4138a	2.00922	
Satisfaction at 24 hours after operation	Control	1.7813c	1.28852	
	Paracetamol	2.8571b	0.64820	0.015
	Dexamethasone	3.7576c	2.15102	

Table 3: Frequency distribution of vomiting rate at 6, 12, and 24 hours after surgery in three groups

		6 hours after operation	**12 hours after operation**	**24 hours after operation**
Group	Vomiting rate	Frequency (%)	Frequency (%)	Frequency (%)
	0	27 (77.1%)	28 (80.0%)	32 (91.4%)
Control	1	8 (22.9%)	6 (17.1%)	3 (8.6%)
	2	0 (0.0)	1 (2.9%)	0 (0.0%)
	0	35 (100%)	٣٤ (97.1%)	35 (100%)
Paracetamol	1	0 (0.0%)	1 (2.9%)	0 (0.0%)
	2	0 (0.0%)	0 (0.0%)	0 (0.0%)
	0	28 (82.4%)	27 (77.1%)	35 (100%)
Dexamethasone	1	6 (17.6%)	8 (22.9%)	0 (0.0%)
	2	0 (0.0%)	0 (0.0)	0 (0.0%)
Chi-square test		8.608	8.166	6.176
Significance level		0.014	0.0٨٦	0.05٦

Table 4: Comparison of the mean narcotic consumption during 24 hours in three group

Groups	**Mean**	**Standard deviation**	***p*-value**
Control	2.3333c	1.51866	
Paracetamol	5.5500a	1.36660	0.041
Dexamethasone	4.5625b	1.96600	

Table 5: Comparison of the mean pain intensity at 6, 12, and 24 hours postoperatively in three groups

Pain Severity		**Mean**	**Standard deviation**	***p*-value**
At 6 hours postoperatively	Control	1.4600a	1.98820	
	Paracetamol	0.4671b	1.37932	0.045
	Dexamethasone	1.4743a	1.92157	
At 12 hours postoperatively	Control	2.4691a	2.16038	
	Paracetamol	0.4299b	0.88403	0.000
	Dexamethasone	1.7509a	1.52128	
At 24 hours postoperatively	Control	0.0580a	0.16903	
	Paracetamol	0.0289a	0.33806	0.145
	Dexamethasone	0.2871a	0.95706	

Osteogenesis Imperfecta: Genetic Overview and the Role of Anesthesiologists

Kamran Mottaghi[1], Rofeideh Fallahinejadghajari[1], Parisa Sezari[1], Mohammadreza Kamranmanesh[1], Masoud Nashibi[1]

Abstract

Osteogenesis Imperfecta (OI) is a rare disorder of type 1 collagen with 13 currently identified types attributable to inherited abnormalities in type 1 collagen amount, structure, or processing.OI is a genetic disorder with skeletal, vascular, and soft tissue involvement with different clinical presentations. Since these patients need different surgical procedure in their lifetime, anesthesiologists are involved with their preoperative care and should be familiar with pathogenesis and anesthetic considerations of osteogenesis imperfecta. Here we represent a case of osteogenesis imperfecta, which was candidate for Video Assisted Thoracic Surgery (VATS) and review the literature.

Keywords: Osteogenesis Imperfecta, Video Assisted Thoracic Surgery

1. Anesthesiology Research Center, Shahid Beheshti University of Medical Sciences, Tehran, Iran

Corresponding Author:
Masoud Nashibi, MD, Assistant Professor, Anesthesiology Research Center, Shahid Beheshti University of Medical Sciences, Tehran, Iran.
E-mail: masoudnashibi@sbmu.ac.ir

Introduction

Osteogenesis Imperfecta (OI) is a rare disorder of type 1 collagen with 13 currently identified types attributable to inherited abnormalities in type 1 collagen amount, structure, or processing (1). OI comprises a heterogeneous group of disorders characterized by susceptibility to bone fractures ranging in severity from perinatal death to a subtle increase in fracture frequency (2). In addition to the skeletal phenotype, common additional extraskeletal manifestations include blue sclera, dentinogenesis imperfecta, vascular fragility, and hearing loss (1). Despite the low prevalence, the wide range of heterogeneity in features and advances in treatment makes OI a disease with special requirements and considerations. OI is a differential diagnosis for child abuse and different specialists, including orthopedist, pediatrist, dentists and even psychiatrists, are involved in treatment procedures to give the affected people a qualified life. Evidently, the role of anesthesiologists in this multidisciplinary approach may not be disregarded. Therefore, anesthesiologists should have proper knowledge about the variable genetic abnormalities and the consequent apparent and invisible features of OI, may affect the perioperative management.

Case presentation

A 44 years old man was brought to the emergency department after falling trauma. He was a known case of osteogenesis imperfecta diagnosed at the age of 18 years, made him disqualified for military service. He had a history of some long bone fractures in the past with minor trauma. His daily performance was acceptable without any respiratory or cardiac symptoms. He was homeless without any relatives so there were limited data about family history.

He weighed 70 kg, was conscious and his hemodynamic parameters were in normal range. He had blue sclera (Fig. 1) without vision impairments. The neck and jaw movements were normal with mallampati score of 2. Apart from poor dentition, the mouth and pharynx were normal. In lung auscultation there was decreased sound in the left hemithorax, congruent with pleural effusion on chest X-ray, besides a prominent aortic arch. Further X-ray studies demonstrated right scapula, humerus, tibia and knee fractures. Lab tests findings showed leukocytosis. The spirometry showed normal pattern. In echocardiography the ejection fraction was 60% and the pulmonary artery pressure was 28 mmHg with mild tricuspid regurgitation. Bone densitometry proved low bone marrow density in spine and hip.

Chest tube insertion was planned in emergency department while the operation team prepared for unexpected hemorrhage and emergent thoracotomy and isogroup cross matched packed RBC was requested for probable event. After proper splinting and padding, the patient was transferred cautiously to operating room for visual assisted thoracoscopic surgery (VATS) to evaluate the source of hemothorax. The difficult airway equipments were prepared as well. The routine OR monitoring alongside temperature monitoring with nasopharyngeal probe attached and two large bore intravenous (IV) access number 18 and 16 were inserted under local anesthesia. He did not receive anything per os (NPO) during the last several hours. For surgical procedure all the intraoperative requirements for difficult intubation, malignant hyperthermia (MH), proper positioning and blood products were prepared beforehand. Total intravenous anesthesia (TIVA) was our choice for general anesthesia with full monitoring. The premedication included midazolam 2 mg, lidocaine 80 mg and fentanyl 150 μg via intravenous rout. The intubation was done with left side double lumen tracheal tube (DLT) number 39 after the induction of anesthesia with 140 mg propofol and 40 mg atracurium. Maintenance of anesthesia provided using propofol infusion to keep the depth of anesthesia in the range of 40 to 60 on cerebral state monitoring. Then the

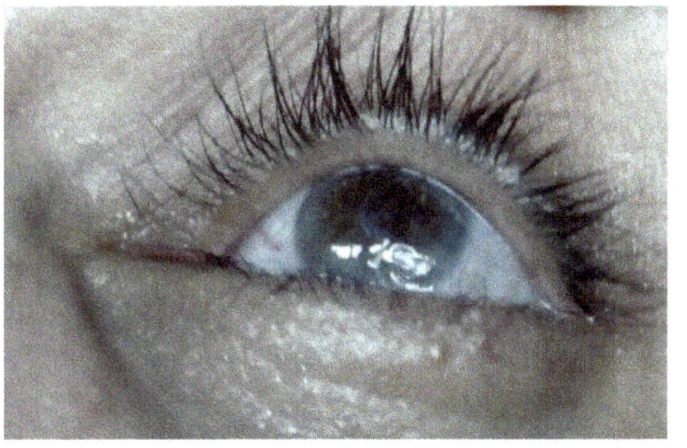

Figure 1. Blue Sclera.

patient changed to right lateral decubitus position (LDP). During procedure there was about 150cc drainage of blood which caused no hemodynamic instability with no rising in temperature and end tidal CO_2. At the end of VATS, DLT changed to 7.5 mm armored tracheal tube and orthopedic surgery began. Orthopedic procedure lasted about 3 hours with minor hemorrhage and at the end patient was awakened and extubated uneventfully.

Discussion

Osteogenesis imperfecta (OI), commonly called "brittle bone disease", is a genetic disorder characterized by increased bone fragility and decreased bone density due to quantitative and/or qualitative abnormalities of type I collagen (3). It is a variable condition with a range of clinical severities (4). Most of the cases of OI are inherited in autosomal dominant fashion with mutations in COL1A1 or COL1A2 genes. Over last few years, twelve genes for autosomal recessive OI have been identified (5). After 2006, mutations were identified in the CRTAP, FKBP10, LEPRE1, PLOD2, PPIB, SERPINF1, SERPINH1, SP7, WNT1, BMP1, and TMEM38B genes, associated with recessive OI and mutation in the IFITM5 gene associated with dominant OI. Mutations in PLS3 were recently identified in families with osteoporosis and fractures, with X-linked inheritance pattern. In addition to the genetic complexity of the molecular basis of OI, extensive phenotypic variability resulting from individual loci has also been documented (6).

Osteogenesis imperfecta is classified into 11 types to date, on the basis of their clinical symptoms and genetic components (7). For simplicity, the objectives of treatment can be reduced to three typical situations: the lethal perinatal form (type II), in which the problem is survival at birth; the severe and moderate forms (types III-IX), in which the objective is 'autonomy' and the mild form (type I), in which the aim is to reach 'normal life' (8). The hallmark feature of OI is bone fragility, with susceptibility to fracture from minimal trauma, as well as bone deformity and growth deficiency. OI has multiple secondary features, including macrocephaly, blue sclera, dentinogenesis imperfecta, hearing loss, neurological defects (macrocephaly and basilar invagination) and cardiopulmonary complications (the major cause of mortality directly related to OI) (9).

Thanks to the genetic discoveries, bisphosphonates therapy and new surgical and rehabilitation method, a new era is developed for life span with rising quality in the population affected by this rare disease. As long as all surgical procedures need anesthesia, anesthesiologist should be aware of all aspects of OI which may interfere with anesthesia in perioperative period. Commonly encountered complications include a difficult airway, intraoperative bleeding due to platelet dysfunction, respiratory compromise due to skeletal deformity, and congenital cardiac anomalies (10). Cardiovascular effects are identifiable in childhood even in mild forms of OI. Aortic dilation is the predominant finding, while valvular abnormalities are infrequent (11). Cautious moving and positioning to avoid further fractures and meticulous monitoring of temperature due to the risk of malignant hyperthermia should not be underestimated. Proper preparation and preoperative assessment is important, as is the choice of anesthetic technique (10). Even though a direct relationship between OI and MH has not been proven (12), TIVA is the choice in OI to reduce the risk of MH during intraoperative period. Succinylcholine and volatile anesthetics are avoided in anesthesia management in OI.Cardiopulmonary assessment can reveal hidden problems especially in mild forms of OI and prevent further complications.

Our patient, regarding to clinical manifestation, was in mild category. Since the airway was not compromised and the team was ready for difficult airway management including surgical tracheostomy, induction with IV anesthetic and nondepolarizing muscle relaxant was performed. The position and movements were carefully supervised by attendants. Certainly, close and full monitoring was the priority of our intraoperative care.

Conclusion

As a result of novel achievements in genetic and cellular studies and uprising hope to treat the patients with rare genetic disorders, anesthesiologists find themselves in new era of required skillful adaptable individuals who can work in dynamic situations (13-16). In addition to the fragile bones and probable difficult intubation, the risk of MH or probable hypermetabolic state, the risk of bleeding and cardiopulmonary complication should never be neglected in the shadow of urgent and emergent procedures.

Acknowledgment

The authors would like to thank the kind help of physicians and nurses, operating room and anesthesiology ward staffs, Loghman Hakim Hospital and Anesthesiology Research Center Shahid Beheshti University of Medical Sciences, Tehran, Iran for their kind help and support.

Conflicts of Interest

The authors declare that there are no conflicts of interest.

References

1. Thomas IH, DiMeglio LA. Advances in the Classification and Treatment of Osteogenesis Imperfecta. Curr Osteoporos Rep. 2016;14(1):1-9.

2. Cho SY, Lee JH, Ki CS, Chang MS, Jin DK, Han HS. Osteogenesis imperfecta Type I caused by a novel mutation in the start codon of the COL1A1 gene in a Korean family. Ann Clin Lab Sci. 2015;45(1):100-5.

3. Renaud A, Aucourt J, Weill J, Bigot J, Dieux A, Devisme L, et al. Radiographic features of osteogenesis imperfecta. Insights Imaging. 2013;4(4):417-29.

4. Balasubramanian M, Wagner BE, Peres LC, Sobey GJ, Parker MJ, Dalton A, et al. Ultrastructural and histological findings on examination of skin in osteogenesis imperfecta: a novel study. Clin Dysmorphol. 2015;24(2):45-54.

5. Stephen J, Girisha KM, Dalal A, Shukla A, Shah H, Srivastava P, et al. Mutations in patients with osteogenesis imperfecta from consanguineous Indian families. Eur J Med Genet. 2015;58(1):21-7.

6. Valadares ER, Carneiro TB, Santos PM, Oliveira AC, Zabel B.

What is new in genetics and osteogenesis imperfecta classification? J Pediatr (Rio J). 2014;90(6):536-41.
7. Womack J. Osteogenesis imperfecta types I-XI: implications for the neonatal nurse. Adv Neonatal Care. 2014;14(5):309-15; quiz 16-7.
8. Monti E, Mottes M, Fraschini P, Brunelli P, Forlino A, Venturi G, et al. Current and emerging treatments for the management of osteogenesis imperfecta. Ther Clin Risk Manag. 2010;6:367-81.
9. Marini J, Smith SM. Osteogenesis Imperfecta. In: De Groot LJ, Chrousos G, Dungan K, Feingold KR, Grossman A, Hershman JM, et al., editors. Endotext. South Dartmouth (MA)2000.
10. Oakley I, Reece LP. Anesthetic implications for the patient with osteogenesis imperfecta. AANA J. 2010;78(1):47-53.
11. Rush ET, Li L, Goodwin JL, Kreikemeier RM, Craft M, Danford DA, et al. Echocardiographic phenotype in osteogenesis imperfecta varies with disease severity. Heart. 2017;103(6):443-8.
12. Erdogan MA, Sanli M, Ersoy MO. Anesthesia management in a child with osteogenesis imperfecta and epidural hemorrhage. Braz J Anesthesiol. 2013;63(4):366-8.
13. Mottaghi K, Safari F, Sezari P, Gholizadeh N, Nashibi M. Anesthetic management of patients with Klippel-Feil syndrome, a case series. J Cell Mol Anesth 2017;2(2):6.
14. Nashibi M, Tajbakhsh A, MahdavipourVahdati S, Safari F, Mottaghi K. Didmoad (Wolfram) Syndrome: Case Report. Journal of Cellular & Molecular Anesthesia. 2016;1(3):126-8.
15. Nashibi M, Tajbakhsh A, Safari F, Mottaghi K. Anesthetic Consideration of Niemann-Pick Disease Type C. Journal of Cellular & Molecular Anesthesia. 2016;1(2):73-7.
16. Safari F, Mottaghi K, Fallahinejadghajari R, Nashibi M. Crouzon Syndrome: a fibroblast growth factor receptor 2 gene mutation. J Cell Mol Anesth. 2017;2(1):15-8.

9

The Effect of Pulsatile Blood Flow during Proximal Graft, on Liver Function in Coronary Artery Bypass Graft Surgery

Seyed Mohammadreza Amouzegar Zavareh[1], Marzieh Lak[1]*

Abstract

Background: Liver dysfunction is a rare complication with high mortality and morbidity rate in coronary artery bypass grafting (CABG) surgery. Pulsatile blood flow probably maintains liver function during cardiopulmonary bypass (CPB).

Methods: In this randomized clinical trial study, 68 patients who underwent CABG surgery were divided into two groups: pulsatile and non-pulsatile groups. We transferred continuous blood flow to pulsatile blood flow during proximal graft by using cardiac contraction.

Results: There was no significant difference in Alanine transaminase (ALT) and alkaline phosphatase (ALP) values at variable times between the groups. In addition, the procedure of ALT and ALP in the case and control groups was not significantly different in three days. There was no significant difference between AST values at variable times in two groups. However, the trend of AST in the case group was significantly increased while it was not significantly different in the control group during the next three postoperative days.

Conclusion: It seems that hemodynamic stability is more important than type of blood flow in maintaining liver function.

Keywords: pulsatile perfusion, cardio pulmonary bypass, liver function

1. Department of Anesthesiology, School of Medicine, Baqiyatallah University of Medical Sciences, Tehran, Iran

Corresponding Author: Marzieh Lak, MD, Baqiyatallah University of Medical Sciences Tehran, Iran.
Email: marziehlak@yahoo.com

Introduction

Liver dysfunction is a rare complication with high mortality and morbidity in coronary artery bypass grafting (CABG) surgery (1). Maintenance of pulsatile circulation during cardiopulmonary bypass (CPB) is simple and is closer to natural physiology (2). According to Pappas and his colleagues who evaluated glutamic oxaloacetic transaminase as a marker of liver function found that pulsatile blood flow preserves liver function. Mathie *et al.* found similar results in canine models and furthers clinical studies showed that pulsatile blood flow improves tissue perfusion and microcirculation with maintenance of liver function and lower blood levels of AST than non-pulsatile circulation (3).

Pulsatile blood flow probably maintains microcirculation in selective arterioles, which are collapsed during non-pulsatile flow. It reduces the increased blood levels of AST, ALT and liver cellular damage (4).

Koning *et al.* stated that pulsatile circulation lead to rapid recovery of microcirculatory perfusion at the end of CPB in CABG surgery. This is the first study with the use of side stream dark field imaging of the sublingual micro circulation which showed maintenance of microcirculatory perfusion during pulsatile blood flow (5).

Methods

This prospective, randomized study was composed of 70 consecutive patients who underwent a CABG surgery. Ethics committee approval was received along with the informed consent of each patient. The same surgical team operated on all of the patients who were randomly divided into two groups. Randomization was stratified using a random table number. Non-pulsatile CPB was performed on 35 patients, and pulsatile flow CPB was carried out on 35 others. We assessed the preoperative liver function of each patient by examining the serum AST, ALT and alkaline phosphatase (ALP).

Patients with a history of renal disease, a history of liver disease and impaired liver function tests, insulin dependent diabetes mellitus (DM), morbid obesity (BMI≥40), redo surgery, needing intra-aortic balloon pump, and valvular heart disease were excluded from the study. All of the participants underwent elective surgeries; emergent cases were not included.

For patients who took anticoagulant medication, the drug was stopped 7 days before surgery. Patients received intramuscular Morphine (5 mg) and oral Lorazepam (1 mg) 1 hour before surgery.

The patients were taken to the operating room under standard monitoring. In addition, vital signs and invasive blood pressure monitoring via left radial artery were recorded. Induction of anesthesia was carried out by Fentanyl (7 µg/kg), Diazepam (0.15 mg/kg), and Atracurium (0.5 mg/kg), if needed to the loss of eyelash reflex by continuous Propofol infusion.

After orotracheal intubation, maintenance of anesthesia consisted of Fentanyl (0.07 µg/kg/min), Midazolam (0.5 µg/kg/min), Atracurium (0.8 µg/kg/min) and, if necessary, Propofol (20–200 mg/h). All patients underwent Mechanical ventilation while ETCO2 was maintained between 35 and 40 mmHg. Central venous catheter (CVC) was inserted in right internal jugular vein. Patient's vital signs, including blood pressure (BP) by the invasive method, prothrombin ratio (PR), core temperature via nasal probe, SPO2 and ET CO2 and CVP were recorded every five minutes. Arterial blood gas analysis (ABG) was performed after installing the arterial line, induction of anesthesia and immediately after the starting and stopping the CPB. Systolic blood pressure was kept between 100 to 110 mm Hg by using beneficial effects of nitroglycerin (TNG) and inotrope agents . After sternotomy and releasing of internal thoracic artery and saphenous vein, Heparin was injected.

Activated coagulation time (ACT) was controlled 3 to 5 minutes after injection of Heparin. In case of ACT≥480s patient were connected to CPB pumps (pump type was Stockert S3 which is a roller Pump, and fluid Prime includes Ringer, Voluven, heparin, sodium bicarbonate, mannitol, Tranexamic acid). Patients were cooled to 32°C to 34°C. During cardiopulmonary bypass mean arterial pressure was maintained between 60 to 80 mm Hg by using noradrenaline or TNG. After completion of the flow (Full Flow) mechanical ventilation was stopped. Transformation of total cross clump to partial clump was started after completing–the distal grafts. In pulsatile group, ventilation resumed with 1/3 of tidal volume and heart was filled by partial clumping of venous cannula accompanied with reduction of 20-30% in venous return.

In this way, the non-pulsatile blood flow was transformed to pulsatile blood flow by using patient's own cardiac contraction. In non-pulsatile group continuous blood flow was kept on. In both groups, temperature was increased to 36-37°C and ventilation was completed after the completion of proximal grafts. After confirming acceptable situation such as Hct≥22, normal electrolytes and acid base status, patients were separated from CPB. Protamine sulfate was administered to reverse the heparin. After completion of surgery, patients transferred to ICU-OH.

Weaning and extubation were performed according to standards of ICU-OH such as full consciousness, hemodynamic stability, control of drainage, and chest X-ray acceptable. Patients' laboratory tests such as serum AST and ALT were measured at the arrival to the ICU-OH and 24 and 48 hours after admission.

Descriptive statistics such as mean, SD and percentage were calculated for the presented data. The Kolmogorov–Smirnov test was used for normality of the data. Chi-square test, repeated measure, ANOVA and t-test were used for determining the association between variables. SPSS® software version 18 (SPSS Inc., Chicago, Ill., USA) was used for data analysis. The significance level for all the tests was considered less than 0.05.

Results

Seventy patients were evaluated in this study. Two patients in control group were excluded due to lack of blood samples to check for liver tests. Total of 33 patients in the control group and 35 patients in the case group were examined. There was no significant difference between the two groups regarding gender, age, BMI, DM, and hypertension (Table 1). In addition, there was no significant difference between the two groups regarding CPB time, cross clamp time, and the number of grafts, systolic and diastolic blood pressure preoperative (Table 2). Table 3 depicts AST mean of the study sample. The average AST of the participants preoperatively, day 1, day 2 and day 3 post-operative was not a significant difference between the two groups (P=0.067, P=0.194, P=0.480 and P=0.726, respectively). But the procedure of AST in the case group were significantly different in three days (P=0.004) but in the control group were not significant (P=0.051) (Table 3, Figure 1)

Average ALT of the participants preoperatively and in the post-operative period was not significantly different between the two groups (P=0.575, P=0.261,

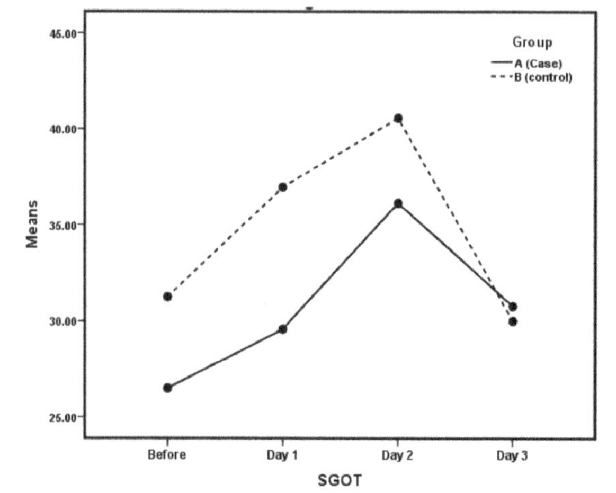

Figure 1. Comparison between mean AST values at Variable Times in Two Groups.

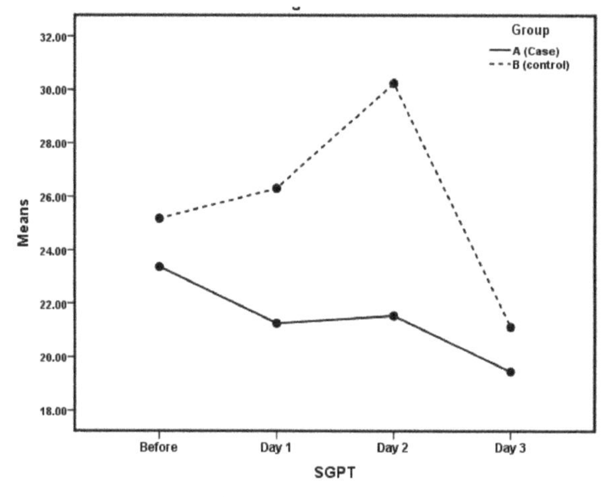

Figure 2. Comparison between mean ALP values at different times in the two study groups.

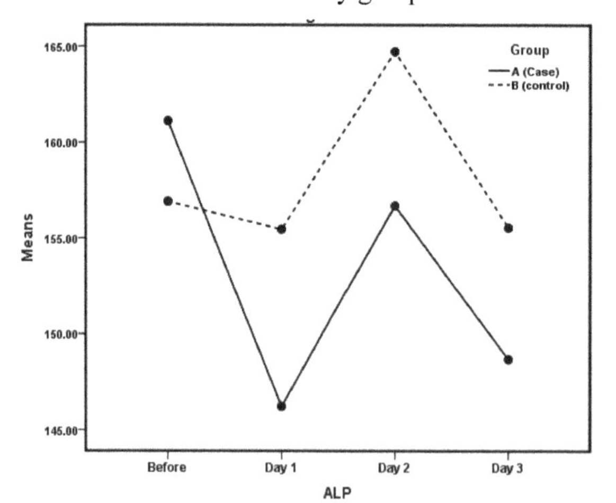

Figure 3. Comparison Between mean ALP values at different times in the two study groups

Table 1: Demographic values and history of comorbidities in the two study groups

		Case n = 35	Control n = 33	P value
Age Mean (±SD)		61.89(±8.98)	62.06(±7.64)	0.931
BMI Mean (±SD)		30.59(±2.97)	30.88(±3.33)	0.773
Gender Frequency (%)	Male	25(71.4%)	27(81.8%)	0.313
	Female	10(28.6%)	6(18.2%)	
Diabetes Mellitus Frequency (%)	Negative	25(71.4%)	17(51.5%)	0.091
	Positive	10(28.6%)	16(48.5%)	
Hypertension Frequency (%)	Negative	13(38.2%)	9(27.3%)	0.339
	Positive	21(61.8%)	24(72.7%)	

Table 2: Comparison between two groups regarding mean CPB (cardiopulmonary bypass) and cross clump times, systolic and diastolic blood pressure and number of grafts

	Case n = 35	Control n = 33	P
CPB Time (hour: minute) Mean (±SD)	1:03(±0:22)	0:58(±0:19)	0.357
Cross Clamp (hour: minute) Mean (±SD)	0:31(±0:14)	0:33(±0:15)	0.620
Systolic (before) mean(±SD)	120.61(±21.48)	112.18(±21.76)	0.110
Diastolic (before) Mean (±SD)	64.29(±15.39)	57.02(±14.18)	0.073
Graft Mean (±SD)	3.45(±0.72)	3.42(±0.61)	0.871

Table 3: Comparison between mean AST values at different times in the two study groups

	SGOT Before	SGOT Day1	SGOT Day2	SGOT Day3	P
Case (n = 35)	26.49(±10.44)	29.57(±10.25)	36.14(±19.11)	30.77(±10.69)	0.004
Control (n = 33)	31.25(±16.44)	36.97(±28.05)	40.56(±26.32)	30.00(±14.44)	0.051
P value	0.167	0.194	0.480	0.726	-

P=0.107 and P=0.583, respectively). In addition, the ALT values in the case and control groups were not significantly different in three days (P=0.104 and P=0.218, respectively) (Table 4, Figure2).

The average ALP of the participants preoperatively in days 1-3 post-operative was not a significant difference between the two groups (P=0.755, P=0.442, P=0.493 and P=0.499, respectively). Procedure of ALP in the case and control groups were not significantly different in three days (P=0.166 and P=0.390, respectively) (Table 5, Figure 3).

Discussion

In this study, we examined 33 patients in control group and 35 patients in case group. There was no significant difference between two groups regarding age, sex, BMI, history of DM or HTN, CPB time, cross clump time and number of grafts. Pre-operative systolic and diastolic blood pressure was not significantly different between two groups. We tried to maintain intra operative and cross clump blood pressure by proper application of several drugs. There was no significant difference in ALT and ALP values at variable times in two groups. In addition, the procedures of ALT and ALP in the case and control groups were not significantly different in three days.

There was no–significant difference in AST values at variable times in two groups. However, the trend of AST was significantly increased in the case group; while this trend was not significantly different in the control group during the next three days. However, due to the P=0.051 in control group, this significant increase could be anticipated. Perhaps increasing the number of samples can resolve this ambiguity.

Given that even a very short time pulsatile flow can be effective on hemodynamics and vital organ function, in this study, we transferred continuous blood flow to pulsatile blood flow during proximal graft by using cardiac contraction. In this way after completion of distal graft, the surgeon turned cross clump to partial clump and after starting of heartbeat, we decreased the venous return 20-30% by partial clumping in venous cannula. This effect on liver function was benchmarked.

In a study by Mori *et al.* on 56 dogs, they did cardiopulmonary bypass with hypothermia in 20 C and total circulatory arrest for 40 minutes. They found that liver blood flow gradually decreased in both groups due to cooling while this effect was more in non-pulsatile than pulsatile group and this difference was significant between two groups before total circulatory arrest but it wasn't significant during rewarming (6).

In an another study by Poswal *et al.* on 100 patients undergone coronary artery bypass grafting (CABG) on CPB with normal left ventricular function, the effect of pulsatile blood flow on the platelet number and function, coagulation state, renal and liver function was studied. They found that the platelet number was decreased in both groups but they were not significant. The hemoglobin concentration was decreased in both groups. The liver enzymes were increased in two groups similarly which was not significant. The increase in AST and ALT levels postoperatively at 24 and 48 hours in non-pulsatile group were higher than pulsatile group (4).

Sabzi *et al.* evaluated the liver function tests on 200 patients undergoing CPB. They saw the significant elevation in Bilirubin and aspartate aminotransferase (AST) and ALP levels on the 3rd day postoperatively. They found a clear relation between hypotension and change in ALP and AST (7).

Bingyangji and Akifundar by studying of 194 article (74 study on animals and 85 clinical trials) in 1952-2006 explained that pulsatile blood flow increases the blood flow of the brain, heart, liver and pancreas significantly and it decreases the inflammatory responses and the mortality and morbidity rate after surgery with CPB. They didn't report any side effects of pulsatile flow (8).

Conclusion

The results of this study suggests that if hemodynamic stability is restored (using vasoactive agents), liver damage and increasing liver enzymes could be prevented in both study groups (*i.e.* surgical operation under CPB with pulsatile and non-pulsatile blood flow). However, pulsatile blood flow has no negligible effect on the liver enzymes changes. Judgment about the effects of this technique on liver function is dependent on the results of further studies.

Acknowledgment

The authors would like to acknowledge the kind help of their colleagues in the operating room and Anesthesiology Department.

Conflicts of Interest

The authors declare that they have no conflict of interest.

References

1. Shahbazi S, Panah A, Sahmeddini MA. Evaluation of factors influencing liver function test in on-pump coronary artery bypass graft surgery. Iran J Med Sci. 2013;38(4):308-13.

2. Hökenek F, Gürsoy M, Bakuy V, Kavala AA, Demir T, Gülcan, F, et al. An evaluation of renal functions in pulsatile and non-pulsatile cardiopulmonary bypass in the elderly. Turk J Thorac Cardiovasc Surg. 2013; 21(3): 610-5.

3. Gravlee GP. Epidural analgesia and coronary artery bypass grafting: the controversy continues. J Cardiothorac Vasc Anesth. 2003;17(2):151-3.

4. Poswal P, Mehta Y, Juneja R, Khanna S, Meharwal ZS, Trehan N. Comparative study of pulsatile and nonpulsatile flow during cardio-pulmonary bypass. Ann Card Anaesth. 2004;7(1):44-50..

5. Koning NJ, Vonk AB, van Barneveld LJ, Beishuizen A, Atasever B, van den Brom CE, Boer C. Pulsatile flow during cardiopulmonary bypass preserves postoperative microcirculatory perfusion irrespective of systemic hemodynamics. J Appl Physiol (1985). 2012;112(10):1727-34. .

6. Mori A, Watanabe K, Onoe M, Watarida S, Nakamura Y, Magara T, Tabata R, Okada Y. Regional blood flow in the liver, pancreas and kidney during pulsatile and nonpulsatile perfusion under profound hypothermia. Jpn Circ J. 1988;52(3):219-27.

7. Sabzi F, Faraji R. Liver Function Tests Following Open Cardiac Surgery. J Cardiovasc Thorac Res. 2015;7(2):49-54.

8. Ji B, Undar A. An evaluation of the benefits of pulsatile versus nonpulsatile perfusion during cardiopulmonary bypass procedures in pediatric and adult cardiac patients. ASAIO J. 2006;52(4):357-61.

Table 4: Comparison between mean ALP values at different times in the two study groups

	ALT Before	ALT Day1	ALT Day2	ALT Day3	P
Case (n = 35)	23.37(±12.79)	21.26(±10.42)	21.54(±10.35)	19.46(±10.29)	0.104
Control (n = 33)	25.19(±13.68)	26.30(±23.35)	30.24(±28.57)	21.12(±14.38)	0.218
P	0.575	0.261	0.107	0.583	-

Table 5: Comparison between mean ALP values at different times in the two study groups

	ALP Before	ALP Day1	ALP Day2	ALP Day3	P
Case (n = 35)	161.11(±57.72)	146.23(±49.61)	158.69(±48.89)	148.69(±40.06)	0.166
Control (n = 33)	156.91(±52.64)	155.45(±48.64)	164.73(±47.21)	155.55(±41.94)	0.390
P	0.755	0.442	0.493	0.499	-

10

Anesthesia for Pediatric Lung Transplantation

Premal M. Trivedi[1], **Erin A. Gottlieb**[1], **Emad B. Mossad**[1]

Abstract

Pediatric lung transplantation is a relatively rare procedure offered to infants, children, and adolescents with end-stage lung disease. Compared to adult lung transplantation, the pre-operative condition of the patients, indications for transplantation, and the conduct of the surgery itself can be quite different. Through this case presentation of a 2-month-old undergoing bilateral lung transplantation, we discuss the unique anesthetic considerations in the management of the pediatric patient, and review the data on the recent era of pediatric lung transplantation. Other concerns relevant to the anesthesiologist such as the disease states leading to transplantation, the ages at which patients most commonly present, and causes of post-operative morbidity and mortality are also presented.

Keywords: Pediatric, Lung, Transplantation, Anesthesia

1. Department of Anesthesiology, Perioperative, and Pain Medicine, Texas Children's Hospital, Division of Pediatric Cardiovascular Anesthesiology, Baylor College of Medicine, Houston, TX, United States of America

Corresponding Author:
Premal M. Trivedi, MD; Department of Anesthesiology, Perioperative, and Pain Medicine, Texas Children's Hospital, 6621 Fannin St, Houston, TX 77030, USA
E-mail: pxtrived@texaschildrens.org

Introduction

The first pediatric lung transplant was performed in 1987 at the University of Toronto in a 15-year-old with familial pulmonary fibrosis (1). Since that time, over 2000 children have received lung transplants worldwide, with an annual number ranging between 99 and 137 over the past decade (2).

While these numbers reflect the consistency in the need for this procedure, they also highlight its relative infrequency. Pediatric lung transplants have accounted for only 5.5% of all lung transplants since 1988 and represent an equally small percentage of all pediatric solid organ transplants (3). This lag has been attributed to the decreased incidence of end-stage lung disease in the pediatric population, a paucity of acceptable donors, and the modest late survival associated with transplantation. Nonetheless, pediatric lung transplantation has become a life-saving option for those with irreversible and progressive pulmonary parenchymal or vascular disease. For the anesthesiologist charged with managing these rare patients, an understanding of the indications that lead to transplantation, their pathophysiology, and the physiology of the transplanted lungs are critical.

To provide a context for the anesthetic management of the child undergoing lung transplantation, we discuss the case of a 2-month-old who underwent bilateral lung transplantation for intractable respiratory failure. Both the unique aspects of this case and pediatric lung transplantation, in general, are presented.

Case Report

A full-term infant who was the product of an uncomplicated gestation and an uneventful delivery presented to our institution at 10 weeks of age for bilateral lung transplant evaluation due to a pulmonary growth abnormality. Imaging on arrival demonstrated hyper-expansion of the right middle lobe causing both mediastinal shift to the left as well as compression of the right upper and lower lobes (Figure 1). This anatomy was reflected clinically with impaired ventilation and intermittent hypotension, presumably due to diminished venous return caused by the compressive effect of the right middle lobe on the right atrium.

Blood gases revealed a compensated respiratory acidosis with $PaCO_2$ levels chronically between 80-100 mmHg despite mechanical ventilation with paralysis and the use of inhaled nitric oxide (iNO, Table 1). Oxygenation, though also impaired, was acceptable with an increased FiO_2. Echocardiography revealed a patent foramen ovale, mild right ventricular hypertrophy, pulmonary hypertension, and normal biventricular function.

Medical management entailed aggressive diuresis and a strategy of differential lung ventilation to minimize the negative effects of the emphysematous right middle lobe. Through this process, the left lung was selectively ventilated via a cuffed oral endotracheal tube (ETT) placed in the left mainstem bronchus, while the right lung was ventilated via the tracheostomy (Figure 2). Using two ventilators, one for each lung, the right lung was ventilated more cautiously using a decreased rate and decreased inspiratory and positive end-expiratory pressures (Table 1). More ventilation that is effective was thereby achieved with less mediastinal shift. Given the infant's irreversible defect in lung growth, however, the patient was ultimately put forward for transplantation. Within 1 week of listing, a suitable organ became available.

As the patient was maintained on differential lung ventilation in the intensive care unit (ICU), a central consideration in our pre-operative evaluation was the safety and feasibility of maintaining this arrangement for transport and in the operating room. Due to concerns about this approach, we opted to trial

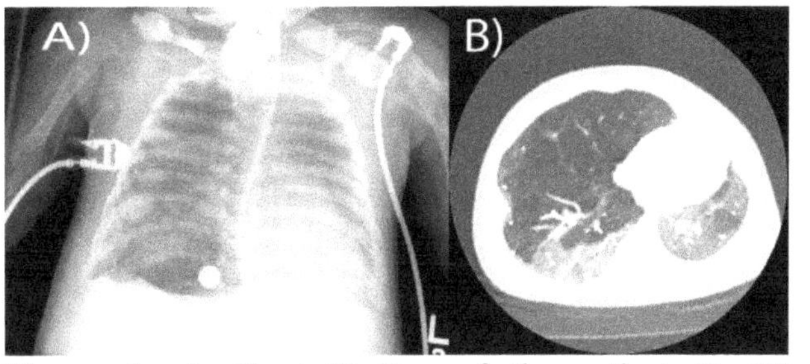

Figure 1. A Chest X Ray of the patient B CT demonstrating hyperexpansion of the right middle lobe, displacement of the mediastinum to the left, and compression of adjacent lung fields.

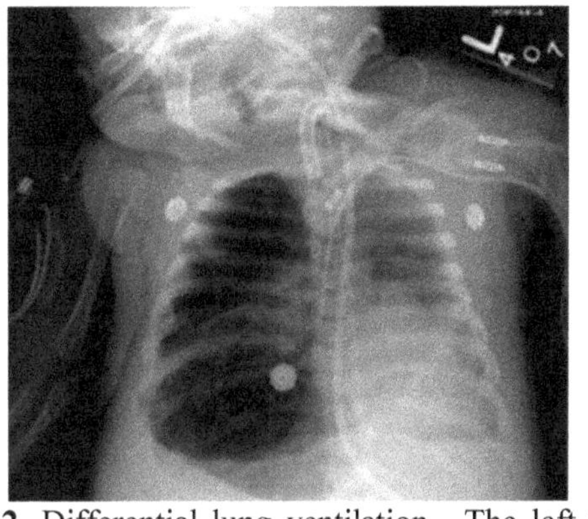

Figure 2. Differential lung ventilation. The left lung is ventilated via an oral ETT placed into the left mainstem bronchus while the right lung is ventilated via the tracheostomy.

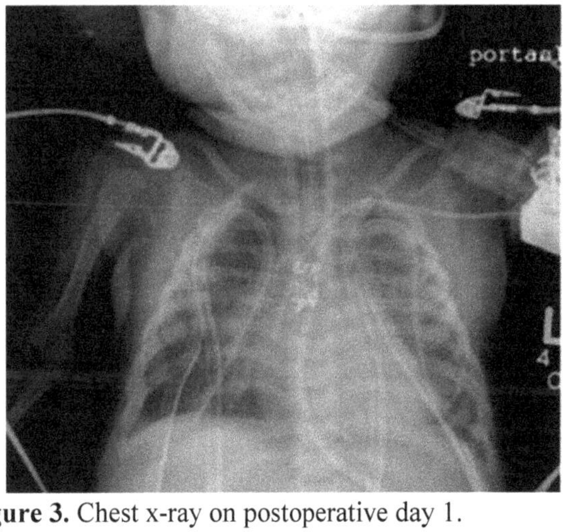

Figure 3. Chest x-ray on postoperative day 1.

the effect of stopping differential ventilation in the ICU in favor of ventilating both lungs through the tracheostomy at lower ventilatory settings. No significant change in hemodynamics or ventilation resulted, and so we proceeded with this traditional means of ventilation (Table 1).

Once in the operating room, the tracheostomy

Table 1: Ventilatory Settings and Blood Gases at Different Times in Management.

Time	*Conduit*	*Ventilator Mode*	*PIP[a] cmH$_2$O*	*Rate*	*PEEP[b] cm H$_2$O*	*FiO$_2$*	*iNO ppm*	*Blood Gas: pH/PCO2/PO2*
1	Tracheostomy	PCV[c]	38	40	5	0.7	20	7.23/121/146
2	*Right lung:* Tracheostomy	SIMV/PC[d]	30	28	5	0.6	5	
	Left lung:							7.35/89/41[e]
	Bronchial cuffed oral ETT	SIMV/PC	38	28	8	0.6	5	
3	Cuffed nasal ETT	PCV	30-33	28	6	1.0	5	7.44/76/332
4	Cuffed nasal ETT	PCV	23	24	5	0.45	20	7.39/46/83

1: Arrival to our institution
2: Morning of transplantation
3: Initial operating room (OR) ventilatory settings
4: Following transplantation and liberation from cardiopulmonary bypass

a: Peak inspiratory pressure
b: Positive end-expiratory pressure
c: Pressure control ventilation
d: Synchronized intermittent mandatory ventilation/pressure control
e: Venous blood gas

Table 2: General goals for ventilation following transplantation (Texas Children's Protocol).

Recruitment maneuvers	< 30 cm H$_2$O
Ventilatory Mode	Pressure Control Ventilation
Peak inspiratory pressure (PIP)	< 25 cm H$_2$O
Positive end expiratory pressure (PEEP)	5
Tidal volumes	Donor-appropriate, < 10 cc/kg
FiO$_2$	0.4-0.5, goal SpO$_2$ > 90%

tube was exchanged for a nasal cuffed endotracheal tube (ETT) to allow a more exposed surgical field. A femoral arterial line was placed and central venous access was obtained. Bilateral cerebral near-infrared spectroscopy monitors (Somanetics INVOS, Troy, Michigan) were also placed to assess cerebral oxygenation. Anesthesia was maintained with isoflurane, fentanyl, and midazolam, and induction immunosuppressive therapy was administered as directed by the transplant service.

When the donor lungs were visualized and deemed acceptable, the recipient dissection was begun via a bilateral thoracosternotomy or "clamshell" incision. Due to the patient's size, tenuous respiratory status, and abnormal lung anatomy, the removal of the patient's lungs and placement of the donor lungs was performed on cardiopulmonary bypass. The transplantation was uneventful: three anastomoses were created in a posterior to anterior fashion with first the bronchi on each side, then the pulmonary veins, and finally the pulmonary arteries.

Prior to weaning from bypass, bronchoscopy was performed to evaluate the bronchial anastomoses and clear the airway of blood and secretions. Vasoactive agents to assist right ventricular function and minimize pulmonary vascular resistance were also initiated and included epinephrine 0.02

mcg/kg/min, milrinone 0.375 mcg/kg/min, prostaglandin E_1 0.025 mcg/kg/min, and inhaled nitric oxide (iNO) at 20 parts per million (PPM). Minimal peak inspiratory pressure, positive-end expiratory pressure, and inspired oxygen concentration were chosen to avoid further injury to the newly transplanted lungs (Tables 1 and 2). To augment ventilation, gentle recruitment maneuvers and suctioning were needed at regular intervals to combat atelectasis and prevent obstruction from bloody secretions.

The patient was successfully weaned on this regimen. Donor lung ischemic time was 6 hours and 47 minutes with a total CPB time of 6 hours and 5 minutes. The anticipated post-bypass coagulopathy was treated with platelets, cryoprecipitate, and recombinant activated factor VII. A total of 3 units of packed red blood cells, 3 units of fresh frozen plasma, 2 units of cryoprecipitate, and 1 unit of apheresis platelets were used during the bypass and post-bypass periods.

On arrival to the ICU, the patient's ABG was pH 7.46, $paCO_2$ 43, and paO_2 275. Chest x-ray demonstrated areas of atelectasis and pulmonary congestion, but symmetric lung fields and a normally positioned heart (Figure 3). In the days following transplantation, evidence of mild graft dysfunction appeared with a subsequent need for increased PIP and a slow wean of FiO_2. The allograft function remained acceptable, however, and progress was made in decreasing PIP and FiO_2 over time.

Discussion

What are the most common indications for pediatric lung transplantation?

The most common indications for pediatric lung transplantation include cystic fibrosis, pulmonary hypertension, interstitial lung disease, and obliterative bronchiolitis (2, 3). Of note, the indications largely correlate with age (Table 3). For those greater than 6 years, cystic fibrosis (CF) was the most common indication between 2000 and 2015 (2). In those who were less than 5 years, pulmonary hypertension, interstitial lung disease, congenital heart disease, and surfactant protein B deficiency led the indications for transplantation (2).

Contraindications to pediatric lung transplantation likely vary among institutions, but absolute contraindications may include systemic disease with major extra-pulmonary manifestations, severe multi-organ dysfunction, left ventricular failure, and severe scoliosis.

What are the characteristics of transplant recipients?

Transplant recipients between 1988 and 2008 had a mean age of 12±5.6 years and a mean weight of 33.6±16.3 kg (3). Adolescents (age≥13) were the group most commonly transplanted (58%), followed by those between 2 to 12 years (31%), with infants (11%) being the group least commonly transplanted (3). On average, 3-5 infants are transplanted annually. When listed, infants tend to be in the ICU and either mechanically ventilated or on extracorporeal membrane oxygenation (ECMO). Some, like our patient, may even have a tracheostomy pre-transplant (Table 4). This is in contrast to older children, many of whom wait at home while listed and are able to oxygenate and ventilate without support.

Median overall waiting times once listed are 5 months with a range of 0-96 months; infants have a significantly shorter waiting time of 1 month, with a range of 0-7 months, perhaps reflecting the small number of infants who are listed as well as the severity of their disease state at the time of listing.

Pre-operative evaluation

Pre-operative assessment should focus on the patient's indication for transplantation, the disease process's current effect on oxygenation and ventilation, and any other end-organ dysfunction that may be present. Of particular concern, regarding co-morbidities are those patients with cystic fibrosis. Given that the mutated gene, the cystic fibrosis transmembrane regulator (CFTR), is expressed in multiple organs, such patients can also present with diverse manifestations including diabetes, pancreatic exocrine insufficiency, and hepatic dysfunction (Table 5). Moreover, patients with end-stage cystic fibrosis often have multi-drug resistant bacteria. If not otherwise stated in the patient's transplant plan, such a history should prompt a discussion regarding the intraoperative antibiotics to be administered during the transplant.

In reviewing previous surgeries, particular attention should be given to prior thoracic procedures.

Table 3: Most Common Indications for Pediatric Lung Transplantation by Age, 2000-2015.

Diagnosis	*Age < 1 year (%)*	*1-5 years (%)*	*6-10 years (%)*	*12-17 years (%)*
Cystic fibrosis	-	4%	50%	67.8%
Idiopathic pulmonary hypertension	12.3%	27.3%	10.2%	7.7%
Non-idiopathic pulmonary hypertension	24.6%	18.2%	3.7%	1.6%
Interstitial lung disease	19.3%	18.2%	12.9%	6.7%
Surfactant protein B deficiency	21.1%	4%	0.5%	-
ABCA3 transporter mutation	7%	4%	0.5%	0.1%
Bronchopulmonary dysplasia	7%	3%	1.4%	0.3%
Obliterative bronchiolitis (non-retransplant)	-	8.1%	12.5%	4.6%
Retransplant	-	7%	4.6%	6.7%

Adapted from the Registry of the International Society for Heart and Lung Transplantation: Nineteenth Pediatric Lung and Heart-Lung Transplantation Report

Table 4: Support status and location of patients prior to lung transplantation at Texas Children's Hospital 2002-2011.

Age	*Tracheostomy*	*Otherwise mechanically ventilated*	*ICU*	*Home*
< 1 year	5/7	1/7	6/7	1/7
1-5 years	5/16	2/16	7/16	9/16
6-11 years	3/21	1/21	4/21	17/21
12-17 years	3/59	2/59	5/59	54/59
Total	16/103 (16%)	6/103 (6%)	22/103 (21%)	81/103 (79%)

Their presence may suggest an increased risk of bleeding and/or a lengthy dissection period during the transplant due to adherent tissues.

Vascular access

It is our institution's preference to use femoral arterial access for lung transplants. This choice has its basis in the clinical observation that radial arterial lines often seem to fail in this population. This may, in part, be due to the clamshell incision that can lead to compression of the subclavian artery, or as is the case in patients with cystic fibrosis, the decrease in systemic vascular resistance that can occur due to dissection-induced bacteremia.

Central venous access is routinely obtained unless a patient has an indwelling peripherally-inserted central catheter. Given the potential for intraoperative bleeding, adequate peripheral access should also be obtained.

Not surprisingly, vascular access may be challenging, particularly in those who have required care in the ICU prior to their transplant. A thorough review of prior invasive lines and any history of major vessel occlusion may assist in planning which vessels to access.

Analgesia: is there a role for a thoracic epidural?

While a thoracic epidural would offer the potential advantages of improved analgesia, earlier mobilization, and earlier extubation, unique risks are present in the setting of lung transplantation that warrant discussion. Because most cases of pediatric lung transplantation are performed using cardiopulmonary bypass (CPB), and thus involve systemic heparinization, the possibility of an associated neuraxial hematoma is theoretically

Table 5: Potential End-Organ Manifestations of Cystic Fibrosis.

Upper airway	• Chronic sinusitis • Nasal polyps
Pulmonary	• Productive cough • Wheezing and/or bronchospasm • Hemoptysis • Pneumothorax • Pulmonary hypertension
Cardiovascular	• Right ventricular dysfunction (cor pulmonale)
Gastrointestinal	• Gastroesophageal reflux • Meconium ileus in the neonate • Distal intestinal obstruction in adults • Intussusception • Fibrosing colonopathy
Hepatobiliary	• Gallstones • Cirrhotic liver disease • Hepatic steatosis
Exocrine pancreas	• Malnutrition • Steatorrhea • Fat-soluble vitamin deficiency
Endocrine pancreas	• CF-related diabetes mellitus
Bone and joints	• Fractures • Arthritis • Osteopenia • Osteoporosis

increased. Moreover, delaying the surgery in the event of a bloody insertion would be detrimental to the donor lungs by prolonging their ischemic time[6].

The age of the patient at the time of transplantation and the presence of other co-morbidities may also influence the decision on whether or not to place an epidural. On average, infants require 24±19 days of postoperative mechanical ventilation because of their accompanying medical issues[4], which would make epidural placement less advantageous; older patients with cystic fibrosis, on the other hand, are commonly weaned from mechanical ventilation within 1-3 days (5).

Consideration, then, needs to be given to the risks and benefits of an epidural as well as to the timing of placement should it be part of institutional practice. At our institution, we do not enough place epidurals due to the potential risk of a bloody tap and the observation that times to extubation and respiratory function do not appear compromised when using intravenous analgesics alone.

The role and impact of cardiopulmonary bypass in pediatric transplantation

In contrast to adult lung transplantation, the use of CPB in pediatric lung transplantation is commonplace. Often times the patient's airway size makes one-lung-ventilation with sequential single lung transplantation impractical; other times the patient's clinical status mandates the use of CPB to ensure a hemodynamically stable dissection and implantation. Disadvantages to CPB include an increased risk of coagulopathy and need for transfusion, and activation of the systemic inflammatory response with potential for allograft injury on reperfusion[8]. Our patient required both CPB and a brief period of aortic cross-clamping for closure of the patent foramen ovale (PFO).

Hemodynamics and fluid management

Assisting right ventricular function is a key

Table 6: Physiologic changes affecting lung function following transplantation.

Anticipated changes influencing lung function	*End-results of these changes*
Vagal denervation and loss of afferent stimuli	• Resting bronchodilation • Less effective cough • Decreased clearance of secretions • Decreased response to hypercapnea • Poor coordination between thoracic and abdominal musculature
Absence of lymphatic drainage	• Decreased lung compliance • Potential for worsening pulmonary edema with volume administration

Table 7: Common Causes of Death in Pediatric Lung Transplant Recipients by Age at Transplantation, 1990-2015.

Cause of death	*0-30 days* (n = 151) No. (%)	*31 days – 1 year* (n = 212) No. (%)	*>1-3 years* (n = 266) No. (%)	*>3-5 years* (n = 128) No. (%)	*>5 years* (n = 140) No. (%)
Bronchiolitis Obliterans	0	24 (11.3)	96 (36.1)	49 (38.3)	65 (46.4)
Infection	23 (15.2)	72 (33.9)	43 (16.2)	22 (17.2)	10 (7.1)
Graft Failure	44 (29.1)	41 (19.3)	70 (26.3)	29 (22.7)	31 (22.1)
Acute rejection	3 (2)	5 (2.4)	6 (2.3)	3 (2.3)	1 (0.7)
Malignancy	0	12 (6.6)	8 (3.0)	4 (3.1)	12 (8.6)
Multiple Organ Failure	16 (10.6)	25 (11.8)	14 (5.3)	5 (3.9)	9 (6.4)
Cardiovascular	22 (14.6)	9 (4.2)	4 (1.5)	1 (0.8)	1 (0.7)
Technical	22 (14.6)	5 (2.4)	6 (2.3)	3 (2.3)	2 (1.4)

Adapted from the Registry of the International Society for Heart and Lung Transplantation: Nineteenth Pediatric Lung and Heart-Lung Transplantation Report

goal in patients undergoing lung transplantation, especially in the pre-bypass period when lung function is marginal. While it would ideal to minimize pulmonary vascular resistance through manipulating oxygenation, ventilation, and pH, this can be challenging due to the intrinsic lung abnormality. As such, one should have inotropes and pressors available to assist contractility as needed and to maintain an adequate coronary perfusion pressure to avoid right ventricular ischemia. Post-bypass, right ventricular function may be hyperdynamic assuming adequate graft function due to normalization in right ventricular afterload compared to the pre-transplant state. Vasoactive agents that can assist right ventricular function post-transplant include epinephrine, milrinone, prostaglandin E_1, and iNO.

Because transplanted lungs lack an intact lymphatic system, caution must be used with the administration of blood products and crystalloid in the immediate post-transplant period to avoid pulmonary congestion and subsequently impaired oxygenation and ventilation (6). This goal is often at direct odds, however, with the need to achieve hemostasis. As evidenced in the patient described, bypass times can often be several hours, leading to deficiencies in platelets, fibrinogen, and clotting factors that require replacement. Given that the transfusion of blood products is, at times, inevitable, one should look carefully for any change in ventilatory compliance and oxygenation that may indicate the onset of pulmonary edema. Such a change may prompt a new strategy towards the use of recombinant factor 7a or another low-volume pro-coagulant like the prothrombin complex concentrates should coagulopathy remain an issue.

Ventilating and oxygenating the newly transplanted lungs

To avoid further injury to the donor lungs, our ventilatory strategy seeks to minimize the peak inspiratory pressures, positive-end expiratory pressures, and FiO_2 necessary to achieve adequate ventilation and oxygenation (Table 2). Common etiologies that may cause an acute increase in airway pressures include obstruction of the airways or ETT with blood or secretions, or airway compression due to surgical manipulation. Frequent suctioning either by suction catheter or with a bronchoscope is often necessary. When deciding what tidal volume is most appropriate with which to ventilate, one should consider the size of the donor patient (as this individual may have been smaller or larger than the recipient), and whether any lobes of the donor lung were surgically resected (as may be the case in significant size-mismatch).

Physiology of the newly transplanted lungs

Transplantation interrupts not only the donor lung's lymphatic drainage, but also its vagal innervation (Table 6). Vagal denervation manifests as resting bronchodilation, decreased ventilatory response to hypercapnea, diminished cough, and reduced mucociliary clearance. Proximal to the anastomosis, however, airway reflexes and mucociliary clearance are retained. Thus, if the upper airway or trachea is to be instrumented as in bronchoscopy, care should be taken to topicalize the airway with local anesthetic as one would in any other patient. Of note, hypoxic pulmonary vasoconstriction and the response to inhaled beta-agonists are preserved in the donor lung.

What are the concerns in the post-operative period following lung transplantation?

Post-transplant complications can be categorized into 3 phases: the immediate phase, representing the first week after transplantation; the early phase, including the first 3 months; and the late phase, entailing the time beyond 3 months.

Immediate and early phase complications

Primary graft dysfunction and ischemia-reperfusion Injury

These represent the most common graft complications following transplantation, occurring in 20-30% (9), and are the leading causes of death within the first 30 days posttransplant (2). The two conditions are inter-related in that primary graft dysfunction is the product of multiple insults of which ischemia-reperfusion injury is a major contributor (8). The clinical spectrum can range from mild hypoxemia with few infiltrates on chest x-ray to severe respiratory distress syndrome (8, 9).

Rejection

Hyperacute rejection is rare as it represents a previous exposure to foreign tissue antigens that are generally screened for. Acute rejection, however, is more common and occurs at a rate comparable to that in adults. The majority of episodes of acute rejection occur in the first 6 months after transplant (10). Infants appear to have a much lower incidence compared to other pediatric age groups, perhaps because of their relatively immature immune systems (11).

Infection

Infection, always a concern following any transplantation, is of greater risk in the lung transplant recipient. Not only is there direct contact of the graft with the external environment, but there is also donor colonization of the airways and a diminished ability to cough due to vagal denervation and potential phrenic nerve injury. Of all age groups, infants are particularly susceptible to severe and fatal viral infections.

Surgical complications

Anastomotic complications, although rare, can involve bronchial dehiscence or pulmonary vascular stenosis. Bronchial stenosis occurs in approximately 10%, and can be treated effectively with serial dilation or angioplasty (10). Issues with the vascular anastomoses can be studied with perfusion lung scans or cardiac catheterization, often performed within the first 24 hours of transplant as a screening tool.

Late phase complications

Issues plaguing the late phases following transplantation include bronchiolitis obliterans (OB), malignancy, and immunosuppressant-related side effects.

Bronchiolitis obliterans

OB is a histiologic diagnosis with a clinical surrogate of decreased forced expiratory volume in 1 second (FEV_1). It is a major cause of death and the need for retransplantation in those who survive 1 year following transplantation, and occurs in nearly 50% of long-term survivors (12).

Malignancy

The overall incidence of malignancy is 5-10%, and is mainly attributable to post-transplant lymphoproliferative disease (PTLD) (10). Primary Epstein-Barr virus (EBV) is a risk factor for PTLD (13). Children may be more susceptible to this complication because they are often seronegative for EBV at the time of transplantation, and can thus acquire a primary EBV infection thereafter.

Immunosuppresant-related side effects

Some of the most common causes of morbidity following pediatric lung transplantation are related to immunosuppressive therapy. Most patients are on a regimen of triple immunosuppression entailing an antimetabolite (azathioprine or mycophenolate mofetil), a calcineurin inhibitor (cyclosporine or tacrolimus), and systemic steroids as maintenance (8). Side effects that are particularly relevant to the anesthesiologist can include hypertension, diabetes, renal dysfunction, and seizures. Within 1 year, the prevalence of hypertension is 42%, renal dysfunction 10%, diabetes 21%, and hyperlipidemia 5% (2). At 5 years, the prevalence increases to 69%, 30%, 31%, and 18%, respectively (2).

What is the survival following transplantation?

Survival has increased over the years due to advances in surgical technique, immunosuppressive regimens, patient selection, and post-transplant care. However, as noted in a recent review of the preceding 2 decades of pediatric lung transplantation, the improved survival is attributable only to an increased 1-year survival (3). Beyond the first year, survival has remained unchanged, and remains low compared to heart and other solid organ transplantations.

The 5-year survival of pediatric lung transplant recipients between January 1990 and June 2014 was 51%, a number comparable to that observed in the adult population during the same period of time (2). Among the different ages of pediatric patients, no significant difference in survival was noted in pair-wise comparisons (3). Survival in the first year post-transplant, however, was lowest in infants, perhaps reflecting the effects of infection on their naïve and suppressed immune systems. Beyond one year, infant survival was comparable to that of other age groups.

The functional status of pediatric lung transplant recipients has been reported to be very good. 86% of those surviving 5 years after transplantation have no activity limitations (2).

What are the major causes of death?

The leading causes of death following pediatric lung transplantation include graft failure, infection, and bronchiolitis obliterans (2) (Table 7). In the first year after transplantation, infection and graft failure account for the majority of deaths, whereas bronchiolitis obliterans is the major cause after the first year. Malignancy and multi-organ system failure are also significant contributors.

Risk factors for increased early and overall mortality **include** preoperative chronic steroid use, pre-transplant ventilatory dependence, and re-transplantation.

An update on our patient

Our patient's postoperative recovery was initially hindered by infectious pulmonary complications, including a CMV pneumonitis and bacterial pneumonia. She was able to overcome these issues, though, and was weaned off the ventilator. Her tracheostomy was decannulated shortly thereafter and she was subsequently discharged home, approximately 3 months after transplantation.

Conclusion

Pediatric lung transplantation has become an accepted therapy for selected patients with otherwise untreatable pulmonary parenchymal or vascular disease, and represents a growing field in medicine. Unique challenges include the limited availability of suitable donor organs, the prevalence of bronchiolitis obliterans, infection, and graft failure following transplantation, and the related effort to maximize survival, growth, and quality of life in these patients.

Anesthesiologists can contribute greatly to the care of these patients in their intraoperative management during the transplantation itself or in the post-transplant period when the patient returns for biopsies, bronchoscopies, or procedures otherwise common to the pediatric population. Care during the transplantation should focus on careful ventilation, oxygenation, and fluid management to optimize graft function. Post-transplant anesthetics, beyond an assessment of graft function, should direct attention to the immunosuppressant-induced and primary disease-related comorbidities present.

Acknowledgment

None

Conflicts of Interest

The authors declare that there are no conflicts of interest.

References

1. Grossman RF, Frost A, Zamel N, et al. Results of single-lung transplantation for bilateral pulmonary fibrosis. N Engl J Med. 1990;322:727-33.
2. Goldfarb SB, Levvey BJ et al. The Registry of the International Society for Heart and Lung Transplantation: Nineteenth Pediatric Lung and Heart-Lung Transplantation Report—2016. J Heart and Lung Transplant. 2016;1196-205.
3. Zafar F, Heinle JS, Schecter MG, et al. Two decades of pediatric lung transplant in the United States: Have we improved? J Thorac Cardiovasc Surg. 2011;141:828-32.
4. Huddleston CB, Sweet SC, Mallory GB, et al. Lung transplant in very young infants. J Thorac Cardiovasc Surg. 1999;118:796–804.
5. Meneloff EN, Huddleston CB, Mallory GB, et al. Pediatric and adult lung transplantation for cystic fibrosis. J Thorac Cardiovasc Surg. 1998;115:404–13.
6. Williams GD, Ramamoorthy C. Anesthesia Considerations for Pediatric Thoracic Solid Organ Transplant. Anesthesiology Clin N Am. 2005;23:709-31.
7. Patterson GA. Bilateral lung transplantation: indications and techniques. Semin Thorac Cardiovasc Surg. 1992;4(2):95-100.
8. Solomon M, Grasemann H, Keshavjee S. Pediatric Lung Transplantation. Pediatr Clin N Am. 2010;57:375-91.
9. King RC, Binns OAR, Rodriguz F, et al.: Reperfusion injury significantly impacts clinical outcome after pulmonary transplantation. Ann Thorac Surg. 2000;69:1681–5.
10. Huddleston CB. Pediatric Lung Transplantation. Current Treatment Options in Cardiovascular Medicine. 2011;13:68-78.
11. Huddleston CB, Sweet SC, Cohen AH, Mendeloff EN, Mallory GB: Bronchiolitis obliterans after pediatric lung transplantation. J Heart Lung Transplant. 1998;17:65.
12. Sundaresan S, Trulock EP, Mohanakumar T, Cooper JD, Patterson GA: Prevalence and outcome of bronchiolitis syndrome after lung transplantation. Ann Thorac Surg. 1995;60:1341–6.
13. Walker RC, Paya CV, Marshall WF, et al.: Pretrans- plantation sero-negative Epstein–Barr virus status is the primary risk factor for post-transplantation lymphoproliferative disease in adult heart, lung and other solid organ transplantation. J Heart Lung Transplant. 1995;14:214–21.
14 Sweet SC. Pediatric Lung Transplantation. Proc Am Thorac Soc. 2009;6:122-7.

Comparison of Adding Neostigmine and Fentanyl to Bupivacaine in Caudal Analgesia in Pediatric Inguinal Herniorrhaphy

Omid Aghadavoudi[1], Amir Shafa[1✉], Zahra Nowrouzi[1]

Abstract

Background: The aim of the present trial was to compare efficacy and adverse effects of neostigmine against fentanyl when used as adjuvant to bupivacaine in caudal anesthesia.

Materials and Methods: A total of 140 children, aged 1-6 year scheduled to elective herniorrhaphy, were enrolled. Exclusion criteria were sacral area infection, history of allergic reactions to local anesthetics, bleeding tendency, neurological or spinal disease and lack of parent consent. Patients were assigned, using permuted block randomization method, into four groups of 35. Children in the first group received a caudal injection of 0.5 ml/kg bupivacaine 0.25% plus fentanyl 1μ/kg. The second group received 0.5 ml/kg bupivacaine 0.25% plus neostigmine 1μ/kg. Patients in the third group received 0.5 ml/kg bupivacaine 0.25% plus combination of fentanyl 1μ/kg and neostigmine 1μ/kg, and those in the fourth group only received 0.5 ml/kg bupivacaine 0.25% concentration. To assess pain intensity, Wong-Baker Scale was used. Time to first analgesic request and the dosage of analgesic agent was recorded. Data were analyzed using SPSS 17.0.

Results: Significant differences were observed among groups in terms of number of patients needing analgesic ($p=0.01$), time to first analgesic request ($p=0.005$) and analgesic dose. ($p=0.05$) The lowest number of requests for analgesia, lowest dose of pethidine and longest time to first analgesic request were in patients receiving combination of bupivacaine, neostigmine and fentanyl.

Conclusion: The present study shows that the combination of fentanyl and neostigmine, could prolong duration of analgesia, and decrease severity of pain when added to bupivacaine.

Keywords: fentanyl, neostigmine, bupivacaine, caudal anesthesia

1. Anesthesiology and Critical Care Research Center, Isfahan University of Medical Sciences, Isfahan, Iran

✉ **Corresponding Author:** Amir Shafa, MD. Assistant Professor of anesthesiology, Isfahan University of Medical Sciences, Isfahan, Iran. Imam Hossein Hospital, Imam Khomeini Ave., Isfahan, Iran.
Email: shafa_amir@yahoo.com

Introduction

Postoperative pain is one the most common problems in surgical patients that can influence their physical and mental health. So, effective pain management is an essential component of postoperative care (1).

Caudal block is one of the technical advancements that is regularly used in children (1-8). This block is safe, effective and easy with less side effects (9-15). It is the most common block technique used in lower abdominal or lower extremity infant surgeries (1, 3, 5, 6, 16-19). In this method, local anesthetics such as bupivacaine have been injected into the caudal canal providing block in the sacral and lumbar nerve roots.

This approach has several advantages: increased intra and postoperative pain relief, decreased use of narcotic and non- narcotic drugs, rapid awakening, and rapid return of bowel function and reduced length of hospital stay (1, 3, 6, 18).

Usually, different additive agents have been used to increase efficacy and to prolong duration of caudal block such as: epinephrine, midazolam, clonidine, neostigmine, ketamine, morphine, tramadol and fentanyl (4-6, 9, 10, 14, 18, 19). But results of these combinations in the field of effectiveness, duration of improvement, hemodynamic changes and side effects have been very different.

Neostigmine is a cholinesterase inhibitor that facilitates transmission of impulses across the neuromuscular junction, used in myasthenia gravis treatment and to reverse the effects of muscle relaxant (11, 18).

Fentanyl is a potent synthetic opioid with many receptors within CNS. It increases pain threshold, inhibits ascending pain pathways and relieves pain in regional or general anesthesia (2, 12, 19).

The aim of the present double-blind randomized clinical trial was to compare efficacy and adverse effects of neostigmine against fentanyl when used as adjuvant to bupivacaine in caudal anesthesia.

Methods

This double-blind, randomized clinical trial was conducted in Imam Hossein pediatric University hospital of Isfahan, Iran.

The protocol of this study was conformed to Declaration of Helsinki, and was approved by the Ethics Committee at Isfahan University of Medical Sciences. Written informed consent was obtained from parents of children, after they were informed about study objectives. The trial was registered in IRCT (IRCT 2017051126866N3).

A total of 140 children, aged 1-6 year and ASA physical status I, who were scheduled to elective herniorrhaphy, were enrolled. Exclusion criteria were sacral area infection, history of allergic reactions to local anesthetics, bleeding tendency, neurological or spinal disease and lack of parent consent.

Demographic characteristics including age, gender, American Society of Anesthesiologists (ASA) class, weight, date and duration of surgery were recorded for each patient.

Caudal anesthesia

Patients were assigned, using permuted block randomization method, into four groups of 35. Children in the first group received a caudal injection of 0.5 ml/kg bupivacaine 0.25% plus fentanyl 1μ/kg. The second group received 0.5 ml/kg bupivacaine 0.25% plus neostigmine 1μ/kg. Patients in the third group received 0.5 ml/kg bupivacaine 0.25% plus combination of fentanyl 1μ/kg and neostigmine 1μ/kg, and those in the fourth group only received 0.5 ml/kg bupivacaine 0.25% concentration.

All children received intravenous midazolam (0.1 mg/kg) as premedication; intubation was performed after induction of anesthesia with fentanyl 2μ/kg, sodium thiopental 6mg/kg and atracorium 0.5mg/kg. The caudal block was performed after intubation and following aseptic technique in lateral position before the onset of surgery. Patients and the researcher who gathered the data were blinded to the solution and patient group.

During surgery, general anesthesia was maintained using inhaled isoflurane (1.2%) in O2 50%, air 50%. Heart rate (HR), SpO2, ETCO2, temperature (T) and blood pressure (BP) was recorded every 15 minutes.

At the end of surgery, intravenous atropine 0.02 mg/kg and neostigmine 0.04 mg/kg was used to reverse neuromuscular block; patients were transferred to recovery after extubation.

Hemodynamic changes and drug side effects (nausea and vomiting) were recorded in recovery room and surgery ward in different time points.

To assess pain intensity, we used the standard pain questionnaire (Wong-Baker Scale). Also, the time to first analgesic request and the dosage of analgesic agent was recorded.

Intravenous pethidine (1-1.5 mg/kg) was administered for patients suffering postoperative pain, and intravenous ondansetrone (0.15 mg/kg) was used for patient with postoperative nausea and vomiting.

Statistical analysis

Data were entered into the Statistical Package for the Social Sciences software version 17.0 (SPSS Inc. Chicago, IL, USA). The data were analyzed using one-way analysis of variance (ANOVA), The Chi-squared test or Fisher's exact test, when appropriate. A *p*-value less than 0.05 were considered as significant.

Results

Baseline characteristics (gender, age, weight, ASA score, duration of anesthesia, surgery) were not significantly different in the four groups (Table 1).

Significant differences were observed among groups in terms of number of patients needing analgesic (p=0.01), time to first analgesic request (p=0.005) and analgesic dose. (p=0.05) The lowest number of requests for analgesia, lowest dose of pethidine and longest time to first analgesic request were in patients receiving combination of bupivacaine, neostigmine and fentanyl (Table 2).

There were no significant differences in preoperative, intraoperative and recovery hemodynamic changes (systolic and diastolic BP, MAP and HR) among the four groups.

Intraoperative and postoperative SpO2 levels were significantly different among the four groups. Furthermore, pre-operative and intraoperative ETCO2 levels were significantly different among the four groups.

We observed significant difference in post-operative Wong-Baker pain score in 15th, 30th, 45th min and 2nd, 4th, 6th and 12th hour between four groups. The lowest pain score was in patients

Table 1: Demographic and surgical profile.

Variable	Bupivacaine and fentanyl (N=34)	Bupivacaine and neostigmine (N=35)	Bupivacaine, fentanyl, and neostigmine (N=36)	Bupivacaine (N=34)	P-value
Age (years) Mean ± SD	2.6 ± 1.4	3.2 ± 1.7	3.1 ± 1.6	3 ± 1.6	0.383
Gender :					
Number (%)	31 (91.2%)	30 (87.7%)	30 (83.3%)	32 (94.1%)	0.498
male	3 (8.8%)	5 (14.3%)	6 (16.7%)	2 (5.9%)	
female					
Weight (kg)	13.3 ± 4.1	13.1 ± 4.1	13.6 ± 4.1	13.8 ± 3.8	0.803
Duration of anesthesia (minute)	61.5 ± 12.9	58.1 ± 6.8	61.9 ± 8.3	59.4 ± 7.8	0.263
Duration of surgery (minute)	47.6 ± 11.9	43.1 ± 8.9	45.7 ± 8.4	44.4 ± 7.5	0.338

Table 2: Comparison of postoperative analgesic administration.

Variable	Bupivacaine and fentanyl (N=34)	Bupivacaine and neostigmine (N=35)	Bupivacaine, fentanyl, and neostigmine (N=36)	Bupivacaine (N=34)	P-value
Patients without need to analgesia (in 12hours), number (%)	22 (64.7%)	18 (51.4%)	۲8 (77.8%)	14 (41.2%)	0.01
Time to first analgesic request (minute)	571.32±212.3	533±226.2	620.97±192.1	433.68±253.6	0.005
Pethidine dose (mg)	2.35±3.6	3.03±3.4	1.5±3.1	4.05±3.8	0.05

receiving combination of bupivacaine, neostigmine and fentanyl ($p<0.001$) (Table 3).

Significant differences were observed in nausea ($p=0.006$) and vomiting ($p=0.12$) among the four groups. Frequency of nausea and vomiting was lowest in patients receiving bupivacaine, and highest in those receiving a combination of bupivacaine, neostigmine and fentanyl (Table 4).

Table 3: Comparison of postoperative pain score (Wong-Baker).

	Bupivacaine and fentanyl (N=34)	Bupivacaine and neostigmine (N=35)	Bupivacaine, fentanyl, and neostigmine (N=36)	Bupivacaine (N=34)	P-value
15 minute	1.65	1.71	1.44	2.29	0.038
30 minute	2.06	2.51	2.11	2.53	0.017
45 minute	2.65	3.31	2.72	3.29	0.029
2 hour	3.12	3.71	2.94	3.94	0.004
4 hour	4.53	5.14	3.33	4.88	0.001
6 hour	3.82	4.34	2.83	5.03	< 0.001
12 hour	2.70	3.20	1.89	4.12	< 0.001

Table 4: Comparison of postoperative nausea and vomiting.

Variable	Bupivacaine and fentanyl (N=34)	Bupivacaine and neostigmine (N=35)	Bupivacaine, fentanyl, and neostigmine (N=36)	Bupivacaine (N=34)	P-value
Nausea Number (%)	6 (17.6%)	2 (5.7%)	7 (19.4%)	0 (0%)	0.006
Vomiting Number (%)	4 (11.8%)	2 (5.7%)	7 (19.4%)	0 (0%)	0.012

Duration of recovery time was not significantly different among the four groups. (p>0.05).

Discussion

Caudal block is one of the most effective methods for postoperative pain management. It is usually performed during lower abdominal and lower extremities surgeries in children, using a local anesthetic, with or without additive agents (1-8, 18, 19).

To the best of our knowledge, this is the first study to compare the efficacy of fentanyl, neostigmine and their combination in caudal block.

The present study shows that the combination of fentanyl and neostigmine, could prolong duration of analgesia, and decrease severity of pain when added to bupivacaine. However, our results indicate that this combination may increase the rate of nausea and vomiting.

Regarding average pain score, the combination of fentanyl and neostigmine resulted in more favorable pain relief when added to bupivacaine.

Some previous studies showed that adding fentanyl to bupivacaine resulted in lower pain score when compared to bupivacaine alone (15-17, 19).

Our present study shows that adding neostigmine to bupivacaine yields better analgesia than bupivacaine alone, which is consistent with prior studies (1, 14, 18), however adding fentanyl to bupivacaine is associated with more frequent nausea and vomiting.

Neostigmine caudal analgesic effect was observed in previous studies through a direct effect on the spinal cord after diffusion from dura to CSF or through peripheral anti-nociceptive effect on surgery site after systemic absorption. Moreover, intra-thecal neostigmine can cause analgesia by preventing the break- down of acetylcholine in the spinal dorsal horn (11, 14).

In our study patients receiving a combination of bupivacaine, fentanyl and neostigmine experienced more nausea and vomiting, in comparison with other groups. Group receiving bupivacaine and fentanyl was associated with more frequent nausea and vomiting than those receiving bupivacaine and neostigmine. Patients receiving bupivacaine alone experienced the least frequent nausea and vomiting among other groups. However, vomiting was controlled with a single dose of ondansetron in each group.

In some studies, increase rates of nausea and vomiting was observed in intra-thecal neostigmine. yet the rate has been higher than our present study, which may be due to higher dose of neostigmine (≥2μ/kg) (14); on the other hand, in other studies vomiting did not increase in patients receiving bupivacaine and neostigmine, compared to those receiving bupivacaine alone (11).

Some limitations of our study are small sample size and short postoperative assessment.

Conclusion

The present study shows that the combination of fentanyl and neostigmine, could prolong duration of analgesia, and decrease severity of pain when added to bupivacaine in caudal anesthesia.

Acknowledgment

None.

Conflicts of Interest

The authors declare that they have no conflict of interest.

References

1. Davoudi M, Kamali AR. A comparison of caudal anesthesia with midazolam and neostigmine co-administered with bupivacaine in reduction of post-operative pain following lower abdominal surgery in pediatrics (2- 8 years old). Arak Medical University Journal. 2011;14(54):27-34.

3. Mirskandari SM, Alavimoghadam SA. Comparision of Caudal Bupivacaine Alone with Bupivacaine-Fentanyl and Bupivacaine-Neostigmine for Caudal Block in Children. Hamedan Medical University Journal. 2006;2(13):55- 9.

3.Gupta P, Grace A. Neostigmine as an adjunct to Bupivacaine, for caudal block in burned children, undergoing skin grafting of the lower extremities. Anesthesia Pediatrica e Neonatale. 2011;9(1):1-16.

4. Naguib M, Gammal M. El, Elhattab Y. S, Seraj M. Midazolam for caudal analgesia in children: comparison with caudal bupivacaine. Can J Anaesth. 1995;42(9):758-64.

5. Xiang Q, Huang D. Y, Zhao Y. L, Wang G. H, Liu Y. X, Zhong L, LuoT. Caudal dexmedetomidine combined with bupivacaine inhibit the response to hernial sac traction in children undergoing inguinal hernia repair. Br J Anaesth. 2013;110(3):420-4.

6. Schnabel A, Poepping D. M, Kranke P, Zahn P. K, Pogatzki-Zahn E. M. Efficacy and adverse effects of ketamine as an additive for paediatric caudal anaesthesia: a quantitative systematic review of randomized controlled trials. British Journal of Anaesthesia. 2011;107(4):601–11.

7. Fernandes ML, Pires KCC, Tibu´rcio MA, Gomez RS. Caudal bupivacaine supplemented with morphine or clonidine, or supplemented with morphine plus clonidine in childrenundergoing infra-umbilical urological and genital procedures: a prospective, randomized and double-blind study.Japanese Society of Anesthesiologists. 2012;26:213–8.

8. Davies K, Wilson G, Engelhardt T. Caudal Additives Do Not Improve the Analgesia Afforded by Levobupivacaine After Hypospadias Repair. Anesthesiology and Pain Medicine. 2012;1(3): 174-7.

9. LocatelliB. G,Frawley G, Spotti A, Ingelmo P, Kaplanian S, Rossi B, Monia L, SonzogniV. Analgesic effectiveness of caudal levobupivacaine and ketaminc. British Journal of Anaesthesia. 2008;100(5):701–6.

10. Hansen TG, Henneberg SW, Walther-Larsen S, Lund J, Hansen M. Caudal bupivacaine supplemented with caudal or intravenous clonidine in children undergoing hypospadias repair: a doubleblind study. British Journal of Anaesthesia. 2004; 92(2):223-7.

11. Ataro G, Bernard M. Effectiveness of Caudal Epidural Block using Bupivacaine with Neostgmine for Pediatric Lower Extremity Orthopedic Surgery in Cure Ethiopia Children's Hospital. Anesthesia & Clinical Research. 2014;5:12.

12. Khatavkar SS, Lonkar SS, Panchal PB, Thatte WS. The efficacy of ropivacaine-fentanyl versus ropivacaine-clonidine for pre-empetive caudal anesthesia in children. Anaesth Pain & Intensive Care. 2016;20(1):54-8

13. Anand VG, Kannan M, Thavamani A, Bridgit MJ. Effect of dexmedtomidine added to caudal ropivacaine in pediatric lower abdominal surgeries. Indian J Anesthesia. 2011; 55 (4) : 340-346.

14. Kaushal D, Singh V, Abbas H, Mallik A, Singh G. Caudal bupivacaine-neostigmine for perioperative analgesia in pediatric patients undergoing infraumbilical surgeries: A prospective, randomized, double blind, controlled study. The Internet Journal of Anesthesiology. 2008;21:1.

15. Solanki N M, Engineer S R, Jansari D B, Patel R J. Comparison of caudal tramadol versus caudal fentanyl with bupivacaine for prolongation of postoperative analgesia in pediatric patients. Saudi J Anaesth. 2016;10(2):154-60

16. Ahuja Sharmila, Yadav Sangeeta, Joshi Nandita, Chaudhary Sujata, Madhu S. V. Efficacy of caudal fentanyl and ketamine on post-operative pain and neuroendocrine stress response in children undergoing infraumbilical and perineal surgery .J Anaesthesiol Clin Pharmacol. 2015;31(1).

17. Achary R, Jena SK, Samal S, Mishra SN. Postoperative analgesia in pediatrics patients through caudal block with bupivacaine and two different doses of fentanyl- A comparative study. J Evol Med Dent Sci. 2013;2:7568-74.

18. Prajapati M, Shah T D, Chadha I, Shah B.J. Caudal neostigmine with bupivacaine for postoperative analgesia in pediatric patient: comparison with bupivacaine alone. Indian Journal of Basic and Applied Medical Research. 2016;5(3):239-47.

19. Goel L, Goel S. A comparison of the efficacy and safety of different doses of fentanyl as adjuvant to bupivacaine for caudal analgesia in children undergoing lower abdominal surgery. Indian Journal of Basic and Applied Medical Research. 2016;5(2):85-90.

12

Comparing the Use of Memantine with Dextromethorphan and Placebo to Reduce Pain before Orthopedic Surgery

Mehrdad Taheri[1]✉, Alireza Mirkheshti[1], Alireza Manafi Rasi[2], Yalda Adili[1]

Abstract

Background: To compare the use of Memantine with Dextromethorphan and placebo to reduce pain after orthopedic surgery.
Materials and Methods: The present study was a double-blind clinical trial including180 patients undergoing elective orthopedic surgery of the lower limbs. Patients were divided randomly into three groups of 60 patients each. The first group (Group M) received 30 mg Memantine orally, the second group (Group D) received 45 mg of Dextromethorphan and the third group (Group P) received only placebo, two and a half hours before the operation. The intensity of pain (VAS score), sedation score, and nausea and vomiting were recorded postoperatively.
Results: In this study, 60 patients were enrolled in each group. The total VAS (Visual Analogue Scale) score was significantly lower among patients receiving Memantine and the satisfaction was significantly higher compared to the Dextromethorphan and placebo groups (P-value <0.001).
Conclusion: The present study results indicate that Memantine has a relatively better outcome compared to Dextromethorphan or placebo in reducing the post-surgical pain among patients undergoing orthopedic surgeries. It also reduced the need for post-surgical opioid use and improved the patients' satisfaction.
Keywords: Memantine, dextromethorphan, pain, surgery

1. Anesthesiology Research Center, Shahid Beheshti University of Medical Sciences, Tehran, Iran
2. Department of Orthopedics, Shahid Beheshti University of Medical Sciences, Tehran, Iran

✉ **Corresponding Author:** Mehrdad Taheri, Anesthesiology Research Center, Shahid Beheshti University of Medical Sciences, Tehran, Iran.
Email: taheri.1352@yahoo.com

Introduction

Pain is defined by the International Association for the Study of Pain as an unpleasant sensory and emotional experience associated with actual or potential tissue damage or described in terms of such damage (1). Acute post surgical pain is one of the most important complications of any surgical procedure and may increase perioperative mortality rate. Post operative pain has negative effects on various body systems such as respiratory, cardiovascular, gastrointestinal and urinary systems and causes metabolic, neurological, and hormonal changes (2). Methods of reducing acute pain after surgery, including preoperative administration of analgesics as well as central and peripheral nerve blocks, each have their usage in reducing the post operative pain. One of pain management procedures to control acute postoperative pain is the use of medical interventions (3, 4).

N-methyl-D-aspartate (NMDA) is a receptor for glutamate neurotransmitter, which is released following a painful stimulus. NMDA is in fact one of several important receptors for rapid transmission in central nervous system and plays an important role in the central sensitization phenomenon (5). Activation of NMDA receptors causes hyperalgesia, neuropathic pain and reduction of opioid receptors' activity. Hyperalgesia and neuropathic pain are due to increase in spinal nerves sensitivity causing higher levels of pain. Reduction in activity of opioid receptors is associated with a decline in their sensitivity. The decrease in sensitivity is known as opioid tolerance and means there is a need for a higher dose to achieve the effects of treatment. So NMDA antagonists can have a role in pain control (6,7), and combined use of opioids and NMDA antagonists will increase the efficacy of opioids and decrease the drug resistance (8). There are different sites for NMDA antagonists to bind and the differences in their potency have been attributed to the difference in binding site and the affinity of the receptors (6, 7). Several studies have shown that NMDA receptor antagonists might have a role in somatic as well as acute and chronic visceral pain control (9, 10).

NMDA receptor antagonists include Ketamine, Methadone, Memantine, Amantadine and Dextromethorphan. Ketamine is a strong receptor antagonist for this receptor. The severity and frequency of adverse symptoms depends on the affinity of drug to NMDA receptor and these symptoms manifest mainly in the central nervous system in the form of hallucinations, lightheadedness, fatigue, confusion, nightmares, headaches and sensory changes in adults, which is more severe when using Ketamine (11, 12).

Memantine is another oral NMDA receptor antagonist which has a non-competitive moderate affinity for this receptor with a rapid onset and fewer side effects. Previous studies have shown that this drug, when administered prior to nerve damage, has the ability to reduce the neuropathic pain (13, 14). Memantine was synthesized for the first time in 1960 and after clinical trials in Germany was used in treatment of dementia, brain diseases and Parkinson disease in the late 1980s. Also after receiving approval from Food and Drug Administration in 2003 this drug is widely used in treatment of Alzheimer's disease, but its use in treatment of chronic pain is relatively new. This drug is different from the first-generation NMDA receptor antagonists like Ketamine since it is better tolerated and causes less hallucinogenic side effects. Several differences may explain why these drugs are significantly different when comparing their clinical side effects. The elimination half-life of Memantine is 60-80 hours compared to a half-life of 2.5 hours for oral or intravenous Ketamine. Faster pharmacokinetics of Ketamine may lead to a sharp increase in drug serum levels and possibly psychotomimetic effects (13-17).

Previous studies had indicated that Memantine might be effective in analgesia, so it was first used in patients with post-surgical neuropathic pain. There is a potential benefit for early treatment, since NMDA channels show a post-surgical increase in activity and might cause neuropathic pain (18,19).

Dextromethorphan and its metabolites are non-competitive NMDA receptor antagonists with low afinity (20). Dextromethorphan is a synthetic derivative of narcotics, but with no narcotic effect (21). Dextromethorphan has a long history of safe use, and it seems that if used in the period immediately before surgery, it reduces the need for analgesic drugs in the post surgical period (22, 23).

In recent years the use of preemptive analgesia has increased worldwide and with substantial progress in understanding pain mechanisms, new therapeutic concepts have emerged. Studies have shown that sensitization of neurons in the dorsal horn of spinal cord after tissue damage, leads to hyperalgesia or allodynia and this process plays a key role in development of chronic pain after a painful stimulation. Thereby reducing the over-stimulation of neurons in the dorsal horn of the spinal cord, with starting the analgesic treatment before tissue damage such as surgical incision, is necessary to reduce the up regulation of central nervous system which is the concept of preemptive analgesia (24).

Numerous studies about the benefits of preemptive analgesia, especially in the last 10 years, have been conducted and all of them have confirmed its benefit. These studies suggest that preemptive analgesia has three objectives: a) reduce the pain caused by the activation of inflammation mechanisms following surgical incision, b) prevent the call memory of the central nervous system to pain, and c) ensure adequate control of postoperative pain to avoid the spread of chronic pain (24).

Preemptive analgesia is an intervention performed before the surgical incision to reduce the establishment of central sensitization and consequently reduces the inflammatory and incisional damage during and after the surgery. The preemptive analgesia can hypothetically prevent the hyperalgesia as well as acute and chronic postoperative pain by reducing the sensitization of central nervous system (24).

The main objective of the present study was to compare the effect of Memantine with Dextromethorphan and placebo in reducing pain after elective orthopedic surgery.

Methods

In this prospective study, 180 patients undergoing elective orthopedic surgery of the lower limbs (calf fracture) aged 18-65 years and physical health status of ASA 1 or 2 were selected and randomly divided into three groups of 60 people each. All patients were visited before and after surgery by an anesthesiologist and entered the study after giving written informed consent. This study was approved by the ethics committee of Shahid Beheshti University of Medical Sciences, Tehran, Iran (sbmu.rec.1393.552). The study was also registered in Iranian Registry of Clinical Trials (IRCT2017062413364N4).

Group (M) received 30 mg oral Memantine group (D) received 45 mg Dextromethorphan and the group (P) was given placebo, about two and a half hours before the start of operation. Only the physician responsible for treatment knew the drug each patient received. The patient and another physician tasked with documenting the post-surgical pain score, the need for analgesics and the patients' satisfaction, were blinded to the drug received by the patient.

The exclusion criteria were ASA physical health status of 3 or 4, diseases of the respiratory system, heart, brain and endocrine glands, any drug consumption in one week prior to surgery, sensitivity to drugs used in the study, a history of mental illness, MAOIs or SSRIs during 4 weeks before the surgery, pregnancy, a history of stroke and finally type 1 and 2 diabetes mellitus. Also all patients developing compartment syndrome were excluded from the study.

All patients went under spinal anesthesia using a number 25 spinal needle and Bupivacaine 0.5 percent. Patients were transferred to recovery after the conclusion of surgery and their VAS score was documented after the return of lower limbs sensation. At this time intravenous PCA pump containing morphine at a concentration of 2.0 mg per ml and transfer rate of 4 ml per hour and a bolus dose of 5.0 ml every 15 minutes was used to control patients' pain. If the patient had a VAS (Visual Analogue Scale) score of over 4 in the recovery or anytime till 48 hours after the surgery, they would receive a 4mg dose of Morphine and the total dose of Morphine was documented. Also at the end of 48 hours the total amount of drugs consumed through intravenous PCA pump was recorded for each patient. The intensity of pain (VAS), sedation score, and nausea and vomiting were recorded 6, 12, 24, 36 and 48 hours after the surgery.

The pain score was assessed on the basis of VAS score, by displaying a scaled ruler to the patient, so that zero equaled no pain and 10 equaled the maximum imaginable pain for patients.

Sedation scores were classified as follow: 0 for restless, 1 for quiet, 2 for sleepy, 3 for confused but with respond to verbal commands, 4 for no response to verbal commands, and 5 for no response to painful stimulus.

Measurement of nausea and vomiting were as follow: 0 for no nausea and vomiting, 1 for mild nausea without the need for medication, 2 for nausea needing medication, 3 for nausea and lack of response to anti-nausea drugs.

At the end of 48 hours post operation patient satisfaction during this period was evaluated based on the following criteria: 0 for absolutely no pain, 1 for sometimes moderate pain, 2 for always moderate pain, 3 for sometimes severe pain, 4 for always moderate pain and sometimes severe pain, and ۵ for always severe pain.

Results

In the present study, 60 patients were enrolled in each group. There was not a significant difference between three groups regarding age and sex (Table 1). Also the type of surgery had no meaningful difference

Table 1: Demographic findings among the three groups of patients entering the study.

Variable	D n=60	M n=60	P n=60	P-value
Age	45.13±11.75	45.68±11.65	42.38±11.64	0.259
Gender				0.914
Female	28 (46.7%)	26 (43.3%)	28 (46.7%)	
Male	32 (53.3%)	34 (56.7%)	32 (53.3%)	
Type of surgery				0.573
Interlock surgery	27 (45.0%)	32 (53.3%)	27 (45.0%)	
Plate surgery	33 (55.0%)	28 (46.7%)	33 (55.0%)	

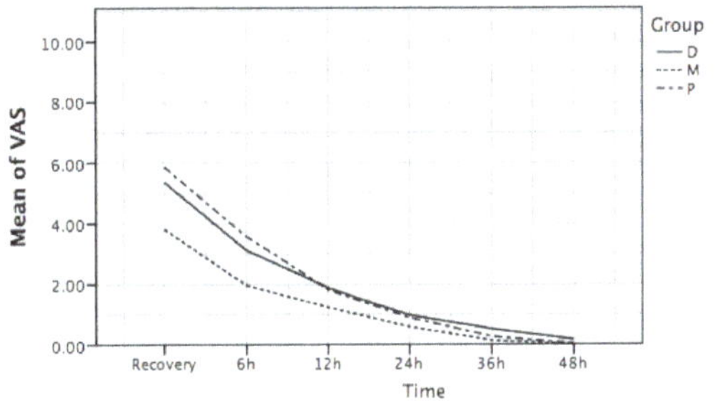

Figure 1. VAS changes in the first 48 hours after the surgery in three groups of patients entering the study.

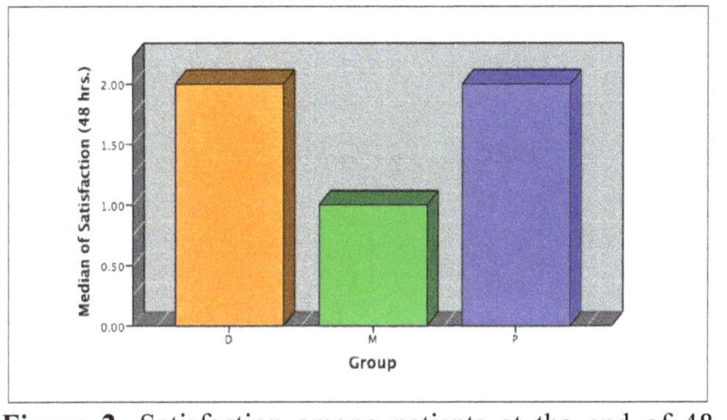

Figure 2. Satisfaction among patients at the end of 48 hours post-surgery.

among the three groups.

The mean VAS score was significantly different among the three groups of patients and was significantly lower in group M compared to group D and group P (P-value <0.001). But this difference was not significant between groups D and P.

The following chart shows changes in VAS score within 48 hours after the surgery. As it can be observed the pain was lower in Memantine group compared to the other two groups.

Table 2 shows the percentage of quiet and restless patients in the three groups. As it can be observed at 6, 12 and 24 hours after the surgery the percent of restless patients was significantly lower in group M compared to group D, but this difference was not statistically significant 36 and 48 hours after the surgery.

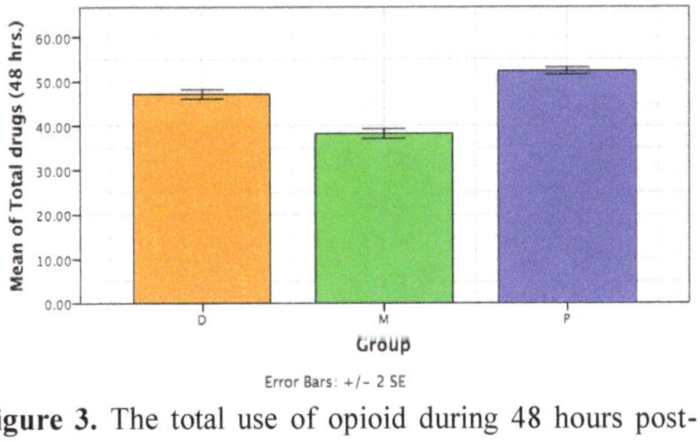

Figure 3. The total use of opioid during 48 hours post-surgery in three groups of patients entering the study.

In 6 and 12 hours post-surgery the number of patients with nausea was lower in group M compared to group D and P, but this difference was not significant in other post-surgical intervals. When comparing the overall satisfaction among patients at the end of 48 hours post-surgery the overall satisfaction was significantly higher in group M compared to groups D and P. There was no significant difference in overall satisfaction between D and P groups (Table 3, Figure 2).

Also the total use of opioid during 48 hours post-surgery was lower in group M compared to group D and P (Table 4, Figure 3).

Discussion

The present study showed that the rate of post-operative pain in group M was lower than group D. Interestingly in group M the pain within 48 hours was significantly lower than Group D, but the difference was more significant during the first 24 hours. This might be due to the half-life of the drugs which makes them less effective after 24 hours.

It should be noted that Memantine as a NMDA

Table 2: The percentage of quiet and restless patients in the three groups entering the study.

Sedation		D n=60	M n=60	P n=60	P-value
6h					<0.001
	Restless	58 (96.7%)	37 (61.7%)	59 (98.3%)	
	Quiet	2 (3.3%)	23 (38.3%)	1 (1.7%)	
12h					0.001
	Restless	33 (55.0%)	14 (23.3%)	17 (28.3%)	
	Quiet	27 (45.0%)	46 (76.7%)	43 (71.7%)	
24h					<0.001
	Restless	13 (21.7%)	2 (3.3%)	2 (3.3%)	
	Quiet	47 (78.3%)	58 (96.7%)	58 (96.7%)	
36h					0.129
	Restless	4 (6.7%)	1 (1.7%)	0 (0.0%)	
	Quiet	56 (93.3%)	59 (98.3%)	60 (100.0%)	
48h					>0.999
	Restless	0 (0.0%)	1 (1.7%)	1 (1.7%)	
	Quiet	6 (100.00%)	59 (98.3%)	59 (98.3%)	
Total					<0.001

antagonist has been used in treatment of many neuropathic pains, but its use in the treatment of acute postoperative pain is not widespread. Oral Memantine has a bioavailability of about 40% and it takes 24 hours to reach a constant plasma level. After a single oral dose the drug reaches Cmax within 6 hours and it has a half-life of 60 to 100 hours. If used as a skin patch it has greater bioavailability of approximately 60% and provides adequate plasma levels for several days (25).

NMDA receptors increase the plasticity of synapses. Only synapses with active NMDA can create plasticity and neuronal pain memory in response to entrance of Ca after unblocking of Mg ++ (26).

Memantine has been indicated to reduce the post-surgical pain in several studies (27). In our study Memantine showed a good potency to reduce the pain during the 48 hours after the surgery, which was significantly better than Dextromethorphan. In fact, Dextromethorphan did not significantly reduce the postoperative pain. Dextromethorphan is a non-competitive antagonist of NMDA receptor with low affinity to these receptors while Memantine has a higher affinity for NMDA receptors, so the difference in analgesic effect of these two drugs is likely to be due to their different affinity for NMDA receptors.

Numerous studies have indicated that Memantine administered after surgery can reduce the chance of chronic post-surgical pain and also prevent phantom

Table 3: Satisfaction among patients at the end of 48 hours post-surgery.

Satisfaction	D n=60	M n=60	P n=60	P-value	P_1*	P_2	P_3
Median (IQR)	2 (1-2)	1 (0-1)	2 (2-2)	<0.001	<0.001	0.699	<0.001
0: Absolutely no pain	0 (0.0%)	17 (28.3%)	0 (0.0%)				
Sometimes moderate pain	17 (28.3%)	37 (61.7%)	12 (20.0%)				
2- Always moderate pain	34 (56.7%)	5 (8.3%)	42 (70.0%)				
3- Sometimes severe pain	9 (15.0%)	1 (1.7%)	6 (10.0%)				
4: Always moderate pain and sometimes severe pain	0 (0.0%)	0 (0.0%)	0 (0.0%)				
5: Always severe pain	0 (0.0%)	0 (0.0%)	0 (0.0%)				

* P_1= P-value for difference between Group D and M
P_2= P-value for difference between Group D and P
P_3= P-value for difference between Group M and P

Table 4: The total use of opioid during 48 hours post-surgery in three groups of patients entering the study.

Opioid	D n=60	M n=60	P n=60	P-value	P_1*	P_2	P_3
The total use of opioid in 48 hours post-surgery	47.17±4.05	38.18±4.30	52.28±2.94	<0.001	<0.001	<0.001	<0.001

* P_1= P-value for difference between Group D and M
P_2= P-value for difference between Group D and P
P_3= P-value for difference between Group M and P

pain after amputation (28-31).

A previous study has indicated that the use of Dextromethorphan syrup 2 to 3 hours before the knee arthroscopic surgery reduces the pain and the need for opioids in first 8 post-surgical hours (8), which is similar to our findings, but the present study indicated that Memantine had a better outcome in reducing the post-surgical pain compared to Dextromethorphan.

In this study, postoperative nausea and vomiting was significantly lower in Memantine group compared to Dextromethorphan group in the first 12 hours after surgery.We also found that after using Memantine the first patient's request for opioid is delayed and also the total post-surgical opioid usage is lower compared to Dextromethorphan or placebo, which can explain the lower incidence of opioid side effects like nausea and vomiting.

It should be noted that in the present study Memantine resulted in significantly higher patient satisfaction, lower post-surgical pain scores and less need for post-surgical opioid use compared to placebo, but there was no difference between placebo and Dextromethorphan. Also the overall satisfaction was higher when comparing Memantine and Dextromethorphan.

Conclusion

The present study results indicate that Memantine has a relatively better outcome compared to Dextromethorphan or placebo in reducing the pain among patients undergoing orthopedic surgeries. It also reduced the need for post-surgical opioid use and improved the patients' satisfaction.

Acknowledgment

We would like to thank the clinical research and development research center, Imam Hossein Medical Center, Tehran, Iran for helping us with financing the present study. This manuscript is the result of the thesis by Dr. Yalda Adili.

Conflicts of Interest

The authors declare that they have no conflict of interest.

References

1. Steven D. Waldman. Pain Management. 2th ed. Philadelphia, Elsevier Saunders; 2011; pp: 50.
2. Wu CT, Yu JC, Liu ST. Preincisional dextromethorphan treatment for postoperative pain management after upper abdominal surgery. World J Surg. 2000;24(5): 512-7.
3. Ong CK, Lirk P, Seymour RA, Jenkins BJ. The efficacy of preemptive analgesia for acute postoperative pain management: a meta-analysis. Anesth Analg. 2005;100(3):757-73.
4. Møiniche S, Kehlet H, Dahl JB. A qualitative and quantitative systematic review of preemptive analgesia for postoperative pain relief.Anesthesiology. 2002;96(3):725-41.
5. Kew JN, Kemp JA. Ionotropic and metabotropic glutamate receptor structure and pharmacology.Psychopharmacology (Berl).2005;179(1):4-29.
6. Flor H, Birbaumer N. Phantom limb pain: cortical plasticity and novel therapeutic approaches. Curr Opin Anaesthesiol.2000;13(5):561-4.
7. Arnstein PM. The neuroplastic phenomenon: a physiologic link between chronic pain and learning. J Neurosci Nurs.1997;29(3):179-86.
8. EntezarySR, FarshadpourS, Alebouyeh MR, Imani F, Emami Meybodi MK, Yaribeygi H. Effects of Preoperative Use of Oral Dextromethorphan on Postoperative Need for Analgesics in Patients With Knee Arthroscopy. Anesth Pain Med. 2013;3(3):e11187.
9. Weinbroum AA, Rudick V, Paret G, Ben-Abraham R. The role of dextromethorphan in pain control. Can J Anaesth.2000;47(6):585-96.
10. Weinbroum AA, Gorodezky A, Niv D, Ben-Abraham R, Rudick V, Szold A. Dextromethorphan attenuation of postoperative pain and primary and secondary thermal hyperalgesia. Can J Anaesth. 2001;48(2):167-74.
11. Lipton SA. Failures and successes of NMDA receptor antagonists: molecular basis for the useof open-channel blockers like memantine in the treatment of acute and chronic neurologic insults. NeuroRx. 2004;1(1):101-10.
12. Muir KW. Glutamate-based therapeutic approaches: clinical trials with NMDA antagonists. Curr Opin Pharmacol. 2006;6(1):53-60.
13. Witt A, Macdonald N, Kirkpatrick P. Memantine hydrochloride. Nat Rev Drug Discov. 2004;3(2):109-10.
14. Schwartzman RJ, Grothusen J, Kiefer RT, Rohr P. Neuropathic central pain: epidemiology, etiology, and treatment options. Arch Neurol. 2001;58(10):1547-50.
15. Johnson JW, Kotermanski SE. Mechanism of action of memantine. Curr Opin Pharmacol. 2006;6(1):61-7.
16. Maier C, Dertwinkel R, Mansourian N, Hosbach I, Schwenkreis P, Senne I, et al. Efficacy of the NMDA-receptor antagonist memantine in patients with chronic phantom limb pain–results of a randomized double-blinded, placebo-controlled trial. Pain. 2003;103(3):277-83.
17. Schwenkreis P, Maier C, Pleger B, Mansourian N, Dertwinkel R, Malin JP, et al. NMDA-mediated mechanisms in cortical excitability changes after limb amputation. Acta Neurol Scand. 2003;108(3):179-84.
18. Chaplan SR, Malmberg AB, Yaksh TL. Efficacy of spinal NMDA receptor antagonism in formalin hyperalgesia and nerve injury evoked allodynia in the rat. J Pharmacol Exp Ther. 1997;280(2):829-38.
19. Sinis N, Birbaumer N, Gustin S, Schwarz A, Bredanger S, Becker ST, et al. Memantine treatment of complex regional pain syndrome: a preliminary report of six cases. Clin J Pain. 2007;23(3):237-43.
20. Javid MJ, Hajijafari M, Hajipour A, Makarem J, Khzaeipour Z. Evaluation of A Low Dose Ketamine in Post Tonsillectomy Pain Relief: A Randomized Trial Comparing Intravenous and Subcutaneous Ketamine in Pediatrics. Anesth Pain. 2012;2(3):107-10.
21. Georg BE, Youssef D, Jocelyne C, Michela R, Adriana W, Alain F, et al. Influence of CYP2D6 Activity on Pre-emptive Analgesia by the N-Methyl-D-Aspartate Antagonist Dextromethorphan in a Randomized Controlled Trial of Acute Pain. Pain Physician. 2013;16:45-56.
22. Woolf CJ, Chong MS. Preemptive analgesia: treating postoperative pain by preventing the establishment of central sensitization. Anesth Analg. 1993;77(2):362-79.
23. Bern J, Peck R. Dextromethorphan: an overview of safety issues. Drug Saf. 1992;7(3):190-9.
24. Pan YS, Hu YF, Tian FB, Xu K. Effects of epidural preemptive analgesia on stress reaction in retroperitoneal laparoscopic adrenalectomy surgery: a randomized controlled study. Int J Clin Exp Med. 2015;8(6):9862-8.
25. Lee SH, Kim SH, Noh YH, Choi BM, Noh GJ, Park WD, et al. Pharmacokinetics of Memantine after a Single and Multiple Dose of Oral and Patch Administration in Rats. Basic Clin Pharmacol Toxicol. 2016;118(2):122-7.
26. Koch HJ, Szecsey A, Haen E. NMDA-antagonism (memantine): an alternative pharmacological therapeutic principle in Alzheimer's and vascular dementia. Curr Pharm Des. 2004;10(3):253-9.
27. Emik U, Unal Y, Arslan M, Demirel CB. The effects of memantine on recovery, cognitive functions, and pain after propofol anesthesia. Braz J Anesthesiol. 2016;66(5):485-91.
28. Nikolajasen L, Gottrup H, Kristensen AGD, Jensen TS. Memantine (a Nmethyl-D-aspartate receptor antagonist) in the treatment of neuropathic pain after amputation or surgery: a randomized double-blinded, cross-over study. Anesth Analg. 2000;91(4):960-6.
29. Maier C, Dertwinkel R, Mansourian N, Hosbach I, Schwenkreis

P, Senne I, et al. Efficacy of the NMDA-receptor antagonist memantine in patients with chronic phantom limb pain-results of a randomized double-blinded placebo-controlled trial. Pain 2003;103(3):277-83.

30. Schley M, Topfer S, Wiech K, Schaller HE, Konrad CJ, Schmelz M, et al. Continuous brachial plexus blockade in combination with NMDA receptor antagonist memantine prevents phantom pain in acute traumatic upper limb amputees. Eur J Pain 2007;11(3):299-308.

31. Hackworth RJ, Tokarz KA, Fowler IM, Wallace SC, Stedje-Larsen ET. Profound pain reduction after induction of memantine treatment in two patients with severe phantom limb pain. Anesth Analg 2008;107(4):1377-9.

13

The Effect of Aqueous Extract of *Malva neglecta* on Expression of Inflammatory Biomarkers Involved in Pain in Synoviocytes and THP-1 Cells as a Model of Monocyte/Macrophage and Human Cartilage Cells in Osteoarthritis

Reza Taherian[1], Mahdi Taherian[2], Hossein Maghsoudi[3]✉, Samaneh Haj-alahyari[3]

Abstract

Background: Osteoarthritis is now considered as an active complex of biomechanical, biochemical and cellular processes, not a mere degenerative disorder. Considering the complications of common treatments of osteoarthritis, including non-steroidal anti-inflammatory drug (NSAIDs) and corticosteroids, establishment of new treatments is crucial. This study aimed to explore the effect of *Malva neglecta* extract on the main inflammatory biomarkers in osteoarthritis.

Materials and Methods: Aqueous extract of *Malva neglecta*, ibuprofen and betamethasone were prepared to investigate their effects on inflammatory biomarkers. Synoviocytes were obtained from the healthy radiocarpal joint cartilage of an 8-month-old Holstein cow. Human monocyte/macrophage (THP-1) cells were also obtained to investigate the effect of *Malva neglecta* extract on inflammatory agents. Lipopolysaccharide (LPS) was used to induce production of inflammatory cytokines in both cells. Real-time PCR was used to investigate the effect of *Malva neglecta* extract on expression profile of TNF-α, IL-1β, COX-2, IL-18 and iNOS. Production of NO and PGE2 was also investigated in THP-1 cells.

Results: *Malva neglecta* extract reduced TNF-α, IL-1β, iNOS, IL-18 and COX-2 expression in synoviocytes. Expression of all of these factors was also reduced by the extract in THP-1 cells. Moreover, production of PGE2 and NO in the LPS-induced THP-1 cells was reduced by Malva neglecta extract. Ibuprofen and betamethasone were more effective in reducing inflammatory agents than the extract.

Conclusion: According to Malva's ability to reduce the pro-inflammatory cytokines in the synoviocytes and THP-1 cells, its potential role as a supplement method to common NSAIDs and corticosteroids was confirmed.

Keywords: Osteoarthritis, *Malva neglecta*, synoviocyte, monocyte/macrophage, cytokine

1. Student Research Committee, School of Medicine, Shahid Beheshti University of Medical Sciences, Tehran, Iran
2. Food and Drug Research Institute, Iran Food and Drug Administration, Ministry of Health and Medical Education, Tehran, Iran
3. Biotechnology Research Center, Payamenoor University, Tehran, Iran

Corresponding Author: Hossein Maghsoudi, PhD. Biotechnology Research Center, Payamenoor University, Tehran, Iran. P.O. Box: 35147-465441, Tehran, Iran.

✉:hossein.maghsoudiadm@gmail.com

Introduction

Osteoarthritis (OA) is one of the most common joint diseases worldwide and has a strong association with aging. Based on the report of Davatchi et.al, the prevalence of OA is about 16% in adults aged between 15-85 in urban areas of Iran (1). OA is beyond a mere degenerative disorder and is now considered as an active complex of biomechanical, biochemical and cellular processes (2). This complex includes activation of macrophages and synoviocytes and also synovial inflammation which is considered as the main cause of joint pain in OA (3, 4). These activated cells contribute to the release of inflammatory cytokines such as TNFα and IL-1β and also up-regulation of iNOS and COX-2 enzymes that produce NO and PGE2, respectively. Mentioned pro-inflammatory factors induce chondrocyte apoptosis and inhibit proteoglycans synthesis which leads to articular cartilage degeneration (5, 6). Although current treatments of OA, including NSAIDs and corticosteroids, can partially relieve the sign and symptoms of this disease, they are often associated with some side effects such as peptic ulcers and gastrointestinal bleeding. Because of the degree of inflammation associated with pain in patients with OA, there is an increasing trend on the plants with anti-inflammatory and analgesic properties. Compared to NSAIDs and corticosteroids, the side effects of such plants are low; hence, these plants can make a substantial contribution to the patients with osteoarthritis.

Malva neglecta (English name Common mallow) is an annual herbaceous species of genus Malva. This plant is widespread in all regions of Iran. Leaf and other parts of this plant are traditionally used in different conditions such as wound healing, stomach, menstrual aches and muscle pain and contains hydroxycinnamic acids, flavonoids, flavonols, proanthocyanidins and anthocyanins (7). Recent researches have focused on the different medical benefits of this plant. Previous studies have reported the antioxidant (7, 8), anti-ulcerogenic (9) and antibacterial activity (10) of *Malva neglecta* extract. Moreover, a recent study reported that *Malva neglecta* aqueous extract has beneficial effects on preventing and treating nephrolithiasis and decreasing tubulointerstitial damage in a dosage-dependent manner (11). Although the effect of this extract on inflammatory agents in chondrocytes was investigated before (11), its effect on synoviocytes, which their involvement in OA is recognized in recent years, is less studied. In this study, we investigated the effect of *Malva neglecta* aqueous extract on joint inflammation through analyzing expression and production of pro-inflammatory factors in synoviocytes and THP-1 cells.

Methods

Malva neglecta extract, corticosteroid and NSAID preparation

Malva neglecta was initially obtained from Iran's center of genetic resources, and then its aqueous extract was prepared according to the available protocols. Betamethasone, a corticosteroid, was applied as an aqueous solution of betamethasone 21-phosphate disodium with a concentration of 1.30 mg/mL, equivalent to betamethasone-base 1.00mg/mL. Ibuprofen, a NSAID, was dissolved in water to a concentration of 1.00 mg/mL at 100°C for five minutes.

Synoviocyte and THP-1 cell culture

Synovial fluid was punctured from the radiocarpal joint cartilage of an 8-month-old Holstein cow and washed out three times by 1 Molar PBS buffer (pH=7.2). Then, it was incubated in collagenase type II at 37°C for 16h. After incubation, it was filtered through 1mm Wire Strainer Screen, which was sterilized, and the wastes resulted from the effect of the collagenase type II were isolated from synoviocyte cells. The tube was centrifuged for 3 min, the supernatant was discarded and the pellet cells were washed four times with HBSS. The supernatant was removed with a pipette and finally deposited cells were incubated in the medium containing DMEM-F12 supplemented with FBS, 50 μg/ml ascorbic acid, 100 u/ml penicillin and 0.25 μg/ml streptomycin, with a density of 5×105 cell in the 22.2 cm plates at a temperature of 37°C, the humidity of 90% and 5% CO_2 to reach cell density of 80-85%. THP-1 cells were obtained from the Pasteur Institute of Iran and were amplified in a sterile medium to the extent necessary. The next steps were accomplished completely identical and separately in the two groups of synoviocyte cells and THP-1 cells.

Cell viability assay

MTT assay and trypan blue were used to investigate the cytotoxic effect of aqueous extract of *Malva neglecta* and also the LC50 of it. MTT, a yellow tetrazole, is reduced to purple formazan by succinate dehydrogenase (SDH) in the mitochondria of living cells. To dissolve the insoluble purple formazan product into a colored solution, Dimethyl sulfoxide (DMSO) was added. The absorbance of this colored solution was measured by a spectrophotometer at a wavelength between 500 and 600 nm.

LPS treatment

To induce inflammatory cytokines, the cells were treated with LPS. 6×10^6 cells were cultured in the medium. After 72h, 100ng LPS was added to each plate. Then, the plates were divided into two group. Group one was incubated for 24h at a temperature of 37°C, the humidity of 90% and 5% CO_2 to investigate the expression of pro-inflammatory cytokines. Group two was incubated for 1h at the same conditions to investigate PGE2 and NO production.

Expression analysis

RNA was isolated and RNA concentration was determined using spectrophotometry method. DNase enzyme was used to isolate RNA. Then, isolated RNA was employed to produce cDNA using RT-PCR method. PCR was used to amplify cDNA and finally, Real-Time PCR was used to determine the expression levels of IL-18, IL-1B, TNF-α, COX-2 and iNOS genes by specific primers.

PGE2 production analysis

ELISA system was used to determine the amount of prostaglandins in the required cells. The production of nitric oxide was determined using biochemical methods.

Grouping of cell cultures

Cultured synoviocyte and THP-1 cells were divided into 5 groups and treated according to table 1.

Statistical analysis

Data are presented as mean±SD. ANOVA analysis was done by REST software version.20 and SPSS software version 20. $P<0.05$ was considered statistically significant.

Ethical considerations

No study with human or animal subjects is performed by any of the authors of this article. The ethical committee of "Research and Technology Chancellor" in Shahid Beheshti University of Medical Sciences approved this study.

Results

Real Time-PCR results were analyed using the Pfaffi or ΔΔC method,

$2^{-\Delta\Delta}$ = Expression Ratio

Ct= ΔΔC Calibrater Δ-C main cytokine Δ

Ct= (ΔΔCt main cytokine – Ct GADPH) – (Ct sample positive – Ct GADPH)

Effect of Malva neglecta extract on COX-2 gene expression in synoviocytes

The results of the expression of inflammatory factors in synoviocytes are depicted in figure 1. COX-2 expression was increased in group 3 (LPS+Cell) up to 100%.

In group 4 (LPS+Extract+Cell), COX-2 expression increased about 51% which was significantly lower than group 3. 18% and 21% upregulation of the COX-2 expression was observed in group 6 (LPS+Corticosteroid+Cell) and 7 (LPS+NSAID+Cell), respectively. Upregulation of the expression of COX-2 in group 4 was significantly higher than groups 6 and 7. In group 5, the placebo was administrated and no change was observed in the expression of COX-2.

Effect of Malva neglecta extract on IL-1β gene expression in synoviocytes

IL-1β expression was increased in group 3 (LPS+Cell) up to 100%. In group 4 (LPS+Extract+Cell), IL-1β expression was increased about 47% which was significantly lower than group 3. Upregulation of the IL-1β expression was about 19% in group 6 and 23% in group 7. Upregulation of the expression of IL-1β in group 4 was significantly higher than groups 6 and 7. In group 5, the placebo was administrated and no change was observed in the expression of IL-1β.

Effect of Malva neglecta extract on TNF-α gene expression in synoviocytes

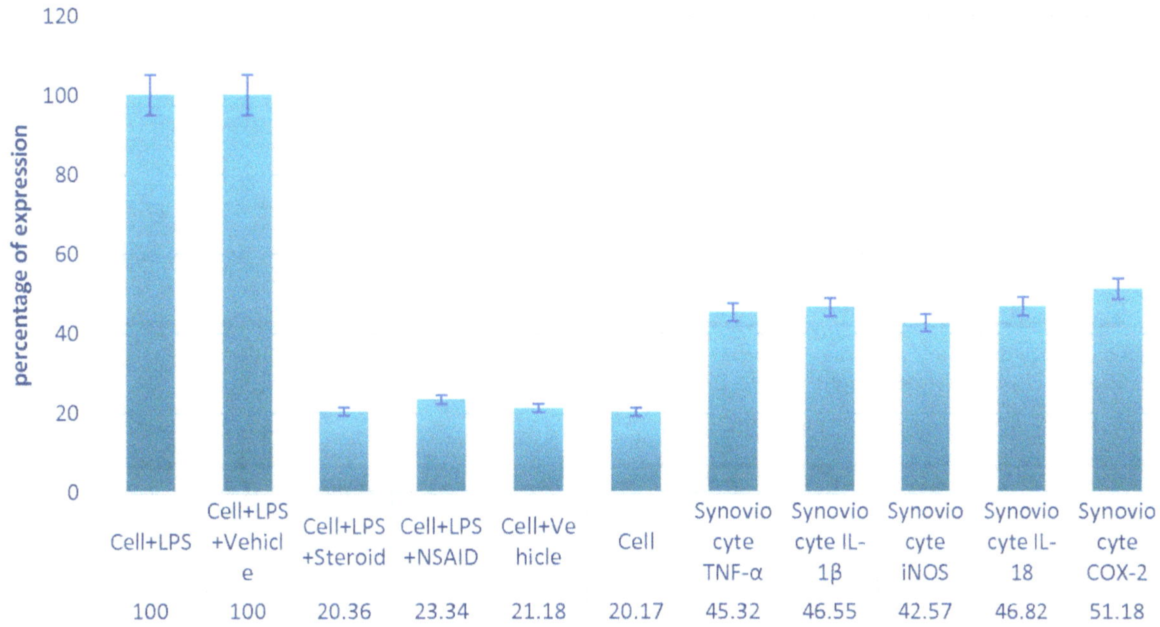

Figure 1. Relative gene expression analysis of proinflamatory cytokines in synoviocytes with Pfaffi method. The data represented as the mean±S.RE.M of three different experiments run in duplicate. The comparisons were done by one-way repeated ANOVA.

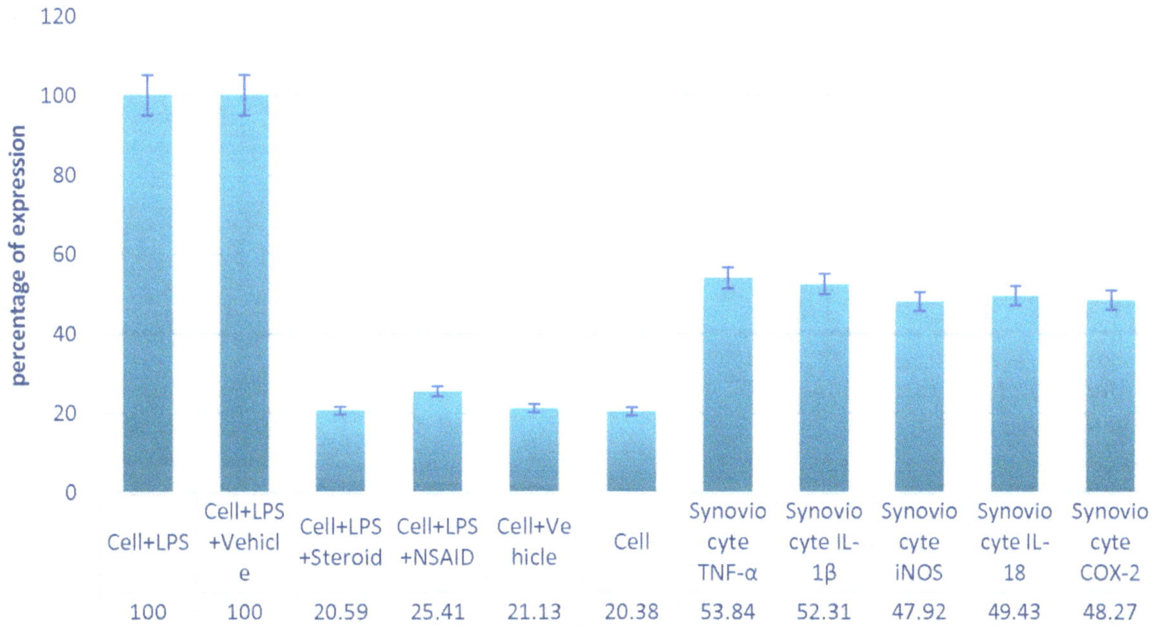

Figure 2. Relative gene expression analysis of proinflamatory cytokines in THP-1 cells with Pfaffi method. The data represented as the mean±S.RE.M of three different experiments run in duplicate. The comparisons were done by one-way repeated ANOVA.

TNF-α expression was increased in group 3 (LPS+Cell) up to 100%. In group 4 (LPS+Extract+Cell), TNF-α expression was increased about 45% which was significantly lower than group 3. Upregulation of the TNF-α expression was about 21% in group 6 and 24% in group 7. Upregulation of the expression of TNF-α in group 4 was significantly higher than groups 6 and 7. In group 5, the placebo was administrated and no change was observed in the expression of TNF-α.

Table 1: Studied groups.

Group	Synoviocyte/THP-1	Malva neglecta extract	Corticosteroid	NSAID	LPS	Placebo (PBS)
1	+	-	-	-	-	-
2	+	+	-	-	-	-
3	+	-	-	-	+	-
4	+	+	-	-	+	-
5	+	-	-	-	+	+
6	+	-	+	-	+	-
7	+	-	-	+	+	-

Studied groups according to receiving different treatments. NSAID: non-steroidal anti-inflammatory drug, LPS: Lipopolysaccharide, PBS: Phosphate-buffered saline.

Table 2: Production of prostaglandin E2 in THP-1 cells.

Group	Logit (%B/B0)	Picogram/ml PGE2
1	1.1	4
2	1.15	4.1
3	2.2	11.8
4	1.9	8.5
5	2.2	11.8
6	1.3	5.5
7	1.5	6.2

Production of prostaglandin E2 in THP-1 cells. PGE2: Prostaglandin E2.

Table 3: Production of nitric oxide in THP-1 cells.

Group	Optical density	Nanomol nitrite
1	0.5	800
2	0.7	1000
3	2.4	2500
4	1.4	1500
5	2.4	2500
6	0.8	1200
7	1.0	1100

Effect of *Malva neglecta* extract on iNOS gene expression in synoviocytes

iNOS expression was increased in group 3 (LPS+Cell) up to 100%. In group 4 (LPS+Extract+Cell), iNOS expression was increased about 43% which was significantly lower than group 3. Upregulation of the iNOS expression was about 19% in group 6 and 23% in group 7. Upregulation of the expression of iNOS in group 4 was significantly higher than groups 6 and 7. In group 5, the placebo was administrated and no change was observed in the expression of iNOS.

Effect of *Malva neglecta* extract on IL-18 gene expression in synoviocytes

IL-18 expression was increased in group 3 (LPS+Cell) up to 100%. In group 4 (LPS+Extract+Cell), IL-18 expression was increased about 47% which was significantly lower than group 3. Upregulation of the IL-18 expression was about 22% in group 6 and 25% in group 7. Upregulation of the expression of IL-18 in group 4 was significantly higher than groups 6 and 7. In group 5, the placebo was administrated and no change was observed in the expression of IL-18.

Effect of *Malva neglecta* extract on COX-2 gene expression in THP-1 cells

The results of the expression of inflammatory factors in THP-1 cells are depicted in figure 2. COX-2 expression was increased in group 3 (LPS+Cell) up to 100%. In group 4 (LPS+Extract+Cell), COX-2 expression increased about 48% which was significantly lower than group 3. 17% and 19% upregulation of the COX-2 expression was observed in group 6 and 7, respectively. Upregulation of the expression of COX-2 in group 4 was significantly higher than groups 6 and 7. In group 5, the placebo was administrated and no change was observed in the expression of COX-2.

Effect of *Malva neglecta* extract on IL-1β gene expression in THP-1 cells

IL-1β expression was increased in group 3 (LPS+Cell) up to 100%. In group 4 (LPS+Extract+Cell), IL-1β expression was increased about 52% which was significantly lower than group 3. Upregulation of the IL-1β expression was about 21% in group 6 and 26% in group 7. Upregulation of the expression of IL-1β in group 4 was significantly higher than groups 6 and 7. In group 5, the placebo was administrated and no change was observed in the expression of IL-1β.

Effect of *Malva neglecta* extract on TNF-α gene Expression in THP-1 cells

Although *Malva neglecta* extract did not change TNF-α expression in group 2, it increased TNF-α expression in group 3 (LPS+Cell) up to 100%. In group 4 (LPS+Extract+Cell), TNF-α expression was increased about 54% which was significantly lower than group 3. Upregulation of the TNF-α expression was about 22% in group 6 and 27% in group 7. Upregulation of the expression of TNF-α in group 4 was significantly higher than groups 6 and 7. In group 5, the placebo was administrated and no change was observed in the expression of TNF-α

Effect of *Malva neglecta* extract on iNOS gene expression in THP-1 cells

iNOS expression was increased in group 3 (LPS+Cell) up to 100%. In group 4 (LPS+Extract+Cell), iNOS expression was increased about 48% which was significantly lower than group 3. Upregulation of the iNOS expression was about 19% in group 6 and 26% in group 7. Upregulation of the expression of iNOS in group 4 was significantly higher than groups 6 and 7. In group 5, the placebo was administrated and no change was observed in the expression of iNOS.

Effect of *Malva neglecta* extract on IL-18 gene expression in THP-1 cells

IL-18 expression was increased in group 3 (LPS+Cell) up to 100%. In group 4 (LPS+Extract+Cell), IL-18 expression was increased about 49% which was significantly lower than group 3. Upregulation of the IL-18 expression was about 20% in group 6 and 27% in group 7. Upregulation of the expression of IL-18 in group 4 was significantly higher than groups 6 and 7. In group 5, the placebo was administrated and no change was observed in the expression of IL-18.

Effect of *Malva neglecta* extract on PGE2 production in THP-1 cells

Production of PGE2 was assessed using ELIZA method, then a standard curve was drawn using different concentrations of PGE2 and the equation proposed by Invitrogen Corporation. Based on the results of this analysis, PGE2 production was significantly higher in groups 3 and 5 compared to other groups (table 2). Production of PGE2 was significantly reduced in group 4 (LPS+Extract+Cell) compared to group 3 about 28%. The reduction in PGE2 production was 53% and 47% in groups 6 and 7 respectively which was significantly higher than the reduction observed in group 4.

Effect of *Malva neglecta* extract on NO production in THP-1 cells

Production of NO was assessed using spectrophotometry, then a standard curve was drawn using different concentrations of standard nitric oxide. Production of NO was significantly higher in groups 3 and 5 compared to other groups (Table 3). Production of NO was significantly reduced in group 4 (LPS+Extract+Cell) compared to group 3 about 40%. The reduction in NO production was 52% and 56% in groups 6 and 7 respectively which was significantly higher than the reduction observed in group 4.

Discussion

According to our knowledge, this is the first study investigating the effects of *Malva neglecta* extract on reducing pro-inflammatory cytokines in synoviocytes. We showed that *Malva neglecta* extract reduces TNF-α gene expression in both LPS-induced THP-1 cells and synoviocytes. Moreover, it can reduce IL-1β, COX-2, IL-18 and iNOS genes expression in synoviocyte cells. These results further confirm the effect of *Malva neglecta* on the reduction of pain and inflammation in OA (12). However, compared to ibuprofen and betamethasone, *Malva neglecta* extract was less effective in reduction of inflammation.

Previous studies have investigated the adverse effects of synovial fluid macrophages in OA. Blom et.al. reported that synovial macrophages induce fibrosis and osteophyte formation in rat models of OA (13). There is a strong association between macrophage count in synovial space and severity and duration of OA (14). These results suggest the role of macrophages in induction and maintaining inflammatory processes in joints involved in OA. It is well known that OA is not exclusively a disease of cartilage. Indeed, studies in humans and animals have led to growing evidence that the synovium also is involved in the disease and its role starts relatively early in OA (4). Several cytokines are produced in OA synovium and are implicated in OA pathology. IL-1β and TNF-α are the primary cytokines in OA pathogenesis, thus suppression of their expression in synoviocytes and macrophages is essential for reducing the cartilage damage (15). Both IL-1β and TNF-α induce production of PGs, NO and matrix metalloproteinases such as collagenase, gelatinase, proteoglycanase etc. leading to cartilage destruction (6, 16). Accordingly, reduction in the production of prostaglandin and nitric oxide is reported in the pain relief and inflammation of OA (17-19). Given that corticosteroids and NSAIDs reduce the expression of genes involved in this matter, they are commonly used as the treatment options in OA.

In this study, we investigated the effect of *Malva neglecta* aqueous extract on bovine synoviocyte and also THP-1 cells. Human THP-1 cells are a proper model for acting as a replacement model for monocytes/ macrophages and now is commonly used in the experimental researches on the inflammatory agents (20). In this study, we showed that *Malva neglecta* extract reduces expression of IL-1β, TNF-α, iNOS, IL-18 and COX-2 in synoviocytes and THP-1 cells which may subsequently lead to a reduction in synovitis and cartilage degeneration. Suppression of the expression of these pro-inflammatory factors, also lead to suppression of COX-2 and iNOS enzymes activity; subsequently leading to a reduction in the NO and PGE2. Compared to groups treated with ibuprofen or betamethasone, reduction in expression or production of inflammatory agents was less when *Malva neglecta* extract was administrated. Therefore, *Malva neglecta* extract has anti-inflammatory properties in OA but it should be used as a supplementary treatment. This extract is reported to be effective in preventing and treating other diseases associated with inflammation and tissue damage such as nephrolithiasis (21). The exact chemical constituents of *Malva neglecta* extract involved in such effects are not fully recognized yet. Studies reveal that *Malva neglecta* contains alkaloids, flavonoids, saponins (22) phenolic compounds (7) and mucilage content (23). Different properties of these components are well recognized; for example, Saponins have antiviral, antifungal and antioxidant effects (24). Thus, anti-inflammatory effect of *Malva neglecta* extract may be due to saponins content presented in this plant.

Conclusion

Malva neglecta extract is effective in reducing expression of inflammatory agents in synoviocytes and monocyte/macrophage implying that this effect can be extended to different cells involved in the pathogenesis of OA. However, this extract cannot be accounted as a replacement of common treatments of OA. Indeed, it may be used as a supplementary treatment to prevent complications of common treatments of OA. Further in-vivo researches should be done to elucidate the effect of *Malva neglecta* extract in treating OA patients.

Acknowledgment

This study is related to the project NO 1395/77494 From Student Research Committee, Shahid Beheshti University of Medical Sciences, Tehran, Iran. We also appreciate the "Student Research Committee" and "Research & Technology Chancellor" in Shahid Beheshti University of Medical Sciences for their financial support of this study.

Conflicts of Interest

The authors declare that they have no conflict of interest.

References

1. Davatchi F, Jamshidi A-R, Banihashemi AT, et al. WHO-ILAR COPCORD study (stage 1, urban study) in Iran. The Journal of rheumatology. 2008;35(7):1384-90.
2. Wang X, Hunter D, Xu J, Ding C. Metabolic triggered inflammation in osteoarthritis. Osteoarthritis and Cartilage. 2015;23(1):22-30.
3. Hill CL, Gale DG, Chaisson CE, et al. Knee effusions, popliteal cysts, and synovial thickening: association with knee pain in osteoarthritis. The Journal of rheumatology. 2001;28(6):1330-7.
4. Blom AB, van den Berg WB. The synovium and its role in osteoarthritis. Bone and osteoarthritis: Springer; 2007. p. 65-79.
5. Goldring MB, Otero M. Inflammation in osteoarthritis. Current opinion in rheumatology. 2011;23(5):471.
6. Goldring SR, Goldring MB. The role of cytokines in cartilage matrix degeneration in osteoarthritis. Clinical orthopaedics and related research. 2004;427:S27-S36.
7. Dalar A, Türker M, Konczak I. Antioxidant capacity and phenolic constituents of *Malva neglecta* Wallr. and Plantago lanceolata L. from Eastern Anatolia Region of Turkey. Journal of Herbal Medicine. 2012;2(2):42-51.
8. Güder A, Korkmaz H. Evaluation of in-vitro antioxidant properties of hydroalcoholic solution extracts Urtica dioica L., *Malva neglecta* Wallr. and their mixture. Iranian Journal of Pharmaceutical Research. 2012;11(3):913-23.
9. Gürbüz I, Özkan AM, Yesilada E, Kutsal O. Anti-ulcerogenic activity of some plants used in folk medicine of Pinarbasi (Kayseri, Turkey). Journal of ethnopharmacology. 2005;101(1):313-8.
10. Seyyednejad SM, Koochak H, Darabpour E, Motamedi H. A survey on Hibiscus rosa—sinensis, Alcea rosea L. and *Malva neglecta* Wallr as antibacterial agents. Asian Pacific Journal of Tropical Medicine. 2010;3(5):351-5.
11. Mirghiasi SM, Akhzari M, Vassaf M, Akbari A, Baghi SMM. The Effect of *Malva neglecta* on the Reduction of Inflammatory Agents in Patients with Osteoarthritis. Molecular Biology: Open Access. 2015;2015.
12. Amiri MS, Jabbarzadeh P, Akhondi M. An ethnobotanical survey of medicinal plants used by indigenous people in Zangelanlo district, Northeast Iran. Journal of Medicinal Plants Research. 2012;6(5):749-53.
13. Blom AB, van Lent PL, Holthuysen AE, et al. Synovial lining macrophages mediate osteophyte formation during experimental osteoarthritis. Osteoarthritis and cartilage. 2004;12(8):627-35.
14. Benito MJ, Veale DJ, FitzGerald O, van den Berg WB, Bresnihan B. Synovial tissue inflammation in early and late osteoarthritis. Annals of the rheumatic diseases. 2005;64(9):1263-7.
15. Aigner T, Kurz B, Fukui N, Sandell L. Roles of chondrocytes in the pathogenesis of osteoarthritis. Current opinion in rheumatology. 2002;14(5):578-84.
16. Chan P-S, Caron JP, Orth MW. Effect of glucosamine and chondroitin sulfate on regulation of gene expression of proteolytic enzymes and their inhibitors in interleukin-1-challenged bovine articular cartilage explants. American journal of veterinary research. 2005;66(11):1870-6.
17. Chaipinyo K, Oakes BW, van Damme MPI. Effects of growth factors on cell proliferation and matrix synthesis of low- density, primary bovine chondrocytes cultured in collagen I gels. Journal of orthopaedic research. 2002;20(5):1070-8.
18. Álvarez-Soria MA, Largo R, Santillana J, et al. Long term NSAID treatment inhibits COX-2 synthesis in the knee synovial membrane of patients with osteoarthritis: differential proinflammatory cytokine profile between celecoxib and aceclofenac. Annals of the rheumatic diseases. 2006;65(8):998-1005.
19. Brenner SS, Klotz U, Alscher DM, et al. Osteoarthritis of the knee–clinical assessments and inflammatory markers. Osteoarthritis and cartilage. 2004;12(6):469-75.
20. Chanput W, Mes JJ, Wichers HJ. THP-1 cell line: an in vitro cell model for immune modulation approach. International immunopharmacology. 2014;23(1):37-45.
21. Saremi J, Kargar-Jahromi H, Pourahmadi M. Effect of *Malva neglecta* Wallr on Ethylene Glycol Induced Kidney Stones. Urology journal. 2015;12(6):2387-90.
22. Mojab F, Kamalinejad M, Ghaderi N, Vahidipour HR. Phytochemical screening of some species of Iranian plants. Iranian Journal of Pharmaceutical Research. 2010:77-82.
23. Pakravan M, Abedinzadeh H, Safaeepur J. Comparative studies of mucilage cells in different organs in some species of Malva, Althaea and Alcea. Pak J Biol Sci. 2007;10(15):2603-5.
24. Francis G, Kerem Z, Makkar HP, Becker K. The biological action of saponins in animal systems: a review. British journal of Nutrition. 2002;88(06):587-605.

Comparison of two methods of bolus and infusion of Tranexamic acid to reduce blood loss in Total Knee Arthroplasty

Mohammadreza Moshari[1], Bahman Malek[1], Mohammadreza Minator-Sajjadi[2], Maryam Vosoghian[1], Mastaneh Dahi[1], Mahshid Ghasemi[1], Razieh Shekari[1]*

Abstract

Background: Until today, many studies conduct to determine the optimal dose and regimen of tranexamic acid to reduce the preoperative and postoperative blood loss in primary total knee arthroplasty. In this study, we were compared two different methods of administration (bolus and infusion).
Materials and Methods: Forty patients were randomized in two groups; all the patients received 500 mg tranexamic acid before tourniquet was turned on. Group (A) consisted of 20 patients (mean age: 64± 6.1 years) received 500 mg tranexamic acid ten minutes before tourniquet was loosened and group (B) (63.5 ± 7.7 years) received 500 mg tranexamic acid IV infusion during 6 hours from the time of tourniquet loosening (total dose of TA 1 g in both groups). Intraoperative blood loss, postoperative drainage (in 6 and 12 hours), blood transfusion (in 48 hours), hematocrit and hemoglobin decrease (6 and 12 hours later) were compared between two groups.
Results: The patients in group (B) had less blood loss intra- and postoperative in 6 and 12 hours, and also had less hemoglobin decrease and packed cell transfusion rate was significantly lower in these patients; compared to group (A).
Conclusion: Our study demonstrated that infusion administration of tranexamic acid in primary total knee arthroplasty was more effective to reduce perioperative blood loss and the demand for blood transfusion in 48 hours.
Keywords: tranexamic acid, total knee arthroplasty, blood transfusion

1. Anesthesiology Research Center, Taleghani Hospital, Shahid Beheshti University of Medical Sciences, Tehran, Iran
2. Taleghani Hospital Clinical Research Development Unit, Shahid Beheshti University of Medical Sciences, Tehran, Iran

***Corresponding Author:**
Razieh Shekari, MD, Anesthesiology Research Center, Shahid Beheshti University of Medical Sciences, Tehran, Iran

Email: razieh.shekari@gmail.com

Introduction

Total knee arthroplasty (TKA) is one of the most common procedures, for treating knee diseases such as end-staged knee osteoarthritis and rheumatoid arthritis (1). The prevalence is increasing greatly in aging societies, and it may cause large amounts of blood loss, ranging from 500 to 2000 ml after a single TKA procedure therefore need for blood transfusion (2-5). As most patients were elderly, blood transfusion may cause more subsequent complications, such as transfusion reactions and even death. So an effective and safe method to decrease intra- and postoperative blood loss would be helpful (6, 7).

There are several suggestions for suppressing perioperative blood loss, including antifibrinolytic agents, intraoperative blood salvage and application of tourniquet (6, 7). One of the pharmacological choices to prevent surgical bleeding is Tranexamic acid (TA), a wildly use synthetical antifibrinolytic agent which prevents the activation of plasminogen to plasmin thus blocks the fibrinolytic action of plasmin on fibrin (8, 9). Many old and recent studies showed that TA can significantly reduce perioperative blood loss and thus need for blood transfusion (6-10), but there is limited information of its effectiveness, safety and method of administration in Iranian patients, so this study is aimed to compare two methods of administration (bolus and IV infusion) of TA in TKA patients.

Methods

The inclusion criteria were: 1) primary knee osteoarthritis, 2) unilateral TKA, 3) ASA I and II. The criteria for exclusion were: 1) ASA III and IV, 2) Pregnancy, 3) Addiction, 4) Autoimmune or inflammatory diseases, 5) Age < 50 years, 6) Severe anemia, 7) Malignant tumors, 8) History of pulmonary thromboemboli, 9) uncontrolled diseases, 10) primary neuropathy, 11) patients who did not cooperate.

The participants of our study were recruited from January 2016 to January 2017, who were randomly classified into two groups. All the patients received 500 mg TA before tourniquet turned on. First group (A) received 500 mg TA 10 minutes before tourniquet was loosened and second group (B) received 500 mg TA IV infusion during 6 hours from the time of tourniquet loosening (total dose of TA 1 g in both groups). Intraoperative blood loss, postoperative drainage (in 6 and 12 hours), blood transfusion (in 48 hours), hematocrit and hemoglobin decrease (6 and 12 hours later) were compared between two groups.

Surgical Procedure

TKA was performed under spinal anesthesia, surgical method was the same in all as a standard midline skin incision, and a medial arthorotmy were obtained. TKA was done same in all cases in both groups. Before the performing the procedure, a tourniquet was used. Each group received TA the way which was mentioned before and then the drainage was placed, incision was sutured and bandaged the tourniquet was loosened.

Post-operative Follow Up

After the operation, the drainage was clamped for 4 hours. Blood transfusion was based on clinical symptoms and laboratory test results. If the Hb was less than 8 g/dl, blood transfusion was concerned. Hb level and the amount of blood drainage were recorded 6 and 12 hours after the procedure. Transfused packed cell was documented in 48 hours after the TKA operation.

Clinical Data Collection

The following data were recorded: 1) Age, 2) Sex, 3) Comorbidity diseases, 4) Intraoperative blood loss (measured by a same anesthesiologist by the net increase in gauze and the liquid of the drainage bottle minus the intraoperative flushing fluid.), 5) Hb, Hct, and Platelets before the surgery, followed by 6 and 12 hours after the surgery, 6) As mentioned previously, the amount of drainage blood 6 and 12 hours after the surgery, 7) Blood transfusion in 48 hours after the surgery. All the data and clinical evaluation were conducted by blinded independent clinicians.

Statistical analysis

SPSS version 21 software was used in order to analyze the data. Patients group were compared using student's T-test but in cases when data was not distributed normally Mann-Whitney U-test was used. When differences were statistically significant, Chi-square test or Fischer's exact test were used in order to compare findings. $P<0.05$ was considered significant.

Results

There were 40 patients with mean age of 63.55±6.9 years (50% males and 50% females) and each group consists of 20 individuals. There were no significant differences between two groups considering age, gender, body mass index, operation time, Hb and Hct values and comorbidities before surgery.

Table 1: Preoperative basic clinical data of patients in the two groups (x ± s).

Basic Data	Infusion Group	Bolus Group	T value	P value
Age	63.5 ± 7.7	64 ±6.1	0.3442	>0.05
Body mass index (BMI)	27.3 ± 1.9	26.9 ± 2.5	0.2653	>0.05
Gender (male/female)	11/9	9/11	0.3622	>0.05
Preoperative hemoglobin (g/dl)	15.25 ± 1.35	14.31 ± 1.61	1.9821	>0.05

Table 2: Comparison of observed postoperative indices between two groups.

Observed indices	Infusion Group	Bolus Group	T value	P value
Intraoperative blood loss (cc)	245 ± 87	322 ± 81	2.897	0.006
Hb decrease in 6 hrs (g/dl)	0.81 ± 0.35	1.35 ± 0.77	2.932	0.007
Hb decrease in 12 hrs (g/dl)	1.031 ± 0.326	1.81 ± 0.87	3.734	0.001
Blood drainage in 6 hrs (cc)	157 ± 46	400 ± 70	9.828	0.000
Blood drainage in 12 hrs (cc)	132.5 ± 37	290 ± 86	6.791	0.000
Blood transfusion rate (cc)	0%	25 % (5/20)	5.714	0.017

The total bleeding (intraoperative blood loss plus the amount of blood drainage in 6 and 12 hours after surgery) (P=0.000), the total postoperative drainage (P=0.000), and drainage in 6 and 12 hours after surgery (P=0.000 for both), intraoperative blood loss (P=0.008) and Hb decrease in 6 and 12 hours (P=0.007 and P=0.001 respectively) significantly differed between the two groups. Blood transfusion (12.5%) was only needed in 5 cases which were in TA bolus group (P=0.047). No deaths or allergic reaction were reported in both groups.

Discussion

TKA causes major perioperative blood loss due to enhanced fibrinolytic activity (2). TA can be used intravenous, intramuscular, local joint cavity injection and as oral route. The results of our study indicated that antifibrinolytic therapy with TA infusion significantly reduced total blood loss compared to bolus administration of TA, which in turn reduced the amount of blood transfusion required.

There were several systemic reviews and meta-analysis that evaluated the role of TA in total hemorrhage following TKA. All of these studies showed that it was significant decrease in the amount of total blood loss in different routes of administering TA. Peng et al. showed that single intravenous dose of TA before tourniquet loosening can significantly reduce post-operative hemorrhage and blood transfusion (11). Lee et al. reported similar results in which TA causes significant decrease in perioperative blood loss without exacerbating complications (5).

Other similar studies also demonstrated that blood loss can be reduced by 20-31%, administering TA in TKA (12).

Maniar et al compared the effect of pre-, intra- and postoperative administration of TA on blood loss which showed that preoperative use of TA is superior to others (13). In another study MacGilirray et al. compared the efficacy of different doses of TA on blood loss in TKA procedures, which showed significant difference between placebo group and TA group (14). Some studies have reported shorter time to peak value in intravenous rather than intramuscular injection or oral route administration. In another study Mutsuzaki et al (15) showed that TA injection via the drainage duct after TKA and also keeping the drainage closed for one hour can reduce 643 ml of blood loss so decreases 21% of allogenic blood transfusion rate.

TA caused no complication in our study; its administration did not increase the risk of thrombosis and reduced local skin ecchymosis after TKA. A meta-analysis by Alshryda et al. reported topical TA is an effective and safe way in order to reduce the need for blood transfusion. There was no higher rate of thromboembolic events in TA group compared to control group (16). In another similar study there were no more risks of complications in patients received TA after TKA (12). Xiao et al. mentioned that as high doses of TA may increase the risk of thrombosis, it is not recommended in patients with a history of PE (17).

Conclusion

Our study demonstrated that infusion administration of tranexamic acid in primary total knee arthroplasty was more effective to reduce perioperative blood loss and the demand for blood transfusion in 48 hours.

Acknowledgment

We would like to acknowledge the kind cooperation of physicians and nurses, operating room, Taleghani Hospital and Anesthesiology Research Center, Shahid Beheshti University of Medical Sciences, Tehran, Iran for their kind support and help.

Conflicts of Interest

The authors declare that they have no conflict of interest.

References

1. Wang G, Wang D, Wang B, Lin Y, Sun S. Efficacy and safety evaluation of intra-articular injection of tranexamic acid in total knee arthroplasty operation with temporarily drainage close. International Journal of Clinical and Experimental Medicine. 2015;8(8):14328-34.
2. Benoni G, Lethagen S, Fredin H. The effect of tranexamic acid on local and plasma brino- lysis during total knee arthroplasty. Thromb Res. 1997;85:195-206.
3. Tan J, Chen H, Liu Q, et al. A meta-analysis of the e ectiveness and safe- ty of using tranexamic acid in primary unilateral total knee arthroplasty. J Surg Res. 2013;184:880–87.
4. Georgiadis AG, Muh SJ, Silverton CD, et al: A prospective double-blind pla- cebo controlled trial of topical tranexamic acid in total knee arthroplasty. J Arthroplasty. 2013;28(8 Suppl.):78–82.
5. Lee SH, Cho KY, Khurana S, Kim KI: Less blood loss under concomitant ad- ministration of tranexamic acid and indirect factor Xa inhibitor following total knee arthroplasty: a prospective randomized controlled trial. Knee Surg Sports Traumatol Arthrosc. 2013;21:2611–17.
6. Zanasi S. Innovations in total knee replacement: new trends in operative treatment and changes in peri-operative management. Eur Orthop Traumatol. 2011;2:21–31.
7. Rajesparan K, Biant LC, Ahmad M, Field RE. The effect of an intravenous bolus of tranexamic acid on blood loss in total hip replacement. J Bone Joint Surg. 2009;91:776–83.
8. Dunn CJ, Goa KL. Tranexamic acid: a review of its use in surgery and other indications. Drugs. 1999;57:1005–32.
9. Lumsden MA, Wedisinghe L: Tranexamic acid therapy for heavy menstrual bleeding. Expert Opin Pharmacother, 2011: 12: 2089–95
10. Lemaire R : Strategies for blood management in orthopaedic and trauma surgery. J Bone Joint Surg Br. 2008;90:1128–36.
11. Peng H, Weng X, Zhai J, Jin J, Lin J, Qian W, et al. Use of intravenous tranexamic acid combined with temporary clamping of drain reduce postoperative blood loss in total knee arthroplasty. Chinese Journal of Orthopaedics. 2014;34:400-5.
12. Shemshaki H, Nourian SMA, Nourian N. Arch Orthop Trauma Surg. 2015;135:573.
13. Maniar RN, Kumar G, Singhi T, et al. Most active regimen of tranexam- ic acid in knee arthroplasty: a prospective randomized controlled study in 240 patients. Clin Orthop Relat Res. 2012;470:2605–12.
14. MacGillivray RG, Tarabichi SB, Hawari MF, Raoof NT. Tranexamic acid to re- duce blood loss after bilateral total knee arthroplasty: a prospective, ran- domized double blind study. J Arthroplasty. 2011;26:24–8.
15. Mutsuzaki H, Ikeda K. Intra-articular injec- tion of tranexamic acid via a drain plus drain- clamping to reduce blood loss in cementless total knee arthroplasty. J Orthop Surg Res. 2012;7:32.
16. Alshryda S, Sukeik M, Sarda P, Blenkinsopp J, Haddad FS, Mason JM. A systematic review and meta-analysis of the topical administration of tranexamic acid in total hip and knee replacement. Bone Joint J. 2014;96(8):1005–15.
17. Yu Xiao. Safety and efficacy of tranexamic acid in total knee arthroplasty © Med Sci Monit. 2015;21:3095-103.

Comparing the Efficacy and Safety of Dexmedetomidine-Lidocaine and Propofol-Fentanyl-Midazolam Combinations during Endoscopic Retrograde Cholangiopancreatography

Mohammad Reza Moshari [1] ✉, Bahman Malek B[1], Maryam Vosoughian[1], Mastaneh Dahi-Taleghani[1], Mahshid Ghasemi[1], Seyed Mohammad Seyed-Alshohadaei[1]

Abstract

Background: Propofol is commonly used for providing sedation in endoscopic retrograde cholangiopancreatography (ERCP). It's simple to use and effective but presents cardiovascular and respiratory adverse effects. Recently, dexmedetomidine has been tried but very little evidence exists to support its use. The aim of this study was to compare the efficacy and safety of combination of dexmedetomidine and lidocaine (DL) with the standard propofol-fentanyl (PF) regimen.

Materials and Methods: After approval of the hospital ethics committee, 63 patients (18-60 years of age) were randomly divided into 2 groups. Thirty-one patients received a PF combination (group PF), and 32 patients received DL combination (group DL). The level of sedation was adjusted to achieve a Ramasy Sedation Scale (RSS) score of 3 (moderate sedation) in both groups of patients. Arterial pressure (MAP), heart rate (HR), and peripheral oxygen saturation (SpO_2) during ERCP and recovery was continuously assessed.

Results: The oxygen saturation (SpO_2) showed high statistical significant differences between both groups throughout the procedure with stability in DL group ($p<0.01$). There was no statistical difference in HR and MAP between the two groups ($p>0.05$). Post-procedural recovery time was significantly shorter in PF group (15.97±3.27 min) compared with (19.38±5.64 min) DL group ($p<0.01$). PONV was 3.2% in PF group, while it was absent in DL group. No drug adverse effect or cardiovascular complications were observed in both groups.

Conclusion: Dexmedetomidine and lidocaine combination as total intravenous anesthesia (TIVA) during ERCP not only did not reported any oxygen desaturation (SpO2<90%) but also showed better stability of oxygen saturation (SpO_2) and less PONV when compared with propofol and fentanyl combination.

Keywords: Dexmedetomidine, Lidocaine, Sedation, ERCP, oxygen saturation.

1. Anesthesiology Research Center, Anesthesia Department, Taleghani Hospital, Shahid Beheshti University of Medical Sciences, Tehran, Iran.

✉ **Corresponding Author:**
Mohammad Reza Moshari, MD, Anesthesiology Research Center, SBMU, Tehran, Iran.

Email: rmoshari@yahoo.com

Introduction

Endoscopic retrograde cholangio-pancreatography (ERCP) has revolutionized the management of many pancreatic and biliary problems with its utility ranging from a diagnostic solution to complex diagnosis and therapeutic intervention (1, 2). It is a complex procedure which requires technical expertise as well as adequate sedation and anesthesia. The procedure time ranges from 30 to 60 minutes, and it is performed with the patient in the prone or semi-prone position. Moderate to deep levels of sedation and analgesia are required to minimize patient discomfort and to facilitate the operation (3).

ERCP is a complicated and long procedure. It requires moderate to deep sedation, and even general anesthesia. The level of sedation depends on the type of ERCP procedure as diagnostic or therapeutic and patient characteristics (4-6). There are various agents available to provide sedation. Current drugs include benzodiazepines (7) with an opioid; most commonly midazolam and diazepam (8), with or without propofol often combine with fentanyl or remifentanil (9). Ketamine has also been used in low doses for moderate sedation. Newer agents such as dexmedetomidine (10) and fospropofol are also being used (11). Combination with Lidocaine never been used. The anti inflammatory and analgesic properties of Lidocaine has also shown in new studies (29).

Recently dexmedetomidine has been used as TIVA in conscious sedation. A few studies have reported the success of dexmedetomidine in combination with ketamine and propofol as safe and effective sedative agent (12, 13). PF-based sedation techniques are effective for ERCP procedures but are not without cardiovascular and respiratory adverse effects (13). The use of dexmedetomidine as the sole anesthetic agent and as the adjuvantanalgesicagenthasbeenpublishedbuthasnotbeeneffective as propofol combined with fentanyl for conscious sedation during ERCP (14). This study was designed to compare the efficacy and safety profile of dexmedetomidine-lidocaine (DL) combination with the standard propofol and fentanyl (PF).

Methods

This study was approved by the ethics committee of Shahid Beheshti University of Medical Sciences at the Taleghani Hospital. The sample was drawn from patients admitted to undergo ERCP. We excluded patients who had ASA physical status Grade III and more, baseline $SpO_2<90\%$, mechanically ventilated patients, patients with comorbid conditions such as diabetes mellitus, hypertension (HTN) or hepatic or renal insufficiency to see the pure effect of both these drugs and to avoid any interaction with any simultaneous drug intake, which could have altered the results. Sixty-three patients with American Society of Anesthesiologist (ASA) classification I and II, aged 18 to 60 years, admitted for diagnostic and therapeutic ERCPs, were enrolled in the study. Patients provided written informed consent for participation in the study.

A detailed pre-operative check-up including general examination and systemic examination of the patient was carried out. On arrival in the Endoscopy Room, all vital parameters such as heart rate (HR), systolic blood pressure (SBP), diastolic blood pressure (DBP), mean arterial pressure (MAP) and oxygen saturation (SpO_2) were recorded. Readings were taken following the loading dose and every 5 min until the completion of the procedure.

This randomized, blind double-dummy clinical trial, with the rater blinded to the intervention, was conducted with patients who were undergoing an ERCP. The intervention was in the form that one group of patients was given dexmedetomidine with lidocaine (DL) and other group received propofol with fentanyl (PF) until achieving Ramasy sedation scale (RSS) score to 3 or 4 as moderate to deep sedation (Table 1). The DL group (n=32) received dexmedetomidine; (200 µg/ 2 ml) which prepared as 2 ml plus 48 ml normal saline total volume 50 ml. patients received loading dose of 1 µg/kg intravenous over 10 min and in 7 min lidocaine 1.5 ml/kg and then followed by 0.5 µg/kg/h infusion until RSS reached to 3-4. Group PF (n=31) received a single dose of midazolam (1mg) and additional fentanyl 1µg/kg and after 2 min patient received propofol 1 µg/kg/h in 60 sec and the followed by0.5 µg/kg/h infusion until RSS reached to 3-4. We used these doses of propofol and dexmedetomidine to preserve sufficient consciousness to allow communication, but provided the necessary degree of sedation to enable surgical comfort and an adequate quality of recovery with no negative effects on hemodynamics and respiratory parameters.

The drug infusion was discontinued if one of the following adverse events was observed: hemodynamic and/or respiratory instability, i.e., hypotension (mean arterial pressure reduction of 30% of its initial value), or apnea longer than 30 seconds, or oxygen desaturation<90%. During the procedure, any of the following complications were noted, recorded and treated accordingly: oxygen desaturation was considered when SpO_2 less than 90% for more than 10s. Both groups were managed by supporting airway and/or assisting ventilation. Bradycardia was considered when HR was less than 50 beats/min and managed with atropine 20 mcg/kg intravenous Hypotension was considered when MAP decreased by >20% of the baseline MAP and managed by fluid bolus or vasopressors. Any cough or gagging was noted and recorded.

Outcome assessed

The primary outcome was defined as the sedation level recorded by the RASS and the requirement of additional sedatives or an analgesic to display signs of insufficient analgesia. The level of sedation was judged adequate when the score on RASS was above or equal to 3, whether the patient tolerated the introduction of the endoscope without the presence of pain, discomfort, or agitation. The secondary outcome was the respiratory maintenance pattern, which was assessed by oxygen saturation (SpO_2).Furthermore, the HR and mean arterial pressure (MAP) were measured by the automated oscillography method. The SpO_2 was monitored by a finger probe. The HR, MAP and SpO_2 were continuously monitored and recorded at 5 min interval. Postoperative nausea and vomiting (PONV) were recorded and managed accordingly. Times of induction, procedure, recovery, and adverse effects were also reported.

Statistical analysis

Data were entered and analyzed using statistical package for social sciences (SPSS) for windows version 21 software (SPSS Inc., Chicago, IL, USA). Data were statistically described in terms of mean± standard deviation (±SD), or frequencies (number of cases) and percentages when appropriate. Numerical data between both groups were done using Student's t-test or Mann-Whitney test, depending on the distribution for independent samples. Categorical data were compared by Chi-square test with continuity correction or Fisher's exact test as applicable. P values less than 0.05 were considered statistically significant.

Results

The study recruited 64 patients scheduled for ERCP over a period of 6 months at a single institution. They were randomized into 2 groups, PF and DL, with 32 patients in each. The data were collected from 32 patients in group DL and 31 patients in group PF. One patient from group PF was excluded from the study because of missing data or procedure termination due to unrelated sedation reasons. Patient characteristics in two groups were shown in table 2. There were no significant differences in the demographic characteristics data between the two groups.

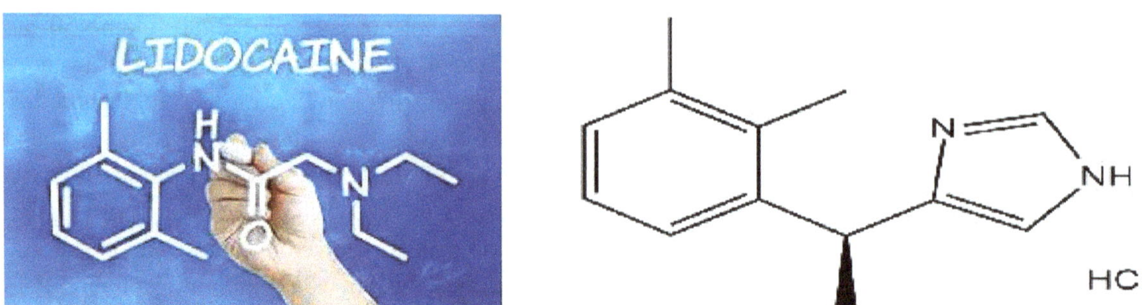

A B

Figure 1.(A) Lidocaine Formula; (B) Dexmedtomidine Formula.

Table 1: Ramsay Sedation Scale.

Score	Term	Description
1	Drowsy	Not fully alert but has sustained awakening (eye opening) to voice (>10s)
2	Light sedation	Briefly awakens with eye contact to voice (< 10s)
3	Moderate sedation	Movement or eye opening to voice (but not eye contact)
4	Deep sedation	Not responsive to voice but movement or eye opening to physical stimulation
5	Unarusable	No response to voice or physical stimulation

Table 2: Characteristics of patients in two groups (n=63).

Variables	Group DL (n=32)	Group PF (n=31)	P-value
Gender (M/F)	19/13	17/14	0.716
Age	51.91±5.96	49.16±8.73	0.152
ASA type (I/ II)	19/13	18/13	0.916
Smoker	7 (21.9%)	13 (41.9%)	0.087

Data were expressed as mean±SD. P value> 0.05 was considered statistically not significant. Group DL; dexmedetomidine with lidocaine, group PF; propofol with fentanyl. ASA; American Society of Anesthesiologists

Table 3: Vital sign during ERCP and recovery time.

Variables	Group DL (n=32)	Group PF (n=31)	P-value
HR (beat/min)	80.31±9.88	77.92±11.85	0.341
MAP (mm Hg)	78.02±5.43	77.86±7.31	0.738
Spo_2	96.02±1.55	94.54±3.01	0.002*
Recovery time	19.38±5.64	15.97±3.27	0.011*
PONV	0 (0)	1 (3.2%)	0.492

HR: Heart rate, MAP: Mean arterial pressure, Spo_2: Oxygen saturation, PONV: Postoperative nausea-vomiting, P-value<0.05 was considered statistically significant

Table 4: Changes of HR between two groups during the ERCP procedure.

HR Time Variable (min)	Group DL (n=32) Mean±SD	Range (min-Max)	Group PF (n=31) Mean±SD	Range (min-Max)	P-value
First	86.25±11.29	70-120	82.26±14.54	65-110	0.220
0-5	86.81±11.29	70-110	82.74±13.77	65-115	0.136
5-10	84.06±9.95	70-105	79.81±14.43	60-120	0.082
10-15	82.41±11.45	70-105	77.58±12.84	60-105	0.144
15-20	81.09±10.91	65-110	76.94±12.29	60-105	0.128
20-25	79.22±9.85	65-110	76.61±10.98	55-100	0.395
25-30	77.81±8.03	65-90	76.29±10.72	60-100	0.292
30-35	75.16±8.93	60-95	76.13±10.22	55-100	0.692
35-40	75.94±8.65	60-95	77.26±9.56	65-100	0.715
Total	80.31±9.88	60-120	77.92±11.85	55-120	0.341

Group DL; dexmedetomidine with lidocaine, group PF; propofol with fentanyl, P-value<0.05 was considered statistically significant

HR, MAP, SpO2, recovery time and POVN were given as mean±SD in Table 3. Patients in DL group significantly showed more stability of SpO2 than patients in PF group (p=0.002).There were no significant differences in MAP and HR values between the two groups (p>0.05). Recovery times were significantly longer in the DL group (p=0.011). Nausea and Vomiting (PONV) were observed in one patient (3.2%) in group PF, while it was absent in DL group but there were no significant statistically

Table 5: Changes of MAP between two groups during the ERCP procedure.

MAP Time Variable (min)	Group DL (n=32) Mean±SD	Range (min-Max)	Group PF (n=31) Mean±SD	Range (min-Max)	P-value
First	82.97±4.37	75-95	81.94±4.60	70-90	0.717
0-5	81.41±5.42	70-95	81.61±5.23	70-95	0.947
5-10	80.19±6.68	65-100	80.48±6.63	70-100	0.861
10-15	79.00±6.96	60-95	78.06±9.10	60-100	0.431
15-20	77.81±6.59	60-95	75.64±7.61	60-95	0.098
20-25	76.56±4.99	60-90	75.48±7.46	65-100	0.158
25-30	76.56±4.99	70-90	76.45±7.09	70-100	0.477
30-35	76.09±3.75	70-80	76.94±8.03	65-100	0.828
35-40	76.56±4.10	70-85	78.23±7.37	65-100	0.415
Total	78.02±5.43	60-100	77.86±7.31	60-100	0.738

Group DL; dexmedetomidine with lidocaine, group PF; propofol with fentanyl, P-value<0.05 was considered statistically significant

Table 6: Changes of SpO_2 between two groups during the ERCP procedure.

SpO2 Time Variable (min)	Group DL (n=32) Mean±SD	Range (min-Max)	Group PF (n=31) Mean±SD	Range (min-Max)	P-value
First	96.53±1.74	99-100	96.26±1.29	94-99	0.401
0-5	96.13±1.74	93-100	95.81±1.70	92-99	0.465
5-10	96.16±1.71	93-99	94.87±3.06	88-99	0.274
10-15	96.16±1.72	92-99	93.81±4.26	85-98	0.064
15-20	96.03±1.69	92-99	93.39±4.24	86-98	0.032
20-25	96.09±1.42	92-99	93.29±3.58	86-98	0.006
25-30	95.94±1.56	92-99	94.06±2.87	88-98	0.015
30-35	95.78±1.36	93-98	95.23±2.67	86-98	0.809
35-40	95.94±1.27	93-98	95.87±1.75	92-99	0.849
Total	96.02±1.55	92-100	94.54±3.01	85-99	0.002

Group DL; dexmedetomidine with lidocaine, group PF; propofol with fentanyl, P-value<0.05 was considered statistically significant

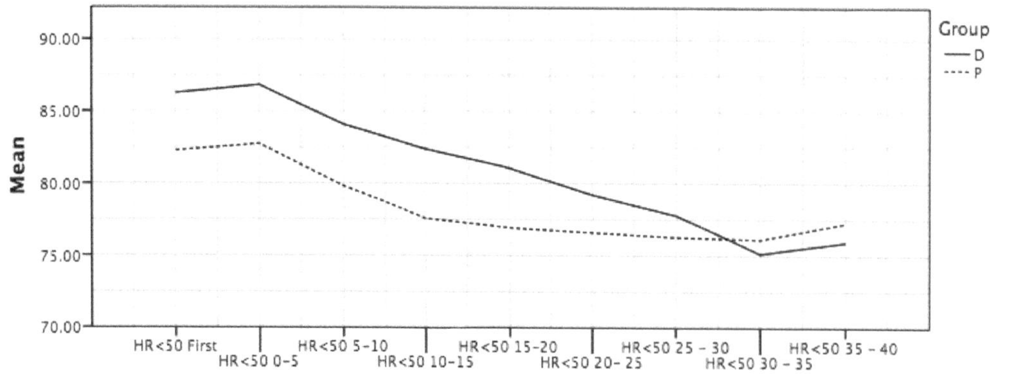

Figure 1.HR during the procedure between two groups.

(p=0.492). there was no event of drug adverse or cardiovascular complication observed in both regimens.

There were no significant differences in HR and MAP between two groups after loading dose in 5,10,15,20,25,30,35 and 40 min during ERCP procedure (Table 4 and 5). The case of oxygen desaturation (SpO2 <90%) was observed in PF groups after the loading dose at 5 to 35 minutes during ERCP procedure. While, it was absent in DL group and no cases in this group presented oxygen desaturation (SpO2 <90%). There is a significant difference in the

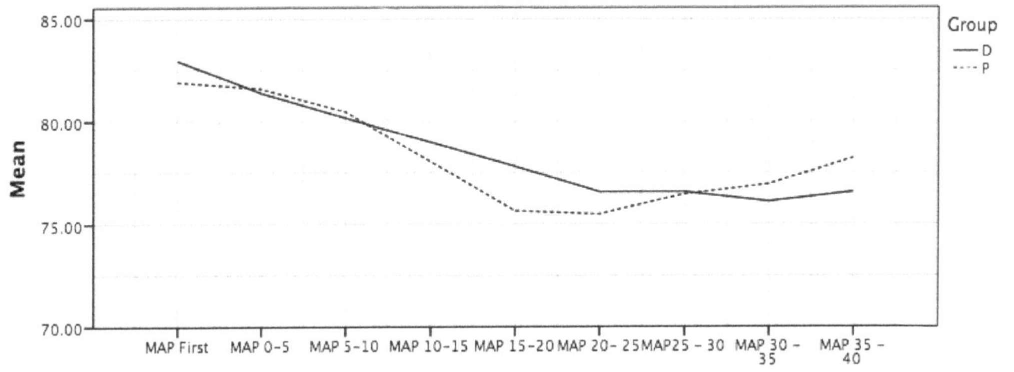

Figure 2.MAP during the procedure between two groups.

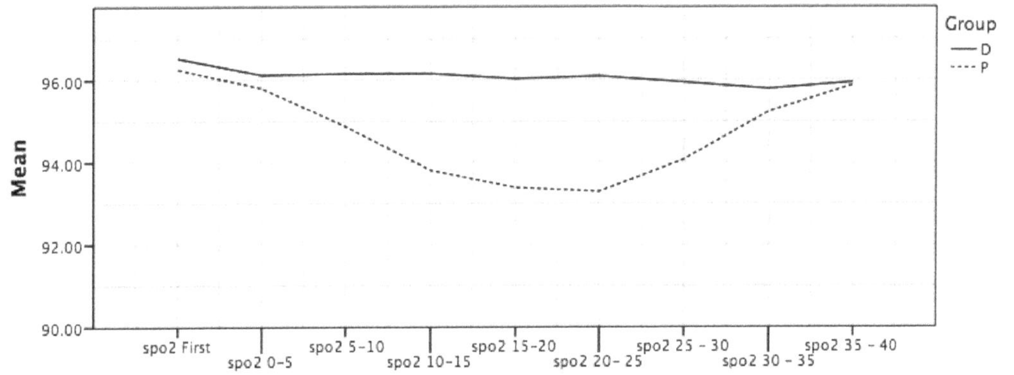

Figure 3.SpO_2 during the procedure between two groups.

oxygen saturation (SpO2) level between the two groups in the 15, 20 and 25 minute of ERCP process (p=0.03, p=0.006 and p=0.015) respectively. Patients in DL group significantly showed more stability (p=0.002) of SpO2 after the loading dose at 5, 10, 15, 20, 25, 30, 35 and 40 min during ERCP procedure (Table 6).

Figures 1 to 3;HR (beats/min), MAP (mmHg), and SpO2 (as Mean±SD), determined at different stages of the study, including baseline (at least 5 minutes before the first drug administration), 5, 10, and 15 minutes after starting sedation, and from 15 minutes until the end of an ERCP (40 min).

Discussion

The goals of this study were to provide adequate steady state of sedation level while maintaining airway reflex, maintain cardiovascular and respiratory status, minimize side effects and pain and ensure patient comfort. Generally, propofol alone or in combination with midazolam or fentanyl is one of the most widely used regimens for sedation during the ERCP (15-17).However, the combination use of sedatives with propofol may produce some additional risks (9, 18). In this study we compared the efficacy and safety of two different methods of moderate sedation; we used dexmedetomidine and lidocaine combination (DL) versus propofol and fentanyl combination (PF) during ERCP procedure.

Many previous studies use dexmedetomidine in combination or single as anesthetic agent during ERCP procedure and they reported different results. Eldesuky Ali Hassan et al. compared the hemodynamic stability, respiratory effect and recovery time in patient, who were randomly assigned in the two groups. Group D received dexmedetomidine as single aesthetic agent, and group K received a combination of ketamine and propofol (Ketofol) as aesthetic agent. MAP and HR in group D were significantly lesser than in the ketofol group. Additionally, time to achieve RSS score and total dose of rescue sedation in both groups were not significantly different. However, patient and endoscopist satisfaction in the ketofol group was significantly higher than in the dexmedetomidine group (4). Furthermore, Ceylan et al. (19) used dexmedetomidine (D) as single aesthetic agent and then evaluated the effects of propofol and dexmedetomidine hemodynamics stability and satisfaction during ERCP procedure. The fifty patients with ASA physical status class I and II were randomized into the two groups. Group P and group D received propofol and dexmedetomidine respectively. All patients were sedated to attain a RSS of 3-4. The mental status examination before and after the procedure as well as pain was evaluated. The blood pressure and heart rate values in group D were significantly lesser than in group P. However, there were no significant differences in patient and endoscopist satisfaction among the two groups.

In combination form of dexmedetomidine, the efficacy of dexmedetomidine with propofol for anesthesia in ERCP procedure was evaluated by Abdalla et al. (20). Sixty patients with ASA physical status class II or III underwent ERCP procedures were randomly assigned into two groups. Group DF received combination of dexmedetomidine and propofol, group K, patients received a loading dose of ketamine 1 mg/kg and followed by 0.5 mg/kg per hour. Group DF during ERCP procedure showed better hemodynamic stability, less nausea and vomiting, as well as shorter recovery time when compared with the combination of ketamine and propofol. However, the negative results of the use of dexmedetomidine for ERCP procedure have been reported; for example, the study of Nagaraj et al. (21) compared the combination of dexmedetomidine and fentanyl with the combination of propofol and fentanyl for procedural sedation in ERCP procedure. The result of study showed that the combination of propofol and fentanyl achieved better overall conditions for ERCP compared to the combination of dexmedetomidine and fentanyl. Other studies used of dexmedetomidine with ketamine or propofol combination for sedation in ERCP procedures and reported that combination of dexmedetomidine gives more respiratory safety and hemodynamic stability (22, 23). The most of studies used dexmedetomidine with ketamine or propofol combination as induction agent for moderate to deep sedation but no study used it with lidocaine combination.

Therefore, in this study we used dexmedetomidine and lidocaine combination (DL) versus propofol and fentanyl combination (PF) during ERCP procedure. In our study there was no event of drug adverse or cardiovascular complication observed in both regimens.

The case of oxygen desaturation (SpO2 <90%) was observed in PF groups after the loading dose at 5 to 35 minutes during ERCP procedure. While, it was absent in DL group and no cases in this group presented oxygen desaturation (SpO2 <90%). There is a significant difference in the oxygen saturation (SpO2) level between the two groups in the 15, 20 and 25 minute of ERCP process (P<0.05). Patients in DL group significantly showed more stability of SpO2. So, the results demonstrate that combination of DL gives more respiratory safety than propofol with fentanyl combination (P<0.01). In contrast to Muller et al. studies which reported, no statistical difference in SpO_2 between the dexmedetomidine as the sole anesthetic agent and propofol group (14). There were no significant differences in MAP, HR values at all-time points between the two groups (P>0.05). Recovery times were significantly longer in the DL group. Nausea and Vomiting (PONV) were observed in one patient (3.2%) in group PF, while it was absent in DL group, this result was consistent with previous study (24).

The most important result from this study was the persistence of oxygen saturation (SpO_2) in patients, who received dexmedetomidine and lidocaine combination (DL). No reported of oxygen desaturation (SpO2<90%) in DL group and more stability of SpO_2 during ERCP procedure in this group is very important because most patients who underwent ERCP are generally elderly and require sedation while in the prone position. This factor may be expected to prevent the risk of arterial hypoxemia (25). Arterial hypoxemia indicate impending respiratory failure or by itself may result in adverse physiological effects including acidosis, hyperkalemia, release of circulating catecholamines, myocardial excitation or depression, arrhythmias, arterial hypertension or hypotension, headache, intracranial hypertension, and agitation or narcosis (26-28).The limitation of this study was we don't measure respiratory rate, as the prone position makes it difficult to accurately count respiratory rate both artificially and automatically. So, the effect on respiratory function was judged only by SpO_2, which may lead to missing subclinical respiratory depression.

Conclusion

Dexmedetomidine with lidocaine is a new combination that has been used in sedation or analgesia for short procedures as ERCP for first time in this study. Compared to other drugs and combinations, it provides similar effects; no event of hypotension or bradycardia but it has an added benefit with less number of postoperative side effects such as nausea and vomiting (PONV) and the most important result from this study was DL combination as total intravenous anesthesia (TIVA) during ERCP not only did not reported any oxygen desaturation (SpO2<90%) but also showed better stability of oxygen saturation (SpO2).

Acknowledgment

None.

Conflicts of Interest

The authors declare that they have no conflict of interest.

References

1. Baillie J. Fifteen years of ERCP. Gastrointestinal endoscopy. 2017;86(2):327-8.
2. NIH state-of-the-science statement on endoscopic retrograde cholangiopancreatography (ERCP) for diagnosis and therapy. NIH consensus and state-of-the-science statements. 2002;19(1):1-26.
3. Dumonceau JM, Riphaus A, Aparicio JR, Beilenhoff U, Knape JT, Ortmann M, et al. European Society of Gastrointestinal Endoscopy, European Society of Gastroenterology and Endoscopy Nurses and Associates, and the European Society of Anaesthesiology Guideline: Non-anesthesiologist administration of propofol for GI endoscopy. Endoscopy. 2010;42(11):960-74.
4. Hossam Ibrahim Eldesuky Ali Hassan. Dexmedetomidine versus ketofol for moderate sedation in Endoscopic Retrograde Cholangiopancreatography (ERCP) comparative study. Egyptian Journal of Anaesthesia. 2014;31:15-21.
5. Lichtenstein DR, Jagannath S, Baron TH, Anderson MA, Banerjee S, Dominitz JA, et al. Sedation and anesthesia in GI endoscopy. Gastrointestinal endoscopy. 2008;68(5):815-26.
6. Demiraran Y, Korkut E, Tamer A, Yorulmaz I, Kocaman B, Sezen G, et al. The comparison of dexmedetomidine and midazolam used for sedation of patients during upper endoscopy: A prospective, randomized study. Canadian journal of gastroenterology = Journal canadien de gastroenterologie. 2007;21(1):25-9.
7. Froehlich F, Schwizer W, Thorens J, Kohler M, Gonvers JJ, Fried M. Conscious sedation for gastroscopy: patient tolerance and cardiorespiratory parameters. Gastroenterology. 1995;108(3):697-704.
8. Zakko SF, Seifert HA, Gross JB. A comparison of midazolam and diazepam for conscious sedation during colonoscopy in a prospective double-blind study. Gastrointestinal endoscopy. 1999;49(6):684-9.
9. Wehrmann T, Riphaus A. Sedation with propofol for interventional endoscopic procedures: a risk factor analysis. Scandinavian journal of gastroenterology. 2008;43(3):368-74.
10. Aantaa R, Jaakola ML, Kallio A, Kanto J, Scheinin M, Vuorinen J. A comparison of dexmedetomidine, and alpha 2-adrenoceptor agonist, and midazolam as i.m. premedication for minor gynaecological surgery. British journal of anaesthesia. 1991;67(4):402-9.
11. Arain SR, Ruehlow RM, Uhrich TD, Ebert TJ. The efficacy of dexmedetomidine versus morphine for postoperative analgesia after major inpatient surgery. Anesthesia and analgesia. 2004;98(1):153-8, table of contents.
12. Nishizawa T, Suzuki H, Sagara S, Kanai T, Yahagi N. Dexmedetomidine versus midazolam for gastrointestinal endoscopy: a meta-analysis. Digestive endoscopy : official journal of the Japan Gastroenterological Endoscopy Society. 2015;27(1):8-15.
13. Goyal R, Hasnain S, Mittal S, Shreevastava S. A randomized, controlled trial to compare the efficacy and safety profile of a dexmedetomidine-ketamine combination with a propofol-fentanyl combination for ERCP. Gastrointestinal endoscopy. 2016;83(5):928-33.
14. Muller S, Borowics SM, Fortis EA, Stefani LC, Soares G, Maguilnik I, et al. Clinical efficacy of dexmedetomidine alone is less than propofol for conscious sedation during ERCP. Gastrointestinal endoscopy. 2008;67(4):651-9.
15. Fanti L, Testoni PA. Sedation and analgesia in gastrointestinal endoscopy: what's new? World journal of gastroenterology. 2010;16(20):2451-7.
16. Amornyotin S. Sedation and monitoring for gastrointestinal endoscopy. World journal of gastrointestinal endoscopy. 2013;5(2):47-55.
17. Amornyotin S. Registered nurse-administered sedation for gastrointestinal endoscopic procedure. World journal of gastrointestinal endoscopy. 2015;7(8):769-76.
18. Bahrami Gorji F, Amri P, Shokri J, Alereza H, Bijani A. Sedative and Analgesic Effects of Propofol-Fentanyl Versus Propofol-Ketamine During Endoscopic Retrograde Cholangiopancreatography: A Double-Blind Randomized Clinical Trial. Anesthesiology and pain medicine. 2016;6(5):e39835.
19. Ceylan G, Yavascaoglu B, Korfali G, Kaya FN, Mogol EB, Turker G. A comparison of propofol and dexmedetomidine on the effects of hemodynamic and cognitive functions in conscious sedation during endoscopic retrograde cholangiopancreatography. Uludag Universitesi Tip Fakultesi Dergis. 2010;36:103-10.
20. Abdalla MW, El Shal SM, El Sombaty AI, Abdalla NM, Zeedan RB. Propofol dexmedetomidine versus propofol ketamine for anesthesia of endoscopic retrograde cholangiopancreatography (ERCP) (a randomized comparative study). Egypt J Anesth. 2015;31:97-105.

21. Nagaraj MC, Geetha CR, Rajavardhan R. Is dexmedetomidine a poor surrogate to propofol for procedural sedation during endoscopic retrograde cholangiopancreatography (ERCP). J Evolut Med Dent Sci. 2013;2:8165-75.

22. Sethi P, Mohammed S, Bhatia PK, Gupta N. Dexmedetomidine versus midazolam for conscious sedation in endoscopic retrograde cholangiopancreatography: An open-label randomised controlled trial. Indian journal of anaesthesia. 2014;58(1):18-24.

23. Tobias JD, Leder M. Procedural sedation: A review of sedative agents, monitoring, and management of complications. Saudi journal of anaesthesia. 2011;5(4):395-410.

24. Kilic N, Sahin S, Aksu H, Yavascaoglu B, Gurbet A, Turker G, et al. Conscious sedation for endoscopic retrograde cholangiopancreatography: dexmedetomidine versus midazolam. The Eurasian journal of medicine. 2011;43(1):13-7.

25. Davis DP, Hwang JQ, Dunford JV. Rate of decline in oxygen saturation at various pulse oximetry values with prehospital rapid sequence intubation. Prehospital emergency care : official journal of the National Association of EMS Physicians and the National Association of State EMS Directors. 2008;12(1):46-51.

26. Pierson DJ. Pathophysiology and clinical effects of chronic hypoxia. Respiratory care. 2000;45(1):39-51; discussion -3.

27. Sarkar M, Niranjan N, Banyal PK. Mechanisms of hypoxemia. Lung India : official organ of Indian Chest Society. 2017;34(1):47-60.

28. Michiels C. Physiological and pathological responses to hypoxia. The American journal of pathology. 2004;164(6):1875-82.

29. Memary H, Mirkheshti A, Ghasemi M, Taheri M, Arhami Dolatabadi A, Kaboudvand A. Effect of Lidocaine Infusion during General Anesthesia on Neutrophil-Lymphocyte-Ratio in Breast Cancer Patients Candidate for Mastectomy; a Clinical Trial. J Cell Mol Anesth. 2016;1(4):146-53.

16

The Effects of 6% Hydroxyethyl Starch Compared with Normal Saline on Controlling Undesirable Hemodynamic Changes Following Spinal Anesthesia in Patients Undergoing Orthopedic Surgery

Siamak Yaghobi[1], Amir Hesam Alirezaei[2], Mahmood Bakhtiyari[3,4], Marzieh-Beigom Khezri[1], Nilofar Massoudi[5]✉

Abstract

Background: The aim of the current study was to compare the effects of normal saline solution and 6% hydroxyethyl starch (HES/HAES) solution on hemodynamic changes after spinal anesthesia in patients undergoing lower limb orthopedic surgery.

Materials and Methods: This randomized clinical trial was performed on 50 patients undergoing surgery, aged 20-60, with physical status of ASA I, II. Before surgery, the hemodynamic status of each patient including systolic and diastolic blood pressure, heart rate, and central venous pressure was measured. Then, the patients were randomly divided into two groups and for the control group, 7 ml/kg 9% (or normal) saline and for the experimental group 6% hydroxyethyl starch were administered. Hemodynamic indices were re-measured after the completion of infusion, and then spinal anesthesia was performed. After anesthesia, hemodynamic indices were measured every 5 minutes for 1 hour and then every 10 minutes for 2 hours. The analysis of variance (ANOVA) for repeated measures was used to evaluate the significant changes in hemodynamic indices.

Results: The mean and standard deviation of systolic and diastolic blood pressure, heart rate, and central venous pressure in the control group were 113.0 (7.3), 73.0 (6.0), 95.6 (5.7), and 5.8 (0.9), respectively, and in the intervention group were 104.8 (5.5), 66.1 (4.2), 95.8 (8.2), and 4.3 (0.9). ANOVA for repeated measures showed that the incidence of decreasing changes in systolic and diastolic blood pressure, heart rate, and central venous pressure of the patients for whom hydroxyethyl starch was prescribed was significantly less than that of the patients for whom normal saline was prescribed.

Conclusion: Hydroxyethyl starch has a more effective role in controlling hemodynamic changes before spinal anesthesia than normal saline.

Keywords: Hydroxyethyl starch, Normal saline, Hemodynamic, Randomized clinical trial.

1. Department of Anesthesiology, School of Medicine, Qazvin University of Medical Sciences, Iran
2. Clinical Research Development Center at Shahid Modarres Hospital, Department of Nephrology, Shahid Beheshti University of Medical Sciences, Tehran, Iran
3 PhD, Department of Community Medicine, School of Medicine, Alborz University of Medical Sciences, Karaj, Iran
4. Department of Epidemiology and Biostatistics, School of Public Health, Tehran University of Medical Sciences, Tehran, Iran
5. Clinical Research Development Center at Shahid Modarres Hospital, Department of Anesthesiology, Shahid Beheshti University of Medical Sciences, Tehran, Iran

✉ **Corresponding Author:** Nilofar Massoudi (MD), Clinical Research Development Center at Shahid Modarres Hospital, Department of Anesthesiology, Shahid Beheshti University of Medical Sciences, Tehran, Iran.

Email: Massodi@sbmu.ac.ir

Introduction

Spinal anesthesia, except for contraindications, is the preferred method of performing numbness in lower limb surgery (1). Spinal anesthesia's benefits such as reduction in blood loss, infection rates, need for transfusion, and thromboembolic events compared with those of general anesthesia have been confirmed in numerous studies (2).

Despite being safe and having many benefits, this anesthetic technique has side effects such as hemodynamic changes, headaches, cauda equine syndrome, and radiculopathy. Among the complications of this anesthetic technique, hypotension is very common in 95% of the patients in line with findings of some researchers (3). The main reason for this event is the block of the sympathetic nervous system following cardiac output reduction and/or vascular resistance reduction. This complication is considered to be a very important and serious complication because it can lead to the limitation of blood supply to vital organs such as the heart and brain (4).

To reduce the adverse effects of hemodynamic changes following spinal anesthesia, especially hypotension, various therapeutic approaches have been studied (5-7). Comparing the effects of three different doses of dihydroergotamine—a family of ergot alkaloids—on hemodynamic changes following spinal anesthesia, Sahmedini et al. (4) Revealed that intravenous injection of this drug at a dose of 5-10 mcg/kg was effective in the treatment of spinal anesthesia-induced hypotension. Baygmohammadi et al. (8), in a double-blind clinical trial, compared the effect of atropine and placebo (normal saline) on hemodynamic changes following spinal anesthesia. The results of this study demonstrated that hemodynamic changes in the atropine-receptor group were significantly lower than those in the placebo-receptor group. McDonnell et al (9), also performed a randomized double- blind clinical trial and determined that both metaraminol and phenylephrine had the same advantages in preventing hypotension due to spinal anesthesia.

In general, one of the recommended methods for preventing hypotension following spinal anesthesia is the administration of crystalloid solutions, including Ringer's solution (10). However, owing to the fact that the administration of high volumes of these solutions can lead to a peripheral edema in cardio-pulmonary patients and then a reduction in oxygen-carrying capacity, it seems that the administration of colloid solutions is the best choice (11). Hydroxyethyl starch (HES) is a colloidal, synthetically adapted polymer of amylopectin, a waxy starch derived from maize or sorghum (Figure 1). Clinically, HES is used for volume alternate to keep on or improve tissue perfusion in patients with sepsis, trauma, shock, or surgical stress (10, 12, 13). In addition to its consequence on continuation of stability of hemodynamic parameters, latest studies have shown that HES may decrease capillary leakage in many pathological circumstances that increase capillary permeability (14).

Neuraxial block is one of the methods that can be used to perform spinal anesthesia in lower limb surgeries. This technique, like any other medical technique, has complications, one of which is hypotension due to decreased intravascular volume of hypovolemia because of patients fasting (15). Therefore, in order to prevent this complication, the use of a solution that can produce more intravascular volume, such as colloidal solutions, is more effective than crystalloid solutions (16). Since there is not enough information about the effect of prescribing colloidal solutions prior to spinal anesthesia in preventing hemodynamic changes in patients undergoing lower limb orthopedic surgery, the aim of the present study was to compare the effects of normal saline and 6% hydroxyethyl starch solutions on hemodynamic changes after spinal anesthesia in patients undergoing lower limb orthopedic surgery.

Methods

This study was a double-blind randomized clinical trial being performed on 50 patients undergoing lower limb orthopedic surgery with spinal anesthesia in Shahid Rajai Hospital in Qazvin. The inclusion criteria of the study included:

- the patient should be a candidate for lower limb orthopedic surgery with spinal anesthesia,
- the age of the patient should be between 20 and 60 years of age, and
- ASA I and II physical status class

The exclusion criteria included:

- the age of the patient should be less than 20 years or more than 60 years,
- the patient should have prohibition of spinal anesthesia, and
- the patient should have hypotension or hypertension

Patients who had undergone a spinal anesthesia in a sequential manner due to lower limb trauma and had inclusion criteria were included in the study, if they were satisfied. Patients were randomly divided into two groups of normal saline and hydroxyethyl starch recipients using colored cards. The procedure of the study was that first before the surgery a CVP cannula (14 gauge) which was positioned into the right antecubital area and in the supine position using regional anesthesia was used to measure systolic and diastolic blood pressure, heart rate, and central venous pressure of each patient (i.e., baseline measurements). Then, the patients were randomly divided into two groups. For control group, 7 ml/kg normal saline and for the experimental group 6% hydroxyethyl starch was administered. These solutions were infused from the peripheral vein and within 10 minutes. After the completion of infusion, systolic and diastolic blood pressure, heart rate, and central venous pressure were measured and then spinal anesthesia at the L3.4 level was performed using a 22-gauge needle and 3 cc of 0.5% Marcaine. After anesthesia, the anesthesia level was measured using the pin-prick technique and systolic and diastolic blood pressure, heart rate, and central venous pressure values were measured every 5 minutes for 1 hour and then every 10 minutes for 2 hours. To describe the results, the mean ± standard deviation and number (percent) were used. An analysis of variance for repeated measures was used to examine the existence of significant changes in these variables over time.

Results

The number of participants in this study was 50 (i.e., 25 participants in the intervention group and 25 participants in the comparison group). 34 (68%) participants were male and the rest were female. The mean (SD) age of the patients was 45.3 (9.07). The gender composition of the participants in the intervention and control group was completely similar (50% male and 50% female). The mean (SD) age of the participants in the intervention and control group was 44.24 (8.81) and 46.36 (9.38), respectively. The independent t-test did not show a significant difference between these means ($P = 0.414$).

The mean (SD) systolic blood pressure at baseline in the intervention and control groups was 104.8 (5.5) and 113.0 (7.3), respectively ($P < 0.001$). The mean (SD) diastolic blood pressure at baseline in the intervention and control groups was 66.1 (4.2) and 73.0 (6.0), respectively ($P < 0.001$). The mean (SD) heart rate at baseline in the intervention and control groups was 95.8 (8.2) and 95.6 (5.7), respectively (P-value 0.921). The mean (SD) central venous pressure at baseline in the intervention and control groups was 4.3 (0.9) and 5.8 (0.9), respectively ($P < 0.001$).

The mean systolic and diastolic blood pressure, heart rate, and central venous pressure based on measurement time are presented in Table 1. To determine the existence of significant changes in these variables over time, the analysis of variance for repeated measures was used. According to Mauchly's test of sphericity, for each of the four outcomes examined, the coefficients of continuous measurements were significantly different, so the Greenhouse-Geisser correction was used to check for significant changes in each of the four outcomes. In addition, due to the significant differences in baseline values of the two groups, these values were considered as covariate in the equation to modify their effect in the comparison of changes between the two groups. In this way, the analysis of variance for repeated measures with the Greenhouse–Geisser correction of sphericity and modulation of the effects of age, gender, and basic parameters of the outcome variables was performed. In the following sections, the results of these tests are presented separately for the outcome variables.

Systolic Blood Pressure: The mean systolic blood pressure based on measurement time and intervention group type (i.e., normal saline and hydroxyethyl starch groups) are presented in Table 1. According to this table, the mean systolic blood pressure significantly increased in both groups after completion of infusion compared with the baseline values and 5 minutes after

Table 1: The status of hemodynamic changes (SBP&DBP) over time in the groups treated with Hydroxyethyl starch and normal saline.

Measurement times	Systolic blood pressure: Intervention group (Hydroxyethyl starch) Mean±SD	Systolic blood pressure: Control group (normal saline) Mean±SD	P-value	Diastolic blood pressure: Intervention group (Hydroxyethyl starch) Mean±SD	Diastolic blood pressure: Control group (normal saline) Mean±SD	P-value
After the completion of infusion	124.92 ± 4.77	116.17 ± 6.68	<0.001	82.16 ± 5.15	76.58 ± 5.84	0.001
20th minute after spinal anesthesia	110.88 ± 6.66	91.75 ± 5.50	<0.001	70.64 ± 4.67	60.17 ± 5.34	<0.001
40th minute after spinal anesthesia	117.16 ± 3.75	97.50 ± 5.99	<0.001	75.88 ± 4.08	64.42 ± 4.34	<0.001
60th minute after spinal anesthesia	120.74 ± 3.02	104.79 ± 6.29	<0.001	52.78 ± 4.33	67.54 ± 2.84	<0.001
80th minute after spinal anesthesia	122.08 ± 2.84	109.13 ± 5.29	<0.001	80.08 ± 3.52	69.67 ± 3.21	<0.001
100th minute after spinal anesthesia	120.44 ± 4.16	110.08 ± 4.77	<0.001	79.56 ± 5.29	69.75 ± 2.80	<0.001
120th minute after spinal anesthesia	121.00 ± 2.63	112.42 ± 4.89	<0.001	79.04 ± 3.90	71.83 ± 4.92	<0.001
140th minute after spinal anesthesia	121.96 ± 2.85	115.25 ± 5.41	<0.001	80.56 ± 4.10	73.96 ± 5.62	<0.001
160th minute after spinal anesthesia	124.92 ± 4.18	116.88 ±5.24	<0.001	81.22 ± 5.50	74.71 ± 6.23	<0.001
180th minute after spinal anesthesia	125.64 ± 3.93	116.71 ± 5.29	<0.001	85.20 ± 5.09	75.79 ± 5.59	<0.001

spinal anesthesia significantly decreased. Then, from the fifth minute to the end of the study, there was a slowdown increase (despite slight reductions at some time points). In Figure 1, changes in mean systolic blood pressure are presented for both groups (i.e., hydroxyethyl starch and normal saline groups). The analysis of variance for repeated measures revealed the following issues:

1) The changes in mean systolic blood pressure of the participants were not statistically significant (P value: 0.082 and F=1.84),

2) The effect of the prescribed drug on the changes in systolic blood pressure was statistically significant (P<0.001 and F=15.36); in other words, in patients treated with hydroxyethyl starch, the systolic blood pressure drop was significantly lower than that of those for whom normal saline was prescribed,

3) Gender had a significant effect on the changes in the mean systolic blood pressure of the participants during the study period (P-value 0.026 and F=2.34); in other words, the decreasing changes in mean systolic blood pressure in females were significantly higher than that of males (P-value: 0.052 and F=1.85);

4) Age had no significant effect on the changes in the mean diastolic blood pressure of the participants during the study period (P-value: 0.532 and F=0.86); and

5) There was no significant interaction between gender and prescribed drugs; in other words, the effect of hydroxyethyl starch on systolic blood pressure changes in males and females did not significantly differ (P value: 0.625 and F=0.752).

Diastolic Blood Pressure: The mean diastolic blood pressure based on measurement time and intervention group type (i.e., normal saline and hydroxyethyl starch groups) are presented in Table 1. According to this table, the mean diastolic blood pressure significantly increased in both groups after completion of infusion compared to the baseline values, and 5 minutes after spinal anesthesia significantly decreased.

Table 2: The status of hemodynamic changes (HR&CVP) over time in the groups treated with Hydroxyethyl starch and normal saline.

Measurement times	Heart Rate			CVP		
	Intervention group (Hydroxyethyl starch) Mean±SD	Control group (normal saline) Mean±SD	P-value	Intervention group (Hydroxyethyl starch) Mean±SD	Control group (normal saline) Mean±SD	P-value
After the completion of infusion	85.16 ± 6.61	91.96 ± 4.93	<0.001	8.24 ± 0.60	4.96 ± 0.81	<0.001
20th minute after spinal anesthesia	88.40 ± 5.02	85.48 ± 12.49	0.28	6.36 ± 0.64	5.75 ± 0.61	0.001
40th minute after spinal anesthesia	86.16 ± 5.35	85.72 ± 9.97	0.84	6.24 ± 0.52	5.75 ± 0.85	0.012
60th minute after spinal anesthesia	83.80 ± 4.09	85.00 ± 6.75	0.45	6.12 ± 0.60	5.75 ± 0.74	0.06
80th minute after spinal anesthesia	82.48 ± 3.39	85.16 ± 5.77	0.051	6.04 ± 0.68	6.17 ± 0.70	0.68
100th minute after spinal anesthesia	81.72 ± 4.86	84.80 ± 6.03	0.052	6.08 ± 0.57	6.13 ± 0.74	0.99
120th minute after spinal anesthesia	81.12 ± 4.18	85.28 ± 4.86	0.002	6.08 ± 0.70	5.83 ± 0.82	0.20
140th minute after spinal anesthesia	79.00 ± 4.58	84.68 ± 5.58	<0.001	6.04 ± 0.54	6.13 ± 0.90	0.85
160th minute after spinal anesthesia	76.78 ± 4.68	84.12 ± 4.76	<0.001	5.80 ± 0.76	6.25 ± 0.99	0.08
180th minute after spinal anesthesia	76.80 ± 3.88	83.40 ± 4.59	<0.001	5.72 ± 0.68	6.33 ± 1.05	0.019

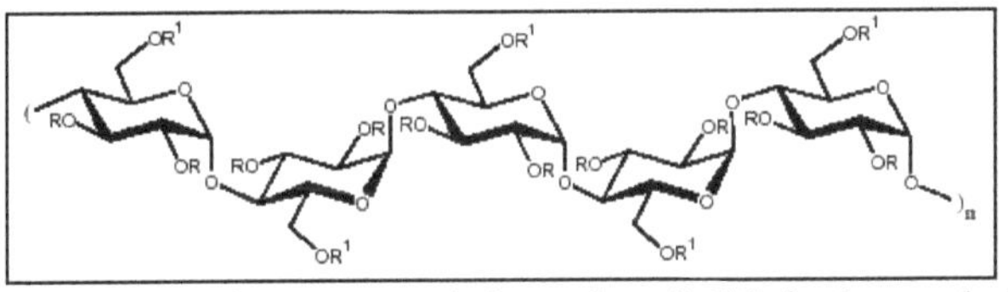

Figure 1. The structural formula of 6% hydroxyethyl starch.

Then, from the fifth minute to the end of the study, there was a slowdown increase (despite slight reductions at some time points). In Figure 2, changes in mean diastolic blood pressure are presented for both groups (i.e., hydroxyethyl starch and normal saline groups). The analysis of variance for repeated measures depicted the following issues:

1) The changes in mean diastolic blood pressure of the participants during the study period were not statistically significant (P value: 0.084 and F=1.89),

2) The effect of the prescribed drug on the changes in diastolic blood pressure was statistically significant (P=0.001 and F=4.05); in other words, in patients

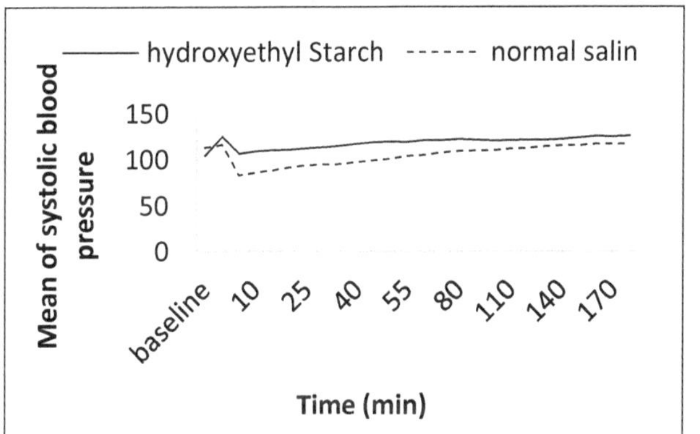

Figure 2. Changes in Mean Systolic Blood Pressure of Groups under Investigation (i.e., hydroxyethyl starch and normal saline groups).

treated with hydroxyethyl starch, the diastolic blood pressure drop was significantly lower than that of those for whom normal saline was prescribed,

3) Gender had no significant effect on the changes in the mean diastolic blood pressure of the participants

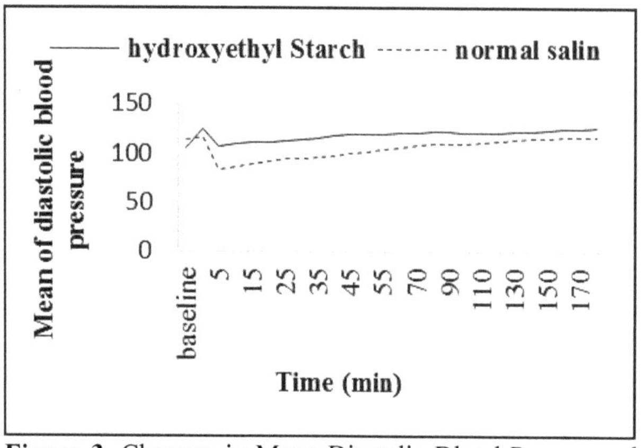

Figure 3. Changes in Mean Diastolic Blood Pressure of Groups under Investigation (I.E., Hydroxyethyl Starch and Normal Saline Groups).

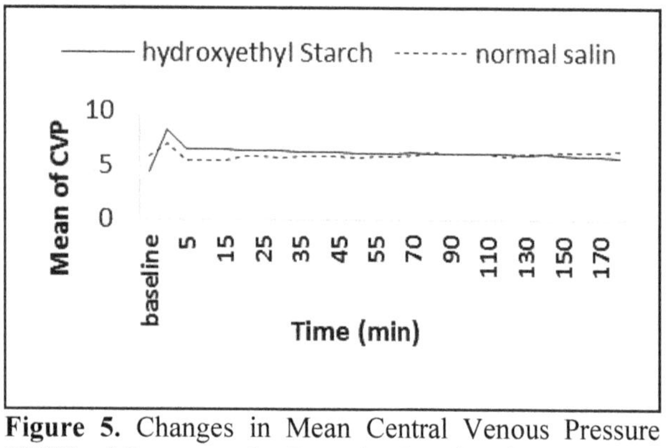

Figure 5. Changes in Mean Central Venous Pressure (CVP) of Groups under Investigation (i.e., hydroxyethyl starch and normal saline groups).

during the study period (P-value = 0.464 and F=0.94); in other words, the changes in mean diastolic blood pressure in males and females did not significantly differ,

4) Age had no significant effect on the changes in the mean diastolic blood pressure of the participants during the study period (P-value: 0.287 and F = 1.26), and

5) There was no significant interaction between gender and prescribed drugs; in other words, the effect of hydroxyethyl starch on diastolic blood pressure changes in males and females did not significantly differ (P value: 0.629 and F = 0.72).

Heart Rate

The mean heart rate based on measurement time and intervention group type (i.e., normal saline and hydroxyethyl starch groups) is presented in Table 1. According to this table, the mean heart rate significantly increased in both groups after completion of infusion compared to the baseline values, and 5

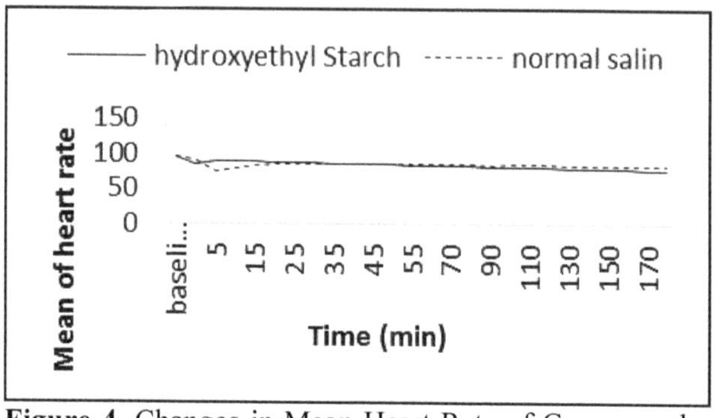

Figure 4. Changes in Mean Heart Rate of Groups under Investigation (I.E., Hydroxyethyl Starch and Normal Saline Groups).

minutes after spinal anesthesia significantly decreased. Then, from the fifth minute to the end of the study, there was a slowdown increase (despite slight reductions at some time points). In Figure 3, changes in mean heart rate are presented for both groups (i.e., hydroxyethyl starch and normal saline groups). The analysis of variance for repeated measures found out the following issues:

1) The changes in mean heart rate of the participants during the study period were not statistically significant (P value: 0.497 and F=0.89),

2) The effect of the prescribed drug on the changes in heart rate was statistically significant (p<0.001 and F=16.58); in other words, in patients treated with hydroxyethyl starch, the heart rate drop was significantly lower than that of those for whom normal saline was prescribed. As it is depicted in the figure, until the thirty-fifth minute, the mean heart rate in the hydroxyethyl starch group was higher than that of the normal saline group, from the 40th minute to the fifty-fifth minute, it was similar in the two groups, and after 50th minute the mean heart rate in the hydroxyethyl starch group was lower than the normal saline group.

3) Gender had no significant effect on the changes in the mean heart rate of the participants during the study period (P-value = 0.394 and F=1.01); in other words, the changes in mean heart rate in males and females did not significantly differ,

4) Age had no significant effect on the changes in the mean central venous pressure of the participants during the study period (P-value: 0.704 and F=0.50), and

5) There was no significant interaction between gender and prescribed drugs; in other words, the effect of hydroxyethyl starch on heart rate changes in males and

females did not significantly differ (P value: 0.101 and F=2.05).

Central Venous Pressure (CVP)

The mean central venous pressure based on measurement time and intervention group type (i.e., normal saline and hydroxyethyl starch groups) is presented in Table 1. According to this table, the mean central venous pressure significantly increased in both groups after completion of infusion compared to the baseline values, and 5 minutes after spinal anesthesia significantly decreased. Then, from the fifth minute to the end of the study, there was a slowdown increase (despite slight reductions at some time points). In Figure 4, changes in mean central venous pressure are presented for both groups (i.e., hydroxyethyl starch and normal saline groups). The analysis of variance for repeated measures revealed the following issues:

1) The changes in mean central venous pressure of the participants during the study period were not statistically significant (P value: 0.596 and F = 5.72),

2) The effect of the prescribed drug on the changes in central venous pressure was statistically significant (P < 0.001 and F = 5.72); in other words, in patients treated with hydroxyethyl starch, the central venous pressure drop was significantly lower than that of those for whom normal saline was prescribed.

3) Gender had no significant effect on the changes in the mean central venous pressure of the participants during the study period (P-value = 0.710 and F = 0.74); in other words, the changes in mean central venous pressure in males and females did not significantly differ,

4) Age had no significant effect on the changes in the mean central venous pressure of the participants during the study period (P-value: 0.656 and F = 0.80), and

5) There was no significant interaction between gender and prescribed drugs; in other words, the effect of hydroxyethyl starch on central venous pressure changes in males and females did not significantly differ (P value=0.462 and F=0.985).

Discussion

In the current study, the effects of hydroxyethyl starch and normal saline on hemodynamic changes after spinal anesthesia in patients undergoing lower limb orthopedic surgery were investigated. The two main options for controlling hemodynamic changes following spinal anesthesia are colloids and crystalloids(17). The role of colloids in improving the hemodynamic changes resulted from spinal anesthesia compared with crystalloids has been confirmed in several studies(18-20).

In this study, hydroxyethyl starch—as one of the known colloidal solutions—was significantly more effective than normal saline—as a standard treatment—in controlling the hemodynamic changes including changes in systolic and diastolic blood pressure, heart rate, and central venous pressure. The mean systolic and diastolic blood pressure drop in patients for whom hydroxyethyl starch was prescribed was significantly lower than that of those for whom normal saline was prescribed. Karinen et al. (21), comparing the effects of crystalloid (lactated Ringer's) and colloidal (hydroxyethyl starch) solutions on hemodynamic changes during spinal anesthesia in cesarean section, showed that the incidence of hypotension after spinal anesthesia in mothers receiving hydroxyethyl starch was lower than mothers receiving lactated Ringer's (38% vs. 62%). In another study, it was demonstrated that immediate infusion of hydroxyethyl starch instantly after spinal anesthesia not only prevented hypertension but also had much more stable effects than lactated Ringer's solution (22). In a clinical trial, Romdhani et al. (23)also compared the effects of hydroxyethyl starch and normal saline on the changes in systolic, diastolic, and arterial blood pressure and heart rate in women who chose cesarean delivery for delivery. In their study, the two groups had just a significant difference in the incidence of hypotension; hence, the incidence of this disorder was significantly lower in the hydroxyethyl starch group than in the other group. However, there was no significant difference between the two groups in terms of preventing heart rate reduction. In a study conducted by Donati et al. (24), there was also no significant difference between the changes in heart rate of the patients receiving hydroxyethyl starch and the control group (no treatment). They attributed this between-groups similarities in heart rate changes to the substantial cardiovascular stability resulted from the selective spinal anesthesia which did not activate a compensatory vagal effect. Meanwhile, in the present study, hydroxyethyl starch was significantly better than normal saline in preventing heart rate reduction.

According to Cook (25), the weaker effect of normal saline in preventing heart rate loss compared with hydroxyethyl starch can be attributed to the weaker ability of this crystalloid solution in maintaining the balance of sympathetic and vagal activity.

The mean of reduction of central venous pressure was also significantly different in the two groups; the hydroxyethyl starch group had totally a lower loss in the mean central pressure. Marhofer et al. (26) also observed that central venous pressure loss of elderly patients, who had been hydrated before spinal anesthesia with hydroxyethyl starch to undergo hip surgery, was significantly less than that of the control group. According to Pollard, one of the reasons for the reduction in central venous pressure after spinal anesthesia is blood loss. For instance, with 10 mL/kg withdrawal blood, the decrease in central venous pressure during spinal anesthesia may be 66% on average. On the other hand, observing the absence of significant changes in the mean central venous pressure during spinal anesthesia, Poon et al. (27) concluded that a significant drop in blood pressure during spinal anesthesia was not due to blood loss during surgery. Based on the results of these two studies and considering the findings of the present study, the mean systolic and diastolic blood pressure drop in the normal saline group was higher than the hydroxyethyl starch group; thus, it can be concluded that the decrease in blood pressure in the normal saline group compared with the hydroxyethyl starch group was probably due to a greater blood loss during surgery.

Conclusion

With regard to the consistency of the results of this study with available sources, it can be determined that the administration of hydroxyethyl starch prior to spinal anesthesia can play a more effective role in controlling hemodynamic changes.

Acknowledgment

The authors would like to thanks Clinical Research Development Center at Shahid Modarres Hospital for his financial support.

Conflicts of Interest

The authors declare that they have no conflict of interest.

References

1. Rai A, Bhutia MP. Dexmedetomidine as an Additive to Spinal Anaesthesia in Orthopaedic Patients Undergoing Lower Limb Surgeries: A Randomized Clinical Trial Comparing Two Different Doses of Dexmedetomidine. Journal of clinical and diagnostic research. J Clin Diagn Res. 2017 Apr; 11(4): UC09–UC12.

2. Park, Y.B., et al., Comparison of Short-Term Complications of General and Spinal Anesthesia for Primary Unilateral Total Knee Arthroplasty. Knee Surg Relat Res. 2017 Jun 1;29(2):96-103.

3. Ahmad, M., M. Ahmad, and N. Atif, haemodynamic preservation in cesarean sections by low dose 0.5% hyperbaric bupivacaine. Journal of Ayub Medical College Abbottabad. 2017;29(2):211-4.

4. Bergenwald L, Eklund B, Kaijser L, Klingenström P, Westermark L. Haemodynamic effects of dihydroergotamine during spinal anaesthesia in man.. Acta Anaesthesiol Scand. 1972;16(4):235-9.

5. Ngan Kee WD, Lee SW, Ng FF, Tan PE, Khaw KS. Randomized double-blinded comparison of norepinephrine and phenylephrine for maintenance of blood pressure during spinal anesthesia for cesarean delivery. Anesthesiology. 2015 Apr;122(4):736-45.

6. Marashi SM, Soltani-Omid S, Soltani Mohammadi S, Aghajani Y, Movafegh A. Comparing Two Different Doses of Intravenous Ondansetron With Placebo on Attenuation of Spinal-induced Hypotension and Shivering. Anesth Pain Med. 2014 Mar 18;4(2):e12055.

7. Pearse RM, Harrison DA, MacDonald N, Gillies MA, Blunt M, Ackland G, Grocott MP, Ahern A, Griggs K, Scott R, Hinds C, Rowan K; OPTIMISE Study Group. Effect of a perioperative, cardiac output-guided hemodynamic therapy algorithm on outcomes following major gastrointestinal surgery: a randomized clinical trial and systematic review. JAMA. 2014 Jun 4;311(21):2181-90.

8. Lim HH, Ho KM, Choi WY, Teoh GS, Chiu KY. The use of intravenous atropine after a saline infusion in the prevention of spinal anesthesia-induced hypotension in elderly patients. Anesth Analg. 2000 Nov;91(5):1203-6.

9. McDonnell NJ, Paech MJ, Muchatuta NA, Hillyard S, Nathan EA. A randomised double-blind trial of phenylephrine and metaraminol infusions for prevention of hypotension during spinal and combined spinal-epidural anaesthesia for elective caesarean section. Anaesthesia. 2017 May;72(5):609-617.

10. Feliu J, Ventura JL, Segura R, Rodas G, Riera J, Estruch A, Zamora A, Capdevila L. Differences between lactate concentration of samples from ear lobe and the finger tip. J Physiol Biochem. 1999;55(4):333-9..

11. Davis AL, Carcillo JA, Aneja RK, Deymann AJ, Lin JC, Nguyen TC, Okhuysen-Cawley RS, Relvas MS, Rozenfeld RA, Skippen PW, Stojadinovic BJ, Williams EA, Yeh TS, Balamuth F, Brierley J, de Caen AR, Cheifetz IM, Choong K, Conway E Jr, Cornell T, Doctor A, Dugas MA, Feldman JD, Fitzgerald JC, Flori HR, Fortenberry JD, Graciano AL, Greenwald BM, Hall MW, Han YY, Hernan LJ, Irazuzta JE, Iselin E, van der Jagt EW, Jeffries HE, Kache S, Katyal

C, Kissoon NT, Kon AA, Kutko MC, MacLaren G, Maul T, Mehta R, Odetola F, Parbuoni K, Paul R, Peters MJ, Ranjit S, Reuter-Rice KE, Schnitzler EJ, Scott HF, Torres A Jr, Weingarten-Abrams J, Weiss SL, Zimmerman JJ, Zuckerberg AL. American College of Critical Care Medicine Clinical Practice Parameters for Hemodynamic Support of Pediatric and Neonatal Septic Shock. Crit Care Med. 2017;45(6):1061-1093.

12. Madhusudan P, Tirupakuzhi Vijayaraghavan BK, Cove ME. Fluid resuscitation in sepsis: reexamining the paradigm. Biomed Res Int. 2014;2014:984082.

13. Nicholson Jp, Wolmarans Mr, Park Gr. The role of albumin in critical illness. Br J Anaesth. 2000 Oct;85(4):599-610.

14. Kaplan SS, Park TS, Gonzales ER, Gidday.JM. Hydroxyethyl starch reduces leukocyte adherence and vascular injury in the newborn pig cerebral circulation after asphyxia. Stroke. 2000;31(9):2218-23.

15. Heesen M, Klimek M, Hoeks SE, Rossaint R. Prevention of Spinal Anesthesia-Induced Hypotension During Cesarean Delivery by 5-Hydroxytryptamine-3 Receptor Antagonists: A Systematic Review and Meta-analysis and Meta-regression. Anesth Analg. 2016;123(4):977-88.

16. Oh AY, Hwang JW, Song IA, Kim MH, Ryu JH, Park HP, Jeon YT, Do SH. Influence of the timing of administration of crystalloid on maternal hypotension during spinal anesthesia for cesarean delivery: preload versus coload. BMC Anesthesiol. 2014 16;14:36.

17. Terkawi AS, Larkin SK, Tsang S, Sheeran JS, Tiouririne M. Effects of hydroxyethyl starch 6 % (130/0.4) on blood loss during cesarean delivery: a propensity-matched analysis. J Anesth. 2016 Oct;30(5):796-802.

18. Upadya M, Bhat S, Paul S. Six percent hetastarch versus lactated Ringer's solution - for preloading before spinal anesthesia for cesarean section. Anesth Essays Res. 2016; 10(1):33-7.

19. Unlugenc H , Turktan M , Evruke IC , Gunduz M , Burgut R , Yapicioglu-Yildizdas H , Isik G. Rapid fluid administration and the incidence of hypotension induced by spinal anesthesia and ephedrine requirement: the effect of crystalloid versus colloid coloading. Middle East J Anaesthesiol. 2015; 23(3):273-81.

20. Ripollés Melchor J, Espinosa Á, Martínez Hurtado E, Casans Francés R, Navarro Pérez R, Abad Gurumeta A, Calvo Vecino JM. Colloids versus crystalloids in the prevention of hypotension induced by spinal anesthesia in elective cesarean section. A systematic review and meta-analysis. Minerva Anestesiol. 2015; 81(9):1019-30.

21. Ueyama H, He YL, Tanigami H, Mashimo T, Yoshiya I. Effects of crystalloid and colloid preload on blood volume in the parturient undergoing spinal anesthesia for elective Cesarean section. Anesthesiology. 1999;91(6):1571-6.

22. Zorko N, Kamenik M, Starc V. The effect of Trendelenburg position, lactated Ringer's solution and 6% hydroxyethyl starch solution on cardiac output after spinal anesthesia. Anesth Analg. 2009 Feb;108(2):655-9.

23. Romdhani C, Trabelsi W, Lebbi A, Naas I, Elaskri H, Gharsallah H, Rachdi R, Ferjani M. Lower incidence of hypotension following spinal anesthesia with 6% hydroxyethyl starch preload compared to 9 ‰ saline solution in caesarean delivery. Tunis Med. 2014; 92(6):406-10.

24. Donati A, Scarcella M, Nardella R, Zompanti V, Sinkovetz L, Iuorio S, Pelaia P. Fluid challenge in patients submitted to spinal block. Minerva Anestesiol. 2007; 73(4):213-8.

25. Cook PR, Malmqvist LA, Bengtsson M, Tryggvason B, Löfström JB. Vagal and sympathetic activity during spinal analgesia. Acta Anaesthesiol Scand. 1990 May;34(4):271-5.

26. Marhofer P, Faryniak B, Oismüller C, Koinig H, Kapral S, Mayer N. Cardiovascular effects of 6% hetastarch and lactated Ringer's solution during spinal anesthesia. Reg Anesth Pain Med. 1999; 24(5):399-404.

27. Poon KS, Wu KC, Chen CC, Fung ST, Lau AW, Huang CC, Wu RS. Hemodynamic changes during spinal surgery in the prone position. Acta Anaesthesiol Taiwan. 2008; 46(2):57-60.

Effect of Acid-Base Balance on Cytokines Serum Levels and Short-Term Outcomes in Kidney Transplant Recipients

Mohammad Fathi[1], Nilofar Massoudi[2*], Navid Noraee[3], Narges-Sadat Ghaemi[2], Dawar Amani[4], Ali Asadirad[4]

Abstract

Background: Control of blood acids and bases can help prevent many potentially life-threatening disorders in end stage renal disease (ESRD) patients. Aim of this study was to assess the effect of acid-base balance on cytokines serum levels and short-term outcomes in kidney transplant recipients.

Materials and Methods: In this randomized clinical trial study, 40 patients with end-stage renal disease aged 18 to 70 who had undergone a kidney transplant from a living donor in Modarres hospital during 2016-2017 were included. The primary outcomes measured in this study were sera levels of cytokine such as IL-2, IL-10, IFN-γ and BUN and Cr serum after the treatment of acidosis in kidney transplant recipients.

Results: Mean±SD of the patient's age was 42±12.6 years. Results showed that there is a significant difference in means of IL-2, IL-10, and IFN-γ between the intervention and control groups over the time (for all $p<0.05$). We also found that correction of acidosis occurred with reduces of IFN-γ to -1.74 in the intervention group compared to the group receiving saline ($P=0.011$); and reduction for IL-2 was -1.37 ($p=0.025$). The concentration of anti-inflammatory cytokine of IL-10 was increased to 2.85 ($P<0.001$).

Conclusion: The results clearly suggest that correction of acidosis in renal transplant patients during surgery helps improve the performance of allograft in the short run; however, more studies are recommended, taking into account the long-term and short-term effects of this intervention.

Keywords: Cytokines, Kidney Transplant, Acid-Base Balance, Clinical Trial

1. Critical Care Quality Improvement Research Center, Shahid Beheshti University of Medical Sciences, Tehran, Iran
2. Anesthesiology Research Center, Shahid Beheshti University of Medical Sciences, Tehran, Iran.
3. Clinical Research and Development Unit at Shahid Modarres Hospital, Department of Anesthesiology, Shahid Beheshti University of Medical Sciences, Tehran, Iran.
4. Department of Immunology, School of Medicine, Shahid Beheshti University of Medical Sciences, Tehran, Iran.

*Corresponding Author: Nilofar Massoudi, MD, Assistant Professor of Anesthesia, Anesthesiology Research Center, Shahid Beheshti University of Medical Sciences, Tehran, Iran.

Email: nilomassoudi@gmail.com

Introduction

Nowadays kidney transplant as the main treatment for end-stage renal failure, has become one of the most common types of transplant and hence a big step in improving the life quality and expectancy. In the history of treatment, the life expectancy of post-transplant patients has greatly increased and the percentage of successful transplants continues to rise (1). From the beginning stages of kidney transplant therapy to now, there have been many changes in anesthesia techniques and surgical methods as well as post-transplant aftercare, which have altogether helped improve longevity of the graft (2). Given the delicacy and importance of anesthesia as well as its important role in the success of transplant, there has been a growing body of literature on this treatment and any attempt to improve the quality of the anesthesia could play a major role in the survival of the patients (3). Patients with kidney failure suffer from chronic metabolic acidosis, hyponatremia, hypokalemia, and hyperchloraemia, which can potentially cause certain arrhythmias including bradycardia, heart block, hypotension, neuromuscular disorders as well as dyspnea and respiratory failure. In this regard, the control of acids and bases help prevent many potentially life-threatening disorders in these patients (4, 5). Given the importance of immunological factors in the transplant success or rejection, it is required to perform certain immunological compatibility experiments before transplantation, which is normally done in the transplant unit. The measurement of serum cytokines is helpful in evaluating the immunological status of the patient and assessing the effects of acidosis correction on immunological parameters. For example TNF- β , IFN- γ and IL-2 are important mediators of transplant rejection. IL-2 is essential in reproduction of T cells and production of efficient CTLs. IFN- γ plays the central role in the formation of delayed-type hypersensitivity response, macrophages infiltration into connective tissue, activation of them and conversion of them into destructive cells (6). The IL-2 and IFN-γ are among the cytokines reinforcing the cellular immune response, and their increased serum levels suggest poor prognosis of the transplantation. This is the fact while IL-10 represents an anti-inflammatory cytokine and inhibits the cellular immune response and, at the same time, increases the probability of a successful transplantation (7). The purpose of the present study was to evaluate the effect of acid-base balance on cytokines serum levels and short-term outcomes in kidney transplant recipients.

Methods

Study design

The present study was a randomized clinical trial with parallel design performed with a 1-1 ratio for the intervention and placebo group in Tehran Shahid Modarres Hospital (is the only governmental facility in north-western Tehran). The study population consisted of all patients with end-stage renal disease who were candidate for a kidney transplant from a living donor, had visited the kidney transplant unit of the hospital from late April in 2016 to early February in 2017, and had undergone a treatment with sodium bicarbonate (intervention group) or placebo (control group). The study participants included 40 patients with end-stage renal disease aged 18 to 70 who had undergone a kidney transplant from a living donor. We used a probabilistic sampling strategy for selection the included participants. To do this, a simple random sampling was considered by using random digit table.

The study inclusion criteria were: A. ASA Class I – II, B. Age range between 18 and 70 years and consent to participate in the study. The exclusion criteria were: A. Patients with end-stage cardiovascular problems, B. Metabolic acidosis with pH less than 7.15, C. Operation duration more than 3 hours, D. Body temperature less than 35 or greater than 38.5°C axilla before or during the operation, E. The need for blood transfusions during the operation, F. age over 70 or under 18 years, G. kidney transplant from a nonliving donor, H. a history of cancer and immunological diseases and immune modulatory medications.

Balanced block randomization techniques were used in the present study to randomly assign the participants in two intervention and control groups. Since blocking was done in 4 units in this study, a series of the random numbers 1 to 6 were produced using STATA to reach the desired sample size. Given that there are in total 6 states to arrange two subjects' in 4 blocks, if the number obtained were more than 6, the next number was produced without considering it. The sequences of balanced block randomization were obtained and put in sealed envelopes numbered with a 5-digit serial number by a third person who was not involved in the study design. All the envelopes (42 persons) had a random 5-digit serial number and were immediately opened after completion of the basic information and tests of the subjects, allocating them to intervention group (receiving sodium bicarbonate) and placebo group (normal saline). The primary outcomes measured in this study were changes of serum cytokine such as IL-2, IL-10, IFN-γ and BUN and Cr serum after the treatment of acidosis in kidney transplant recipients. The baseline clinical and demographic data of the patient such as age, sex, weight, time elapsed since the last hemodialysis, start time of base ESRD and ABG, the ABG when opening the clamp and registration of TOF from the end of the induction to the end of operation were all entered in the patient's information form.

Treatment of metabolic acidosis

The study was conducted as follows: before induction of anesthesia, a catheter no.18 was implanted for fluids and medication. Invasive monitoring of blood pressure was performed under local anesthesia after Allen's test using an artery catheter no.20 through the radial artery of the nondominant hand. The same catheter was used to take arterial blood samples at the beginning of operation and on opening the clamps. First, the patients were preoxygenated with 100% oxygen for 3 minutes; then, based on a medical indication, midazolam with a dosage of 0.02 mg per kg and fentanyl 2μ/Kg were used. For induction of anesthesia, thiopental sodium with a dosage of 5 mg per kg was used. For muscle relaxation, atracurium with a dosage of 0.5 mg per kg was injected slowly. For maintenance of anesthesia, isoflurane with a dosage of 0.6-1% was used together with nitrous oxide at a ratio of 50%. During operation, if necessary, additional dosages of Atracurium were used. It is noteworthy that the last dose of Atracurium was administered while opening the clamp. After induction, central venous line was implanted through the right jugular vein. During the operation, the central venous pressure (CVP) was obtained at 10-12 cmH_2O and the patient's temperature was kept constant at 36°C and the patients in both groups were administered IV Lasix with the same dosage of 3 mg per kg and intravenous mannitol with a dosage of 0.5 g per kg. During this process, none of the patients included in the study required any blood infusion. Similarly, saline fluid at a rate of 50 ml per kilogram of body weight was used in all cadaver donors. Arterial blood samples of all the subjects were sent to the laboratory to analyze Arterial pH, arterial bicarbonate (HCO3), BE (Base Excess) and Pressure of Arterial carbon dioxide (PaCO2) after induction of anesthesia. Other blood samples were sent to the laboratory on opening the clamps. During the first week after transplantation, BUN, Cr and 24-hour urine volume were measured and the blood samples were taken and sent to immunology laboratory to check for the pre-induction immunologic markers before induction and once after opening the clamps. Blood samples and serum were taken from all the study participants at appropriate times (before correction of acidosis, after correction of acidosis and 7 days after operation) to measure the cytokines (IL-2, IL-10, IFN-γ).

The cytokines were measured using ELISA according to the instructions of the manufacturer's kit in the Laboratory of Department of Immunology, Shahid Beheshti University of Medical Sciences. A sample size of 21 patients in each group will be sufficient to detect a clinically important difference between the intervention and control group, using a two-tailed t-test of the difference between means, a power of 80%, and a significance level of 5%. The calculation is based on the assumption that the measurements on main variables are normally distributed.

ELISA assay

Levels of IFN γ, IL-2, and IL-10 in serum were measured using specific ELISA kits (Mabtech, Nacka Strand, Sweden), according to the manufacturer's instructions. All measurements were carried out in duplicates. OPD was used as chromogenic substrates for horseradish peroxidase (HRP). Color intensity in samples/standard wells was measured at 492 nm using an Anthos 2020 microplate reader (Anthos, Wals, Austria). Values of each protein of interest in a sample were calculated by extrapolation from standard curves generated in parallel with kit-provided standards. The level of sensitivity of the kits was 4-400 pg ml-1 for IFNγ, / IL-2 and 2-200 pg ml-1 for IL-10. Furthermore, to prevent the information bias due to measurement error, all the devices are calibrated regularly.

Statistical analysis

Continuous baseline demographic and clinical data are presented as mean ± standard deviation and grouped data as frequencies and percentages. Chi-square test or Fisher's exact test were used to determine the independence of the two categorical variables. Repeated measures of ANOVA were employed to investigate the mean differences of immune factors such as IL-2, IL-10 and IFN-γ between the groups over the time. To investigate the association between the treatment of metabolic acidosis and changes in serum Cr and BUN as well as immune factors such as IL-2, IL-10 and IFN-γ, the generalized estimation equation (GEE) method was undertaken. The GEE is a widely used estimation method for marginal (i.e., population-averaged) modeling of repeated data. In brief, GEEs use the generalized linear model to estimate more efficient and unbiased regression parameters relative to ordinary least squares regression, in part because they permit specification of a working correlation matrix that accounts for the form of within-subject correlation of responses on dependent variables of many different distributions, including normal, binomial, and Poisson (8). All analyses were done using STATA statistical software (version 13MP).

Ethical committee of Shahid Beheshti University of Medical Sciences (IR.SBMU.RAM.REC.1394.390;IRCT2015092712203N4) approved this study.

Results

In the present study, we used data from 40 ESRD patients candidate for receiving a kidney transplant from a living donor visiting Shahid Modarres Hospital in Tehran in 2016. As the figure below shows, finally and after excluding, in each group, 15 people failing to meet the inclusion criteria and 2 more ones who were lost to follow up, 20 patients were examined and analyzed.

In this study, the mean and standard deviation of age of the patients was 42±12.6 years. Of those examined, 29 ones (72.5%) were male and the rest were females (11 participants equivalent to 27.5%), respectively. The basic clinical information for the subjects in both groups is presented in Table 1.

The independent t-test determining the difference of the mean serum creatinine between the two groups shows that from the first to sixth day, there is no significant difference between the mean serum creatinine in the two groups and that the difference was observed only on the seventh day (P = 0.038).

In this study, generalized estimation equations models (GEE) was used to evaluate the effect of treatment on outcomes of creatinine and BUN concentrations in serum. The models are presented in Table 2.

The results showed that, the treatment of patient's acidosis did not affect serum creatinine levels. In other words, although the decrease in serum creatinine over time is statistically significant (p <0.001), this reduction is not attributable to the treatment of acidosis in kidney-transplant patients and there was no difference in the creatinine reduction between the intervention and control group. The results also show that correction of acidosis in kidney-transplant patients resulted in a significant reduction in BUN serum levels in the intervention group compared to the control group (Coefficient= -0.25, 95% CI:-0.5, -0.01). It should be noted, however, that the interaction effects between treatment and time were also significant and this means that treatment at different times would have different effects. Similarly, on investigating 24-hour urine volume within 7 days after transplantation in the intervention group (treatment of acidosis with bicarbonate) and control group (saline), the results of independent t-test showed that there was no statistically significant difference in average urine output between the control group (7870±478cc) and the intervention group (6973±445mL) (P =0.17). It should also be said that, following the investigation of the first-to-seventh-day urinary output in the two groups, the urine output was within the normal range in all the days except for the first day (due to intense hydration) and no statistical difference was observed (p> 0.05). Figure 2 shows the changes in the mentioned outcomes during 7 days after transplantation.

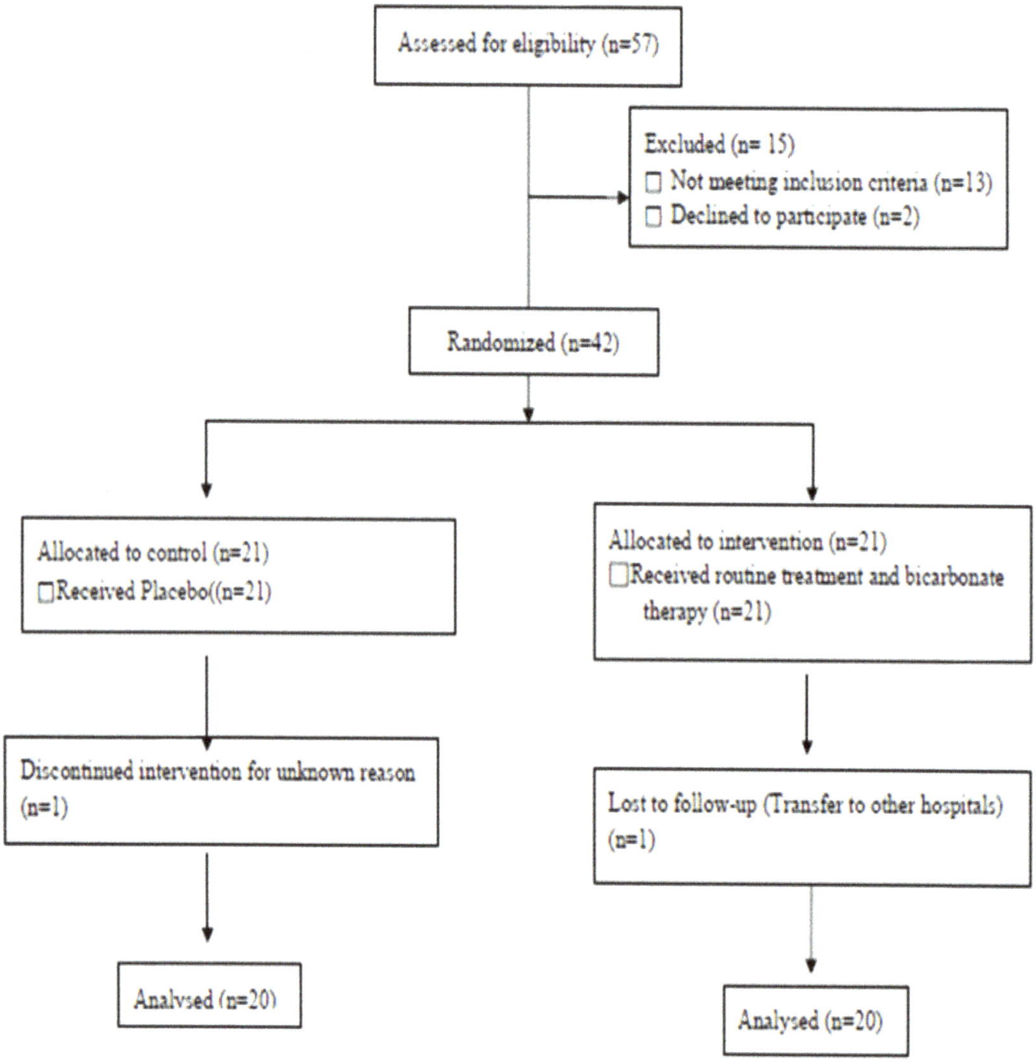

Figure 1. Flowchart of the studied participants.

The repeated measures of ANOVA showed that there is a significant difference in means of IL-2, IL-10, and IFN-γ between the intervention and control groups over the time (Table 3). Also, the mean changes of the factors under study over time and following the treatment of acidosis were statistically significant, in a way that with respect to the factors IFN-γ and IL-2, these changes were decremental in the intervention group and fairly incremental in the control group, while the changes of the factors IL-10 were contrary to those above. In all the models above, Mauchly's Test of Sphericity was meaningful; accordingly, Greenhouse-Geisser statistic was used.

The changes of the three factors examined are shown in Figure 3. In this figure, the time 1 represents that before the transplant, the time 2 represents the first day after the transplant and the time 3 represents the seventh day after the transplant.

For more tangible results in this study, GEE modeling approach was used to evaluate the effect of treatment on immunological factors. The results are given in Table 4. The results show that the time factor and its interaction with the type of treatment has a significant impact on the outcome under study and this means that the treatment has different effects in different times (the P interaction value is < 0.001 for all outcomes as shown in Table 4).

The table shows that correction of acidosis in

Table 1: Baseline characteristics and clinical data.

Baseline Variables	Intervention group Mean (SD)	Control group Mean (SD)
Arterial PH	7.29±0.09	7.30±0.07
Arterial HCO3 (mmol/l)	16.4±4.1	16.6±2.71
Arterial PaCO2 (mmol/l)	32.3±7.3	30.1±3.73
Base excess (mEq/l)	-10.6±4.29	-8.35±3
BUN(mg/dl)	72.8±24.3	85±27.3
Cr(mg/dl)	3.54±1.48	3.9±1.56
IFN-γ(pg/ml)	8.41 (7.09-11.82)	9.14 (8.23-10.7)
IL-10 (pg/ml)	5.75 (3.51-9.17)	3.83 (2.71-7.84)
IL-2 (pg/ml)	7.34 (5.69- 7.88)	6.94(5.73-8.15)

Table 2: Results for the model of generalized equations structural analysis for investigation of the effects of acidosis treatment on Cr and BUN outcomes.

Outcomes	Variables	Coefficient,% 95 CI	P-value
Cr	Group	-0.009 (-0.26, 0.24)	0.93
	Time	-0.15 (-0.18, -0.12)	<0.001
	Interaction *	-0.015 (-0.05, -0.02)	0.42
BUN	Group	-0.25 (-0.5, -0.01)	0.041
	Time	-0.08 (-0.11, -0.05)	<0.001
	Interaction	0.049 (0.01, 0.08)	0.013

*Group time

Table 3: Results of repeated measures of ANOVA on evaluating the effects of acidosis treatment on outcomes IL-2, IL-10, IFN-γ.

Factors		Mean square	F	P value
IFN-γ	Group	91.59	6.29	0.017
	Factor	8.6	3.8	0.041
	Group * Factor	82.4	36.3	<0.001
IL-2	Group	56.84	4.9	0.033
	Factor	9.3	5.1	0.008
	Group * Factor	32.1	17.5	<0.001
IL-10	Group	245.01	12:54	0.001
	Factor	25.1	6.85	0.002
	Group * Factor	118.7	32.1	<0.001

patients reduces the IFN-γ by a factor of -1.74 in the intervention group compared to the group receiving saline (P=0.011). Also, the results showed that the levels of IL-2 was decreased after the treatment by a factors of -1.37 in intervention group compared to control group (p=0.025). The concentration of anti-inflammatory cytokine of IL-10 was incremental by a factor of 2.85 in intervention group compared to control group (P<0.001).

Discussion

The results of this study indicate that treatment of metabolic acidosis during the operation in patients undergoing kidney transplantation is effective in improving the outcome of transplant and the performance of kidney in these patients. In addition, it can enhanced in terms of functional factors, including BUN serum and the factors linked with the cellular immunity of the transplant, including the cytokines IL-2, IL-10, IFN-γ.

In the past two decades, the short-term outcomes of transplant have considerably improved,

Table 4: Results of GEE model on evaluating the effects of acidosis treatment on immunological factors.

Outcomes	Variables	Coefficient,% 95 CI	P-value
IFN-γ	Group	-1.74 (-3.09, -0.39)	0.011
	Time	-0.44 (-1.04, -0.03)	0.033
IL-2	Group	-1.37 (-2.57, -0.17)	0.025
	Time	-0.45 (-0.89, -0.004)	0.048
IL-10	Group	2.85 (1.29, 4.41)	<0.001
	Time	0.65 (0.01, 1.31)	0.044

but the corresponding long-term outcomes have hardly enhanced (9). Chronic renal transplant dysfunction is among the most common reasons leading to graft loss, which is evaluated by measuring kidney function over time. Several studies have been conducted to evaluate short-term and long-term performance of transplant. In these studies, the function of the kidneys is evaluated through clinical indices such as serum creatinine, glomerular filtration rate, and creatinine clearance. Moreover, the slope of the regression line of each of the above indices is determined, in terms of time, as the rate of progression in the transplant population and the patients with chronic kidney disease (10-12). In this study, to investigate the performance of transplant allograft within 7 days from the transplantation, the metabolic acidosis factor and its impact on the transplant outcome have been taken into account with emphasis on immune factors associated with transplant rejection besides the factors mentioned above.

Metabolic acidosis, occurring because of reduced serum concentrations of CO_2, can have adverse effects leading to rejection, depending on the patient's condition and the type of transplant. In a study conducted by Park et al, there was reported a risk of rejection following the increased serum concentrations of CO_2 at approximately 74 (13). In various studies, the prevalence of metabolic acidosis in kidney transplant patients was reported even up to 58 percent, and it is essential to address it considering the effects of this phenomenon on the outcome of kidney transplantation (14). Acidosis in kidney transplant patients is particularly important because, in addition to adverse effects on the hemodynamic system, it increases the production of cytokines and the activity of neutrophils in the body, which is ultimately detrimental to the transplant (15). Similarly, certain studies have addressed the role of post-transplant acidosis in mineral metabolism disorder in the body and its effect on the outcome of transplantation (14).

The present study suggests that short-term treatment of acidosis with bicarbonate sodium in the intervention group (compared to control group) leads to a reduction in BUN serum concentration with a coefficient of -0.25 within seven days after the transplantation, indicating the proper functioning allograft in this period. It should be noted that monitoring of metabolic acidosis in patients with ESRD should be done on a regular basis at least 1 year after transplantation. It important in order to maintain serum concentrations of CO_2 higher than 21 mEq/l, because the interaction of various factors such as metabolic acidosis caused by improper functioning of allograft, immune factors related to transplantation and the patient's condition may lead to acute rejection (16, 17). The results also suggest that treatment of acidosis does not significantly increase creatinine clearance in the intervention group compared to the control group and that both groups gradually witnessed an increase in clearance. However, in this study, reduced serum creatinine was not helpful in the treatment of metabolic acidosis, which is not the case for the studies by other researchers (18). The present study shows that the cytokines IFN-γ and interleukin 2 underwent a reduction after the treatment and correction of metabolic acidosis in patients while IL-10 began increasing. The study by Ori et al. evaluating the effects of correction of acidosis on cytokine secretion in patients with chronic kidney problem showed that the treatment of acidosis in CKD patients leads to decrease desecration of IL-10 but other chemokine including IL-1 β, IL-2, IL-6, TNF α, IFN γ, IL-1ra did not change significantly compared to before the transplant (19). In other study

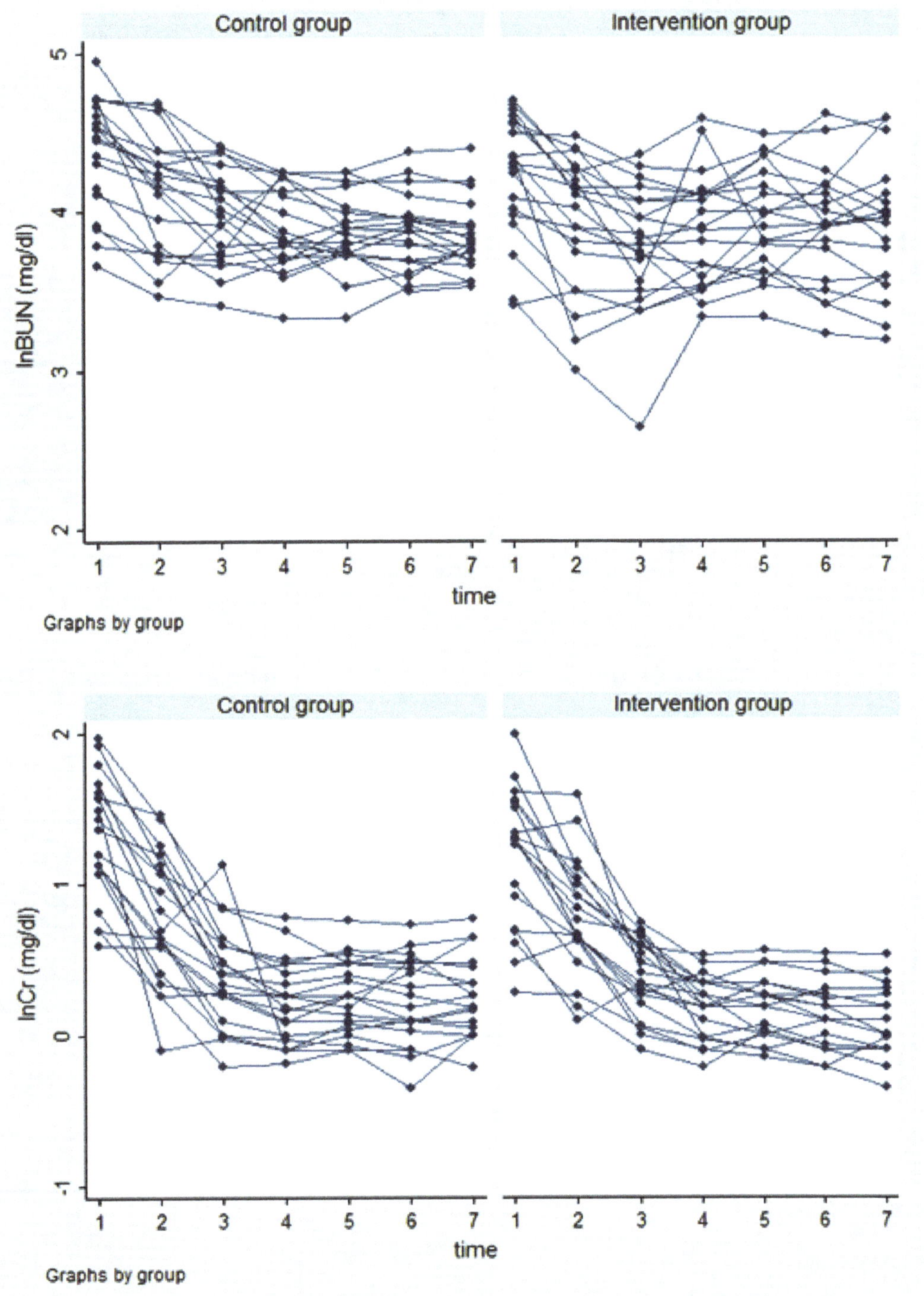

Figure 2. The changes of serum creatinine and BUN during seven days after kidney transplant.

on chronic antibody-mediated rejection and improper performance of allograft, it was shown that in this type of patients, the graft survival can greatly improve simply by regulating the IFNγ secretion (20).

The present study clearly demonstrates that treatment of metabolic acidosis in kidney transplant patients during anesthesia within seven days after transplantation leads to improved outcome of a transplant by reducing the secretion of IL-2 and Interferon Gamma. It should be noted, however, that the outcome of transplant is not affected by treatment of renal tubular acidosis alone and that

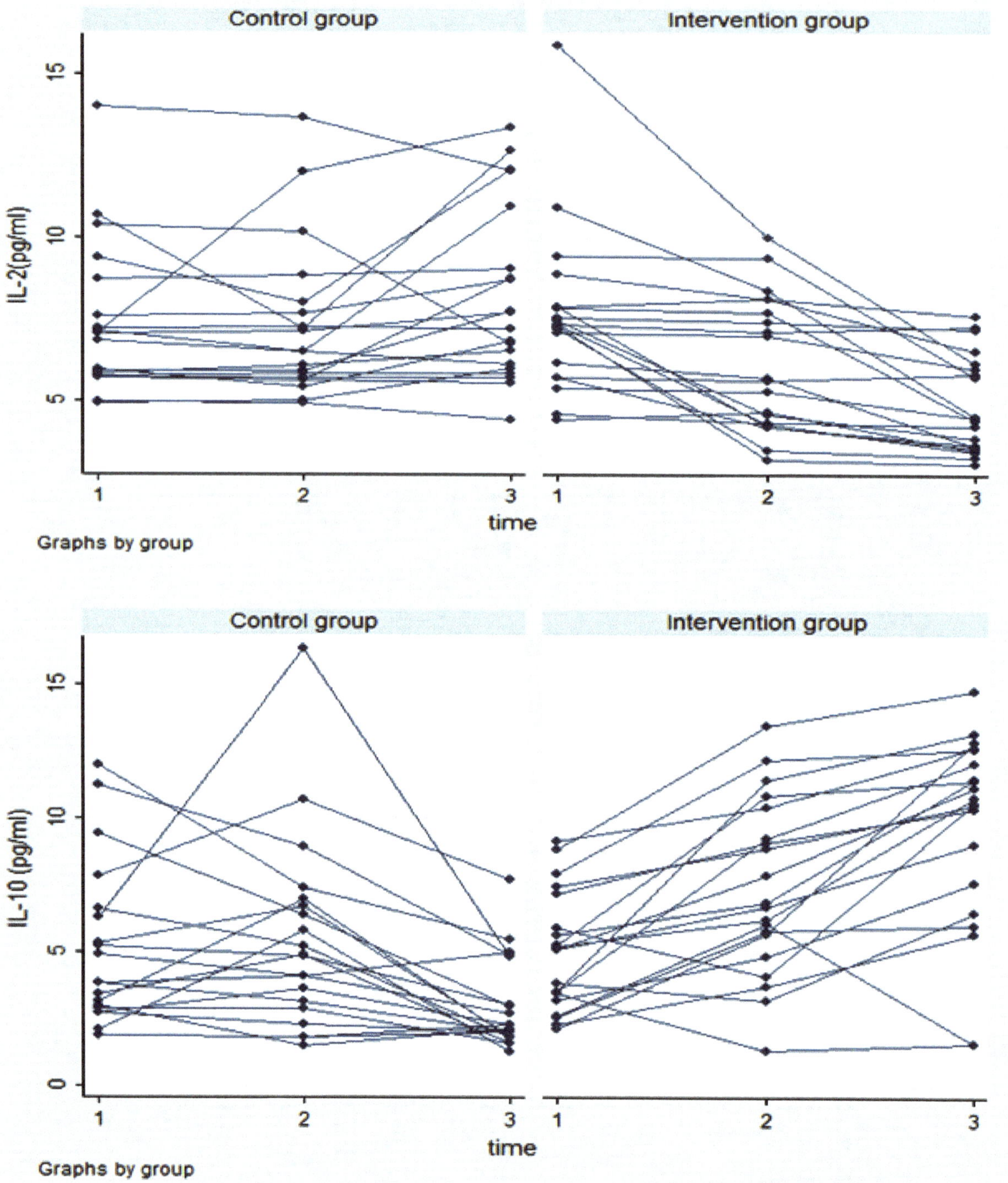

Figure 3. Change pattern of IL-2 and IL-10 during seven days after kidney transplantation.

immunosuppressive regimen, immune factors, personal characteristics and type of the graft are all effective in transplant rejection (17). For example, in a study on the effects of Interferon Gamma on the outcome, the researchers recommended that Pre-transplant determination of the numbers of IFN-γ-producing donor-specific memory cells be performed to predict acute rejection of transplanted cells and then the transplantation be carried out (21).

Despite the fact that metabolic acidosis is a common problem in kidney transplantation and can have negative effects, there is little information on this topic (22). The first issue is lack of awareness about the exact prevalence of acidosis in kidney transplant patients and how it changes over time. The second issue is that there are not still extensive studies with sufficient sample size to make sure that the patients benefit from the correction of this disorder. The other issue is the uncertainty as to what extent of Acidosis should undergo treatment and what the ideal stage of this treatment is. Among the strengths of the present study is that it is the first to have addressed the effect of Acidosis correction on the outcome of kidney transplantation in patients. Although the results clearly suggest that correction of acidosis in renal transplant patients during surgery helps improve the performance of allograft in the short run, it is recommended that more extensive studies are carried out taking into account the long-term and short-term effects of this intervention and its cost-effectiveness for full investigation of the various aspects of correction of metabolic acidosis in kidney transplant patients.

Conclusion

Although the results clearly suggest that correction of acidosis in renal transplant patients during surgery helps improve the performance of allograft in the short run, but it is recommended that more studies be carried out taking into account the long-term and short-term effects of this intervention.

Acknowledgment

The authors would like to acknowledge the Clinical Development Unite (CRDU), at Shahid Modarres Hospital, Shahid Beheshti Medical Sciences, Tehran, Iran for consultation. This project was funded by Anesthesiology Research Center, Shahid Beheshti Medical Sciences, Tehran, Iran.

Conflicts of Interest

The authors declare that they have no conflict of interest.

References

1. Neuberger JM, Bechstein WO, Kuypers DR, Burra P, Citterio F, De Geest S, et al. Practical Recommendations for Long-term Management of Modifiable Risks in Kidney and Liver Transplant Recipients: A Guidance Report and Clinical Checklist by the Consensus on Managing Modifiable Risk in Transplantation (COMMIT) Group. Transplantation. 2017;101(4S Suppl 2):S1-S56.

2. Gondos A, Döhler B, Brenner H, Opelz G. Kidney graft survival in Europe and the United States: strikingly different long-term outcomes. Transplantation. 2013;95(2):267-74.

3. Spiro MD, Eilers H. Intraoperative care of the transplant patient. Anesthesiol Clin. 2013;31(4):705-21.

4. Witham MD, Lamb EJ. Should chronic metabolic acidosis be treated in older people with chronic kidney disease? Nephrol Dial Transplant. 2016;31(11):1796-1802.

5. Dobre M, Rahman M, Hostetter TH. Current status of bicarbonate in CKD. J Am Soc Nephrol. 2015;26(3):515-23.

6. Chen W, Bai J, Huang H, Bi L, Kong X, Gao Y, et al. Low proportion of follicular regulatory T cell in renal transplant patients with chronic antibody-mediated rejection. Sci Rep. 2017;7(1):1322.

7. Trojan K, Zhu L, Aly M, Weimer R, Bulut N, Morath C, et al. Association of peripheral NK cell counts with Helios+ IFN- γ–Tregs in patients with good long- term renal allograft function. Clin Exp Immunol. 2017;188(3):467-79.

8. Wang Y, McDermott S, Mann JR, Hardin JW. Preventing intellectual disability during pregnancy: what are the potentially high yield targets? J Perinat Med. 2016 1;44(4):421-32.

9. Karthikeyan V, Karpinski J, Nair RC, Knoll G. The burden of chronic kidney disease in renal transplant recipients. Am J Transplant. 2004;4(2):262-9..

10. Kukla A, Adulla M, Pascual J, Samaniego M, Nanovic L, Becker BN, et al. CKD stage-to-stage progression in native and transplant kidney disease. Nephrol Dial Transplant. 2008;23(2):693-700.

11. Gill JS, Tonelli M, Mix CH, Pereira BJ. The change in allograft function among long-term kidney transplant recipients. J Am Soc Nephrol. 2003;14(6):1636-42.

12. Massarweh NN, Clayton JL, Mangum CA, Florman SS, Slakey DP. High body mass index and short-and long-term renal allograft survival in adults. Transplantation. 2005;80(10):1430-4.

13. Park S, Kang E, Park S, Kim YC, Han SS, Ha J, et al. Metabolic Acidosis and Long-Term Clinical Outcomes in Kidney Transplant Recipients. J Am Soc Nephrol. 2017;28(6):1886-97.

14. Yakupoglu HY, Corsenca A, Wahl P, Wüthrich RP, Ambühl PM. Posttransplant acidosis and associated disorders of mineral metabolism in patients with a renal graft. Transplantation. 2007;84(9):1151-7.

15. Kellum JA, Song M, Li J. Science review: extracellular acidosis and the immune response: clinical and physiologic implications. Crit Care. 2004;8(5):331-6.

16. Keven K, Ozturk R, Sengul S, Kutlay S, Ergun I, Erturk S, et al. Renal tubular acidosis after kidney transplantation—incidence, risk factors and clinical implications. Nephrol Dial Transplant. 2007;22(3):906-10.

17. Chinen J, Buckley RH. Transplantation immunology: solid organ and bone marrow. J Allergy Clin Immunol. 2010;125(2 Suppl 2):S324-35.

18. Katalinić L, Blaslov K, Đanić-Hadžibegović A, Gellineo L, Kes P, Jelaković B, et al. METABOLIC ACIDOSIS--AN UNDERESTIMATED PROBLEM AFTER KIDNEY

TRANSPLANTATION? Acta Clin Croat. 2015;54(4):486-91.
19. Ori Y, Zingerman B, Bergman M, Bessler H, Salman H. The effect of sodium bicarbonate on cytokine secretion in CKD patients with metabolic acidosis. Biomed Pharmacother. 2015;71:98-101.
20. Shiu KY, McLaughlin L, Rebollo-Mesa I, Zhao J, Burton H, Douthwaite H, et al. Graft dysfunction in chronic antibody-mediated rejection correlates with B-cell–dependent indirect antidonor alloresponses and autocrine regulation of interferon-γ production by Th1 cells. Kidney Int. 2017; 91(2): 477–492..
21. Slavcev A, Rybakova K, Svobodova E, Slatinska J, Honsova E, Skibova J, Viklicky O, Striz I. Pre-transplant donor-specific Interferon-gamma-producing cells and acute rejection of the kidney allograft. Transpl Immunol. 2015;33(2):63-8..
22. Messa PG, Alfieri C, Vettoretti S. Metabolic acidosis in renal transplantation: neglected but of potential clinical relevance. Nephrol Dial Transplant. 2016;31(5):730-6.

18

Treacher Collins Syndrome; Anesthetic considerations and Molecular Findings

Shahram Sayyadi[1], Morteza Jabbari Moghadam[1], Alireza Mirkheshti[1], Elham Memary[1], Dariush Abtahi[1], Sohrab Salimi[1], Ardeshir Tajbakhsh[1*]

1. MD, Anesthesiology Research Center, Shahid Beheshti University of Medical Sciences, Tehran, Iran

*Corresponding Author: Ardeshir Tajbakhsh, MD, Assistant Professor, Anesthesiology Research Center, Shahid Beheshti University of Medical Science, Tehran, Iran;

Email: ardeshir.tajbakhsh@gmail.com

Abstract

Treacher Collins Syndrome (TCS) is a rare disease with mandibulofacial dysostosis. The deformities accompanied by this syndrome could cause especial challenges for anesthesiologist. On the other hand Treacher protein is well recognized in the pathogenesis of this syndrome. In this report we want to present a successful management of a patient with Treacher Collins syndrome and also describe new advances in the molecular aspect of this disease.

Keywords: Treacher Collins Syndrome, Mandibulofacial Dysostosis, Anesthesia, Treacher Protein

Introduction

Rare genetic disorders are great challenges for Treacher Collins Syndrome (TCS, OMIM number 154500) is named after Edward Treacher Collins, an ophthalmologist from London who described this disorder in 1900 (1, 2). In 1949, Franceschetti and Klein described more features and coined the term mandibulofacial dysostosis. It is an autosomal dominant disorder of craniofacial morphogenesis with high penetrance and variable expressivity. It has the frequency of 1 in 50 000 live births and about 60%-90% of them are *de novo* mutations in treacle gene (TCOF1) (1, 2). Up to 130 mutations are reported for this gene and most of them are deletions (1). Treacle protein is essential for proper development of cranial neural crest cells (CNCC) (2). Other mutations are found like POLR1C and POLR1D in which the pattern would be autosomal recessive. TCOF1 is located in chromosome 5q31.3-32 and encodes a serine/alanine rich nucleolar phosphoprotein (treacle protein) which is responsible for the craniofacial development, proliferation, and differentiation of neural crest cells by affecting ribosomes (3, 4). This gene is responsible for 80% of the cases. POLR1C and POLR1D encode subunits of RNA polymerases I and III which are also essential for ribosome biogenesis.

This syndrome contains a congenital malformation of the 1st and 2nd branchial arches (5). The craniofacial abnormalities involve underdevelopment of zygomatic arch, mandible, hard palate and oral cavity (3). These deformities could result in choanal stenosis or dysphagia. These patients also have ocular abnormalities including antimongoloid slanting of the palpebral fissures, and abnormalities if external and middle ear structures resulting in hearing loss. Microcephaly and behavior abnormalities also reported in several cases. These abnormalities could involve: Hypoplastic malars, mandibular hypoplasia, micrognathia, pharyngeal hypoplasia, cleft palate, obstructive sleep apnea, choanal stenosis or atresia, tooth agenesis, conductive hearing loss, microtia, preauricular Tags, eyelid coloboma (6), strabismus, dacrostenosis, microphthalmia, macrostomia, High arch palate, psychomotor delay (2). In spite of heterogeneity of clinical presentations there has not been any explanation for it. The variety of epigenetic factors, gene modifiers and the role of non-mutated genes are proposed (1). The diagnosis is made by thorough clinical evaluation, detailed history and identification of characteristic physical findings. In some cases X-Rays could be helpful.

There is not any clinical therapy for this syndrome. Therefore, early intervention is important to ensure that affected child could reach his/her potential. These interventions include speech therapy, special social support and genetic counseling. Surgery might be indicated in patients with cleft palate, zygomatic or orbital reconstruction, external and inner ear reconstruction.

Brief Report

A 24-year- old boy (153 cm; 45 kg) with TCS was scheduled due to revision of strabismus under general anesthesia. He did not have any past medical or surgical history except characteristic facial appearance of TCS (Fig 1). Thyromental distance was 35 mm and open mouth was one finger. The Mallampati score of four was detected. Preoperative laboratory tests were all within normal limits and no abnormal findings were shown on chest radiograph or electrocardiograph. In the operating room, his vital signs were within normal limits and standard monitoring was applied. Due to anticipated difficult airway, oral flexible fiber optic was performed by administering premedication with Amp Atropine 0.5 mg IV and Amp Fentanyl 50 μgr IV. Spray As You Go (SAYGO) technic was performed for analgesia of airway tract. The trachea was successfully intubated with an ID 6.0 mm armored endotracheal tube.

Discussion

All of the proteins in a cell are synthetized by ribosomes, which in term are constructed by transcription of ribosomal RNA (rRNA) by RNA polymerase I and III. This is called ribosome biogenesis. Ribosome biogenesis is a metabolically expensive and complex task for the cell therefore this process is highly regulated by, and integrated with, cell growth, proliferation and differentiation (8). By accepting its great importance, it is surprising that ribosomopathies like Treacher Collins Syndrome exhibit specific clinical phenotype including craniofacial, axial, or limb skeleton as well as hematopoiesis or organogenesis (8).

Watt *et al.* described a zebra fish model for treacher Collins syndrome and proposed the mechanism of the three genes involved in this syndrome (8). They discovered that POLR1C and POLR1D are spatiotemporally and dynamically expressed specially in craniofacial development. In addition, these genes cause disruptions in biogenesis of ribosome resulting in Tp53-dependent neuroepithelial cell death and deficiency of migrating neural crest cells. Their model also showed that genetic inhibition of Tp53 could suppress this phenomenon and there for could be a gate for the treatment of this syndrome (8).

There has not been any correlation between phenotype and genotype although Teber et al. proposed a lower frequency of conductive hearing loss in patients with mutations of the 3′ part of the open reading frame of TCOF1, which do not confirmed by Vincent et al (4, 9). On the other hand, patients with mutations in POLR1D seemed to have a milder phenotype.(9) Vincent et al. reviewed 146 patients with this syndrome and found that 4% of them were affected with this syndrome but do not have ant mutation in these three genes therefore there could be more genes involved in this syndrome yet to be found (9).

As mentioned above these patients may require anesthesia in different stages of their life. The most important anesthetic consideration for these patients is airway management. It is particularly important due to smaller oropharynx, limited mouth opening, mandibular hypoplasia and hypo plastic larynx.

Anesthesiologist should consider effect of age on the condition of anatomy. This is mentioned in literature that the difficulty with intubation could be increased by advanced age (6). different methods of airway management is proposed including: Direct Laryngoscopy, Fiber optic Bronchoscopy, light wands, blind nasal intubation, Supra Glottic Airway Devices, video laryngoscopy, retrograde intubation and tracheostomy. Shin et al. reported airway management with I-Gel (6). Tsujimoto et al. used McGRATH MAC which turned Cormack-Lehane classification grade four ,with Macintosh blade no. 3, to one (10). Goel et al. described difficulties encountered when using Intubating LMA or light wand due to anterior placement of glottis and posteriorly protruded tongue (11). They also recommended a modified direct laryngoscopy when to additional technics is readily available. It includes (a) maintaining spontaneous breathing with deeper plane of anesthesia (b) Forward lift of both angles of mandible to conquer retrognathia and (c) a good backward upward and rightward pressure (BURP) by a professional assistant (11). Lin et al, described a case in which ventilation could not be adequate with LMA and they had the patient ventilated through endoscopic mask and perform nasal fiber optic intubation. They also had difficulty in extubating the patient which they overcome by Cook airway catheter exchanger and at last they decided to perform tracheostomy (12).

Another view indicated that most of the cases are caused by TCOF1 gene that could be detected by prenatal testing in embryos. Therefore prenatal diagnosis and genetic counseling could help parents to make intelligent decisions and reducing the incidence of TCS (13).

The last efforts of Sakai et al. have considerably interesting results (14). They ameliorate the features of these syndromes by using antioxidant supplementation in mouse models that could be a gate to treatment of this genetic abnormality in humans.

Conclusion

Treacher Collins Syndrome could be a challenge for anesthesiologists due to anticipated difficult airway management. Many approaches have been described with successful outcomes. Hence the gold standard would be awake flexible fiberoptic bronchoscopy and intubation. Also new findings in genetic aspect of this syndrome could be a path for definite treatment of TCS and prevent dysostosis in emberyonic period.

Acknowledgment

The authors would like to thank the kind help of physicians and nurses, operating room and

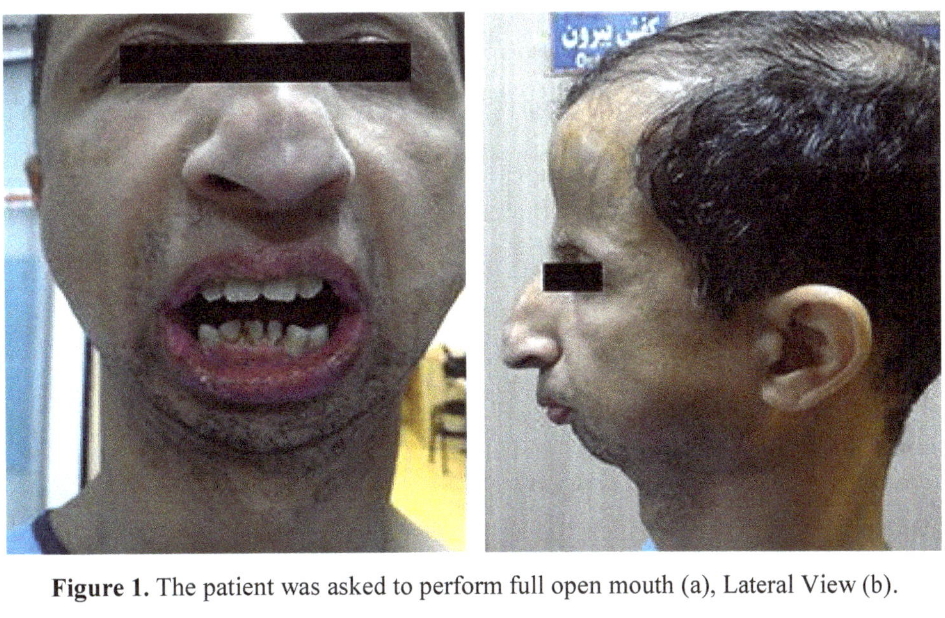

Figure 1. The patient was asked to perform full open mouth (a), Lateral View (b).

anesthesiology ward, Imam Hossein General Hospital, Shahid Beheshti University of Medical Sciences, Tehran, Iran for their kind help and support. And also Professor Marie Vincent from "Centre Hospitalier Universitaire de Nantes" due to generously provide us her new findings in this field.

Conflicts of Interest

The authors declare that there are no conflicts of interest.

References

1. Ulusal S, Gurkan H, Vatansever U, Kurkcu K, Tozkir H, Acunas B. A case of treacher collins syndrome. Balkan journal of medical genetics: BJMG. 2013;16(2):77-80.

2. de Peralta MS, Mouguelar VS, Sdrigotti MA, Ishiy FA, Fanganiello RD, Passos-Bueno MR, et al. Cnbp ameliorates Treacher Collins Syndrome craniofacial anomalies through a pathway that involves redox-responsive genes. Cell death & disease. 2016;7(10):e2397.

3. Vincent M, Genevieve D, Ostertag A, Marlin S, Lacombe D, Martin-Coignard D, et al. Treacher Collins syndrome: a clinical and molecular study based on a large series of patients. Genetics in medicine : official journal of the American College of Medical Genetics. 2016;18(1):49-56.

4. Marsh KL, Dixon J, Dixon MJ. Mutations in the Treacher Collins syndrome gene lead to mislocalization of the nucleolar protein treacle. Human molecular genetics. 1998;7(11):1795-800.

5. Soh J, Shin HW, Choi SU, Lim CH, Lee HW. Easy airway management using the i-gel supraglottic airway in a patient with Treacher Collins syndrome. Korean journal of anesthesiology. 2014;67(Suppl):S17-8.

6. Renju R, Varma BR, Kumar SJ, Kumaran P. Mandibulofacial dysostosis (Treacher Collins syndrome): A case report and review of literature. Contemporary clinical dentistry. 2014;5(4):532-4.

7. Noack Watt KE, Achilleos A, Neben CL, Merrill AE, Trainor PA. The Roles of RNA Polymerase I and III Subunits Polr1c and Polr1d in Craniofacial Development and in Zebrafish Models of Treacher Collins Syndrome. PLoS genetics. 2016;12(7):e1006187.

8. Teber OA, Gillessen-Kaesbach G, Fischer S, Bohringer S, Albrecht B, Albert A, et al. Genotyping in 46 patients with tentative diagnosis of Treacher Collins syndrome revealed unexpected phenotypic variation. European journal of human genetics : EJHG. 2004;12(11):879-90.

9. Tsujimoto T, Tanaka S, Yoshiyama Y, Sugiyama Y, Kawamata M. Successful intubation using McGRATH MAC in a patient with Treacher Collins syndrome. Middle East journal of anaesthesiology. 2014;22(5):523-5.

10. Goel L, Bennur SK, Jambhale S. Treacher-collins syndrome-a challenge for anaesthesiologists. Indian journal of anaesthesia. 2009;53(4):496-500.

11. Lin TC, Soo LY, Chen TI, Lu IC, Hsu HT, Chu KS, et al. Perioperative airway management in a child with Treacher Collins syndrome. Acta anaesthesiologica Taiwanica : official journal of the Taiwan Society of Anesthesiologists. 2009;47(1):44-7.

12. Shete P, Tupkari J, Benjamin T, Singh A. Treacher Collins syndrome. Journal of oral and maxillofacial pathology: JOMFP. 2011;15(3):348-51.

13. Sakai D, Dixon J, Achilleos A, Dixon M, Trainor PA. Prevention of Treacher Collins syndrome craniofacial anomalies in mouse models via maternal antioxidant supplementation. *Nature communications*. 2016;7:10328.

19

The Relationship between s100β and Cerebral Oximetry Trend in Patients Undergoing CABG with Cardiopulmonary Bypass

Kamal Fani[1], Mona Hashem-Aghaei[1], Hossein Ali Jelveh-Moghaddam[1], Golnar Radmand[1], Mahnoosh Foroughi[2], Samira Rajaei[3], Ali Dabbagh[1*]

Abstract

Background: Coronary artery bypass grafting (CABG) is among the most common cardiac surgery procedures carried out on heart pump. However, there are always risks for potential neurologic and neurocognitive insults in CABG. One of the biomarker of central nervous system (CNS) is s100β that shows damage. Cerebral oximetry using near-infrared spectroscopy (NIRS) developed for CNS monitoring especially in cardiac surgery. This study was designed to find the relationship between serum levels of s100β and cerebral oximetry in CABG patients.

Materials and Methods: In an observational study, 44 adult patients (40-75 years) entered the study for elective CABG. Serum levels of s100β were assessed at two times during cardiopulmonary bypass (CPB); i.e. just after aortic clamping and immediately after aortic declamping; while the results were compared with right and left cerebral oximetry readings NIRS. It was measured at baseline, during start of cardiopulmonary bypass (CPB), during aortic clamping, and finally at off-clamping the aorta. Repeated Measures ANCOVA (analysis of covariance), multiple linear regression models and Spearman correlation coefficient with scatter plot were used for data analysis. P value less than 0.05 considered significant.

Results: There was no linear correlation between s100β and NIRS according to correlation coefficients. The only positive linear relationship between s100β and right NIRS was observed among patients whose s100β was more than 10 (spearman correlation coefficient= 0.792; P value=0.006).

Conclusion: This study failed to demonstrate a relationship between on-CPB NIRS numbers and serum s100β in adult patients undergoing CABG during the bypass interval; further studies are suggested to evaluate potential predictive value of NIRS in brain ischemia related to CABG.

Keywords: Cardiopulmonary bypass, cerebral oximetry, near infrared spectroscopy, S100 Calcium Binding Protein beta Subunit

1. Anesthesiology Research Center, Cardiac Anesthesiology Department, Shahid Beheshti University of Medical Sciences, Tehran, Iran
2. Cardiovascular Research Center, Shahid Beheshti University of Medical Sciences, Tehran, Iran
3. Department of Immunology, School of Medicine, Tehran University of Medical Science, Tehran, Islamic Republic of Iran

Corresponding Author: Ali Dabbagh, MD, Professor, Anesthesiology Research Center, Taleghani Hospital, Velenjak, Chamran Exp Way, Tehran, Iran;

Email: alidabbagh@yahoo.com; alidabbagh@sbmu.ac.ir

Introduction

Cardiac diseases impose a great burden on human health and coronary artery diseases are one of the most important titles in this category. Coronary artery bypass grafting (CABG) is among the most common therapeutic options for coronary artery disease (CAD) with an annual number of 400,000 in the US (1-3).

Coronary artery bypass grafting is often performed as on pump surgery. There are a number of drawbacks for CABG when using cardiopulmonary bypass (CPB) including the risk for potential neurologic and neurocognitive insults mainly due to hypoperfusion state, embolic events and inflammatory response. A number of cellular and subcellular biomarkers used for assess the effects of CPB on different organ functions (2, 4-9). The commonly used biomarkers tracking the trend of potential central nervous system (CNS) damage in patients undergoing cardiac surgery with or without CPB is s100β (10-14). On the other hand, a number of CNS monitoring instruments developed to monitor and to help CNS protection during a range of procedures especially cardiac surgery. Cerebral oximetry using near-infrared spectroscopy (NIRS) is mentioned as a relatively novel and common monitoring system (14-19). There is still uncertainty regarding the net predictive value of cerebral oximetry regarding cerebral tissue oxygenation (14, 20). In other words, if cerebral oximetry is valid and reliable monitor for cerebral perfusion, and s100β increases with hypoperfusion and hypoxic injuries in the brain, then there might be a direct relationship between serum levels of s100β and cerebral oximetry readings.

This observational study was designed and implemented to find any potential relationship between serum levels of s100β (considered as one of the CNS neuromarkers of cerebral injury) and cerebral oximetry readings to find out whether the readings of cerebral oximetry by NIRS are in concordance with serum levels of s100β.

Methods

Protocol of the study was confirmed by the Institutional Ethics Committee, Shahid Beheshti University of Medical Sciences, Tehran, Iran.

For each patient, before commencement of the study, written informed consent was obtained. The study was performed from 1st of April 2017 to the end of November 2017; in cardiac surgery operating room, Shaheed Modarres Hospital affiliated by Shahid Beheshti University of Medical Sciences.

All patients entered the study after written informed consent was taken based on the Institutional Ethics protocols. Patients were aged 40-75 years and patient with emergency procedures were excluded. All were managed by the same surgical, anesthesiology and perfusion team and all were transferred to the same adult cardiac ICU. Likewise, each clinical steps in anesthesia, surgery, cardiopulmonary bypass and ICU care strictly followed standard institutional protocols; including range of temperature manipulation, protocols for anesthetic drugs, organ protection and CPB and blood transfusion guidelines including during CPB.

There was a particular NIRS management protocol which was strictly employed. This protocol was adopted from the protocols described by Denault et al. (21), Murkin et al. (18, 19) and discussed in detail in a number of texts (22). Right and left cerebral oximetry readings NIRS were measured at baseline, at the start of CPB, during aortic clamping, and finally at off-clamping of the aorta.

Human s100β ELISA kit was used (IBL-America; Immuno-Biological Laboratories; Minneapolis, MN; United States). Samples for assessment of serum levels of s100β were collected at two times during CPB (at the time of aortic clamping and immediately after aortic declamping) through the following steps; Non-heparinized blood was drawn from the arterial line of the bypass circuit, then they were centrifuged at 2500 G for 10 minutes at 4°C, the samples were refrigerated at -18°C inside the stat laboratory of the operating room, afterwards, they were transferred using ice box at -70°C to the immunology laboratory, after collecting all the samples, they were defrosted for to undergo ELISA testing. We recorded the right and left side NIRS, arterial blood gas analyses (ABG), blood sugar, temperature and s100β at baseline point, at the starting point of CBP and at the "off-clamp time" for each patient. To prevent s100β release from other sources as much as possible, we never used cell saver in any of the patients (23).

All quantitative variables demonstrated as mean±SD; also, qualitative variables demonstrated as percentage. To compare quantitative variables in 2 different times, paired t-test or non-parametric Wilcoxon test were used if needed. Repeated Measures ANCOVA (analysis of covariance) was used to adjust the effects of confounding variables (e.g. the baseline values) on comparing variables in different times. The mean differences of variables (between two times), which had significant confounders, are presented in table 4 at different levels of confounder variable. Multiple linear regression models were used for assessing the effect of other variables on the difference of s100β levels between two times and the best models were selected using forward, backward and stepwise methods. The mean difference of s100β at different levels of PaO2 and blood sugar are presented in Table 5. The Spearman correlation coefficient with scatter plot was used to evaluate the linear correlation between NIRS and s100β values. All of the statistical tests were two-tailed at α= 0.05 and SPSS version 18 (SPSS Inc, Chicago, IL, United States) was used for data entry and analysis.

Results

A total of 44 patients including 15 (34.1%) female and 29 (65.9%) male were entered to this study. The main characteristics of patients and the results of diagnostic assessments are presented in Table 1.

The right and left side NIRS, ABG, blood sugar and temperature were evaluated at baseline, on-CBP, aortic clamping and off-clamp times for each patient; while s100β was measured during CPB just at the time of aortic clamping and at aortic declamping (Table 2). The both side NIRS at off-clamp time were significantly more than on-CBP (right side: P value=0.003; left side: P value =0.007). Also the patients had higher PaO_2 (P value<0.001) on CBP rather than off-clamp time. The blood sugar, temperature and s100β at off-clamp time were more than on-CBP (P values: <0.001, 0.002 & 0.002, respectively; Table 2). After adjusting the effect of baseline values just the differences of PaO_2 and temperature remained significant (P value=0.005 & 0.004, respectively).

Table 1: Main characteristics of study patients and results of diagnostic assessments (N= 44)

N= 44	
Age	57.20±13.24
Gender	
Female	15 (34.1%)
Male	29 (65.9%)
Underlying Disease	
Drug History	17 (38.6%)
Cerebrovascular Accidents	1 (2.3%)
Hypertension	7 (15.9%)
Others	6 (13.6%)
None	13 (29.5%)
Carotid Doppler Result	
Normal	27 (61.4%)
Non-significant Stenosis	17 (38.6%)
Significant Stenosis	0 (0.0%)
Ejection Fraction (EF; mean±SD)	51.82 ± 8.83
Pulmonary Artery Pressure (PAP± mean±SD)	32.42 ± 17.34
Time of cross clamp (minutes; mean±SD)	63.82 ± 23.18
Cardiopulmonary Bypass (CPB) time(minutes; mean±SD)	106.86 ± 33.44
Number of used packed cells (mean±SD)	1.41 ± 1.30

The mean differences of on-clamp and off-clamp times for NIRS and temperature were also presented at different levels of their baseline values. The results show that for patients with 60 ≤baseline NIRS ≤69, off-clamp NIRS was more than on-CBP (right side: P value = 0.010; left side: P value=0.025). And for patients with baseline temperature>35, the off-clamp temperature was significantly more than

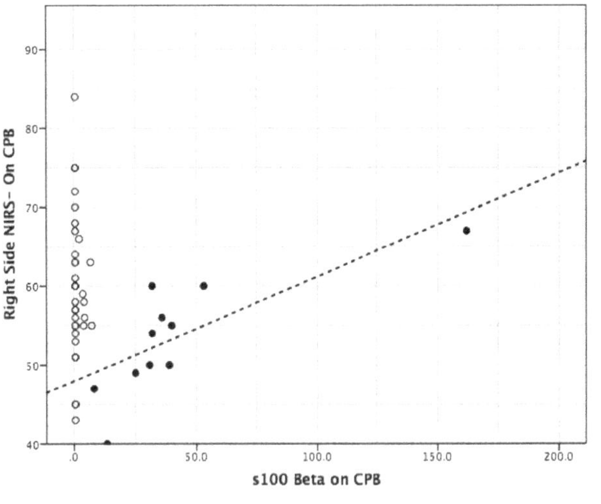

Figure 1. Correlation between s100β and right sided on-CPB NIRS.

Table 2: Results of Outcome Variable Assessments

	Baseline	On-CPB	Off-clamp	difference	P-value	P_{adj}^{*}
NIRS						
Right Side	63.36±10.04	58.22±9.00	62.84±9.66	4.61±9.71	0.003	0.613
Left Side	64.02±10.67	58.98±7.30	62.89±9.76	3.91±0.007	0.007	0.692
HCT	40.57±6.97	24.05±5.04	24.29±3.05	0.25±5.49	0.764	0.266
$PaCO_2$	37.59±8.50	36.77±5.87	35.34±5.44	1.43±5.85	0.112	0.912
PaO_2	227.55±134.16	386.00±69.51	316.05±58.69	69.95±95.81	<0.001	0.005
Blood Sugar	143.93±56.93	162.57±47.04	179.39±46.87	16.82±29.50	<0.001	0.004
Temperature	35.66±1.14	33.80±1.52	34.84±1.26	1.04±2.12	0.002	0.051
s100β	---	11.72±27.05	39.38±58.85	27.66±56.94	0.002	---

* P_{adj}: p-value of difference between on-CPB and off-clamp Adjusted for the baseline value.

Table 3: Difference of NIRS and Temperature between on-CPB & off-clamp at different groups of their baseline values

	Difference between on-CPB & off-clamp values (mean ± SD)	P value
Right side NIRS (Baseline)		
≤59	3.47±10.20	0.209
60-69	6.72±9.80	0.010
≥70	2.73±9.10	0.344
Left side NIRS (Baseline)		
≤59	2.23±9.28	0.403
60-69	5.15±9.47	0.025
≥70	3.64±8.69	0.195
Temperature (Baseline)		
≤35	1.25±2.54	0.068
>35	0.93±1.88	0.015

Table 4: Difference of s100β between on-CPB & off-clamp at different groups of confounders

	Difference (mean ± SD)	P value
PaO_2 (baseline)		
≤102	3.43±32.69	0.690
103-322	10.79±27.43	0.149
>322	71.70±75.32	0.003
Blood Sugar (baseline)		
≤105	28.11±49.27	0.044
106-155	1.84±31.35	0.823
>155	58.79±70.73	0.008

on-CBP (P value=0.015; Table 3).

The patients with PaO_2>322 had higher off-clamp s100β rather than on-CBP time (P value=0.003). Also for patients with blood sugar≤105 or >155, the s100β at off-clamp was more than on-CBP time (P value=0.044 and 0.008, respectively; Table 4).

There was no linear correlation between s100β and NIRS according to correlation coefficients (Table 5). However, the scatter plots showed that there could be a positive linear relationship between s100β and right NIRS among the patients whose s100β>10 (spearman correlation coefficient= 0.792; P value=0.006; Table 5 and Figure 1).

Our follow up for potential neurologic complications was a short time follow (i.e. less than 2 weeks); while in this time period we did not discover any evidence of new onset major clinical neurologic injury as a consequence of operation.

Discussion

The results of the current study demonstrated that in the majority of the measurements, there was no significant correlation between intraoperative s100β

Table 5: Correlation between s100β and NIRS

	Right side NIRS		**Left side NIRS**	
	CC*	P-value	CC*	P-value
s100β (all values)				
On CBP	-0.235	0.124	-0.201	0.190
Off-clamp	-0.058	0.706	-0.165	0.285
	Right side NIRS		**Left side NIRS**	
	CC*	P value	CC*	P value
s100β>10				
On CBP	0.792	0.006	0.567	0.087
Off-clamp	-0.123	0.574	-0.124	0.573

* Spearman Correlation Coefficient.

and NIRS readings in adult cardiac surgery patients. There are many studies measuring serum levels of S100β which focus on cerebral emboli; on the other hand, cerebral oximetry may not be a particularly good monitor for the microembolies that are seen during cardiac surgery. It might be a good monitor for a very large, global embolic phenomenon of the brain, although this would be an extraordinarily rare event. This limitations of cerebral oximetry, as described in our study, could be one of the main reasons for our results.

To our knowledge, this study is the first one assessing such a correlation during the intraoperative period. However, in another study by Harilall et al, the authors found a highly significant relationship between postoperative s100β and intraoperative interventions based on intraoperative clinical interventions suggested by Murkin et al. (18, 19) and Denault et al (21, 22); though, our sample size was twice the sample size of that study (24). The only significant correlation was between on-CPB NIRS numbers and s100β; however, none of the other ones had significant correlation; which suggests a re-thinking about the predictive value of NIRS as a surrogate outcome for assessment of cerebral function and prevention of ischemia. On the other hand, it seems that more sophisticated studies are needed before we could say the final word about this predictive value of NIRS (4, 14).

NIRS explains the balance of the demand/supply of oxygen in the frontal cortex of the brain and is used to assess relative adequacy of cerebral perfusion during hypoperfusion state of CPB with undetermined validity to predict neurologic events. In a number of studies, NIRS was demonstrated as a useful instrument for assessment of cerebral autoregulation; suggesting NIRS as a "means for individualizing MAP during CPB" (25-27). However, this is not a constant finding in all studies; in fact, at times, there is even controversial evidence about correlation of NIRS pathologic findings and postoperative cognitive dysfunction; for example Kok et al. showed high proportion of cognitive dysfunction in CABG patients with low incidence of abnormal NIRS findings (20). Also, Vranken et al have explicitly claimed in their review that there is lack of "clear evidence for a defined desaturation threshold requiring intervention during CPB" (14). In concordance with the two latter studies, the results of our study demonstrated at the neuromarker levels that NIRS readings failed to have a strong correlation with s100β during CPB in adult patients undergoing CABG.

There were a number of limitations in our study which are mentioned here:

1. We had a limited sample size due to budgetary limitations; also, we checked s100β for two times; while, more frequent assessments with a resulting area under curve (AUC) of s100β would be possibly more decisive. Taking into account the inter-individual variability of cerebral oxygen saturation (ScO2) readings and the high variability of biomarkers in the setting of cardiac surgery, a correlation analysis, comparing NIRS values and s100 β levels in two time points could be improved if we could assess and analyze the AUC of perioperative desaturation (in comparison to baseline) and analyzing the time course of s100 beta (up to its maximum that occurs typically 12 to 24 hours after surgery).
2. Our patient population included only the adult patients while the pediatric patients should be assessed in different studies especially considering the type of operations in pediatric population; i.e. congenital heart diseases in the this patients group with more susceptible brain tissue (28, 29)
3. Another limitation of the current study was measuring only s100β; in fact, s100β is a neuromarker that shows neuronal cell damage; while other neuromarkers including neuronspecific enolase (NSE), glial fibrillary acidic protein (GFAP) and

brain-derived neurotrophic factor (BDNF) were studied in other studies but we did not assess them here; meanwhile, our sample size was pretty larger than the sample size of study by Sanchez-de-Toledo et al (29)

4. There are studies demonstrating a heterogeneity of non-brain sources for S100B during surgery; though in the context of surgery there is well documented release of S100B from non-cerebral tissues, this marker was chosen to assess the predictive value of NIRS in brain ischemia since it is the most commonly studied one; however, supplementary studies including cognitive testing or brain imaging could add to our knowledge regarding the predictive value of NIRS in the perioperative period

5. Finally, this study was an observational one and combined interventions in future designs could lead us to more precise determination of the NIRS role as a surrogate outcome and a valid and reliable monitor for potential CNS ischemia and injury.

Conclusion

In brief, this study failed to demonstrate a relationship between on-CPB NIRS numbers and serum s100β in adult patients undergoing CABG during the bypass interval. Further studies are suggested to evaluate potential predictive value of NIRS as a surrogate index in brain ischemia assessment.

Acknowledgment

This research has been financially supported by Anesthesiology Research Center, Cardiac Anesthesiology Department, Shahid Beheshti University of Medical Sciences, Tehran, Iran; research award number: 7129. Also, the authors would like to acknowledge the kind help of all physicians and nurses of cardiac surgery operating room, Modarres Hospital, Shahid Beheshti University of Medical Sciences, Tehran Iran. Besides, the kind help of administrative personnel of Anesthesiology Research Center, Shahid Beheshti University of Medical Sciences is highly acknowledged.

Conflicts of Interest

The authors declare that they have no conflict of interest.

References

1. Alexander JH, Smith PK. Coronary-Artery Bypass Grafting. N Engl J Med. 2016;374(20):1954-64.
2. Dabbagh A, Rajaei S, Bahadori Monfared A, Keramatinia AA, Omidi K. Cardiopulmonary Bypass, Inflammation and How to Defy it: Focus on Pharmacological Interventions. Iran J Pharm Res. 2012;11(3):705-14.
3. Ferasatkish R, Dabbagh A, Alavi M, Mollasadeghi G, Hydarpur E, Moghadam AA, et al. Effect of magnesium sulfate on extubation time and acute pain in coronary artery bypass surgery. Acta Anaesthesiol Scand. 2008;52(10):1348-52.
4. Salameh A, Dhein S, Dahnert I, Klein N. Neuroprotective Strategies during Cardiac Surgery with Cardiopulmonary Bypass. International journal of molecular sciences. 2016;17(11).
5. Warren OJ, Watret AL, de Wit KL, Alexiou C, Vincent C, Darzi AW, et al. The inflammatory response to cardiopulmonary bypass: part 2--anti-inflammatory therapeutic strategies. J Cardiothorac Vasc Anesth. 2009;23(3):384-93.
6. Warren OJ, Smith AJ, Alexiou C, Rogers PL, Jawad N, Vincent C, et al. The inflammatory response to cardiopulmonary bypass: part 1--mechanisms of pathogenesis. J Cardiothorac Vasc Anesth. 2009;23(2):223-31.
7. Dabbagh A, Bastanifar E, Foroughi M, Rajaei S, Keramatinia AA. The effect of intravenous magnesium sulfate on serum levels of N-terminal pro-brain natriuretic peptide (NT pro-BNP) in elective CABG with cardiopulmonary bypass. J Anesth. 2013;27(5):693-8.
8. Aryana P, Rajaei S, Bagheri A, Karimi F, Dabbagh A. Acute Effect of Intravenous Administration of Magnesium Sulfate on Serum Levels of Interleukin-6 and Tumor Necrosis Factor-alpha in Patients Undergoing Elective Coronary Bypass Graft With Cardiopulmonary Bypass. Anesth Pain Med. 2014;4(3):e16316.
9. Foroughi M, Rahimian H, Dabbagh A, Majidi M, Hekmat M, Beheshti M, et al. Postoperative N-terminal pro-brain natriuretic peptide level in coronary artery bypass surgery with ventricular dysfunction after perioperative glucose-insulin-potassium treatment. J Cardiothorac Vasc Anesth. 2012;26(4):631-6.
10. Kawata K, Liu CY, Merkel SF, Ramirez SH, Tierney RT, Langford D. Blood biomarkers for brain injury: What are we measuring? Neuroscience and biobehavioral reviews. 2016;68:460-73.
11. Chong ZZ, Changyaleket B, Xu H, Dull RO, Schwartz DE. Identifying S100B as a Biomarker and a Therapeutic Target For Brain Injury and Multiple Diseases. Current medicinal chemistry. 2016;23(15):1571-96.
12. Zheng L, Fan QM, Wei ZY. Serum S-100beta and NSE levels after off-pump versus on-pump coronary artery bypass graft surgery. BMC cardiovascular disorders. 2015;15:70.
13. van Boven WJ, Morariu A, Salzberg SP, Gerritsen WB, Waanders FG, Korse TC, et al. Impact of different surgical strategies on perioperative protein S100beta release in elderly patients

undergoing coronary artery bypass grafting. Innovations (Philadelphia, Pa). 2013;8(3):230-6.

14. Vranken NPA, Weerwind PW, Sutedja NA, Severdija EE, Barenbrug PJC, Maessen JG. Cerebral Oximetry and Autoregulation during Cardiopulmonary Bypass: A Review. J Extra Corpor Technol. 2017;49(3):182-91.

15. Moerman A, De Hert S. Recent advances in cerebral oximetry. Assessment of cerebral autoregulation with near-infrared spectroscopy: myth or reality? F1000Research. 2017;6:1615.

16. Green DW, Kunst G. Cerebral oximetry and its role in adult cardiac, non-cardiac surgery and resuscitation from cardiac arrest. Anaesthesia. 2017;72 Suppl 1:48-57.

17. Saidi N, Murkin JM. Applied neuromonitoring in cardiac surgery: patient specific management. Semin Cardiothorac Vasc Anesth. 2005;9(1):17-23.

18. Murkin JM, Arango M. Near-infrared spectroscopy as an index of brain and tissue oxygenation. Br J Anaesth. 2009;103 Suppl 1:i3-13.

19. Murkin JM. NIRS: a standard of care for CPB vs. an evolving standard for selective cerebral perfusion? J Extra Corpor Technol. 2009;41(1):P11-4.

20. Kok WF, van Harten AE, Koene BM, Mariani MA, Koerts J, Tucha O, et al. A pilot study of cerebral tissue oxygenation and postoperative cognitive dysfunction among patients undergoing coronary artery bypass grafting randomised to surgery with or without cardiopulmonary bypass*. Anaesthesia. 2014;69(6):613-22.

21. Denault A, Deschamps A, Murkin JM. A proposed algorithm for the intraoperative use of cerebral near-infrared spectroscopy. Semin Cardiothorac Vasc Anesth. 2007;11(4):274-81.

22. Dabbagh A. Postoperative CNS care. In: Dabbagh A, Esmailian F, Aranki S, editors. Postoperative Critical Care for Cardiac Surgical Patients. 1 ed: Springer-Verlag; 2014. p. 245-56.

23. Ishida K, Gohara T, Kawata R, Ohtake K, Morimoto Y, Sakabe T. Are serum S100beta proteins and neuron-specific enolase predictors of cerebral damage in cardiovascular surgery? J Cardiothorac Vasc Anesth. 2003;17(1):4-9.

24. Harilall Y, Adam JK, Biccard BM, Reddi A. The effect of optimising cerebral tissue oxygen saturation on markers of neurological injury during coronary artery bypass graft surgery. Heart Lung Circ. 2014;23(1):68-74.

25. Ono M, Joshi B, Brady K, Easley RB, Zheng Y, Brown C, et al. Risks for impaired cerebral autoregulation during cardiopulmonary bypass and postoperative stroke. Br J Anaesth. 2012;109(3):391-8.

26. Ono M, Brady K, Easley RB, Brown C, Kraut M, Gottesman RF, et al. Duration and magnitude of blood pressure below cerebral autoregulation threshold during cardiopulmonary bypass is associated with major morbidity and operative mortality. J Thorac Cardiovasc Surg. 2014;147(1):483-9.

27. Joshi B, Ono M, Brown C, Brady K, Easley RB, Yenokyan G, et al. Predicting the limits of cerebral autoregulation during cardiopulmonary bypass. Anesth Analg. 2012;114(3):503-10.

28. Tina LG, Frigiola A, Abella R, Tagliabue P, Ventura L, Paterlini G, et al. S100B protein and near infrared spectroscopy in preterm and term newborns. Frontiers in bioscience (Elite edition). 2010;2:159-64.

29. Sanchez-de-Toledo J, Chrysostomou C, Munoz R, Lichtenstein S, Sao-Aviles CA, Wearden PD, et al. Cerebral regional oxygen saturation and serum neuromarkers for the prediction of adverse neurologic outcome in pediatric cardiac surgery. Neurocrit Care. 2014;21(1):133-9.

The Effects of Selenium Supplementation on Clinical Outcomes in Mechanically Ventilated, Non-Surgical/ Traumatic Critically Ill Patients

Kamran Heidari[1], Reza Goharani[2], Masoome Lakestani[1], Mohammadreza Hajiesmaeili[2]*

Abstract

Background: Selenium presents anti-inflammatory and antioxidant properties which plays a critical role in nutrition of patients following devastating conditions. Furthermore, several lines of evidence reported that most of patients who admitted to intensive care unit (ICU) have lower plasma levels of selenium. Therefore, this study was designed to define the impact of selenium supplementation on clinical outcomes of mechanically ventilated non-surgical/traumatic critically ill patients.

Materials and Methods: This study was conducted on 105 subjects hospitalized in ICU of Shohadaye Haft-e Tir Hospital, Tehran, Iran. Here the acute physiologic assessment and chronic health evaluation (APACHE) II score of patients was documented on the day of their ICU admission. The patients were divided to two groups based on block randomization technique and were assigned to receive selenium or placebo. Then the effect of selenium supplementation was evaluated based on the APACHE II score, the occurrence of ventilator associated pneumonia (VAP), length of ICU stay and the rate of mortality.

Results: The acquired data revealed no significant difference between two experimental groups based on the demographical information. Also it was demonstrated that selenium supplementation of critically ill patients was associated with better APACHE II score, fewer length of ICU stay and fewer mortality rate. Incidence of VAP indicated no significant difference between groups.

Conclusion: The obtained data of this single center clinical trial showed that selenium supplementation could improve clinical outcomes of critically ill patients.

Keywords: Selenium supplementation; APACHE II score; ventilator associated pneumonia; mortality rate; length of ICU stay

1. Emergency Medicine, Skull Base Research Center, Loghman Hakim Hospital, Shahid Beheshti University of Medical Sciences, Tehran, Iran
2. Anesthesiology Research Center, Neurocritical Care Research Center, Loghman Hakim Hospital, Shahid Beheshti University of Medical Sciences, Tehran, Iran

*Corresponding Author: Mohammadreza Hajiesmaeili, MD, Loghman Hakim Hospital, Kamali St. Kargar Ave. Tehran, Iran.

Email: mrhajiesmaeili@sbmu.ac.ir

Introduction

Critical illnesses are characterized by a life-threatening production of reactive oxygen species (ROS) and other radical species that lead to oxidative stress. Oxidative stress is related to release of metalloproteins, copper and iron ions, production of nitric oxide and activation of phagocytes (1). It established that critical illnesses are accompanied by immunosuppression which is correlated with the role of ROS (2). Since oxidative stress is associated with the severeness of diseases which occurs following the elevated level of ROS or declined in antioxidant defenses, therefore managing production of ROS is a crucial strategy in treating illnesses (3).

An essential element, selenium, which is found in a bunch of proteins calls selenoproteins presents anti-inflammatory and antioxidant properties. It has been proposed that antioxidant properties of selenium are mediated via glutathione peroxidase enzymes activation which results in products with less toxicity to protect organism against free radicals causing oxidative stress (4). Hence, selenium probably plays fundamental roles to improve devastating condition (5). Nevertheless, in several parts of the world such as the Europe and Australasia it has been reported that owing to low soil content, peoples are prone to low baseline selenium status (6). In addition, a number of studies reported that selenium deficiency is common among Iranian people (7-10). Furthermore, reduced dietary intake, which occurs during critical illnesses, can further impair the selenium status. In such situation, acute illness combined with selenium deficiency might worsen oxidative stress and related damages (5, 6).

Several lines of evidence reported that most of patients who admitted to intensive care unit (ICU) have lower plasma levels of selenium and glutathione peroxidase activity. Moreover, plasma selenium concentrations are inversely associated with the severity disease (5, 6). Therefore, the aim of the present study was to investigate the effects of selenium supplementation on clinical outcomes in mechanically ventilated, non-surgical and non-traumatic critically ill adult patients.

Methods

This study was a prospective single center clinical trial conducted on 105 subjects hospitalized in ICU, Shohadaye Haft-e Tir Hospital (teaching hospital of Iran University of medical sciences, Tehran, Iran). Patient who signed the written informed involved in the study. The investigation was carried out in accordance with the declaration of Helsinki and approved by the ethics committee of Shohadaye Haft-e Tir Hospital.

The inclusion criteria were patients with age of more than 18 years who received mechanical ventilation more than 3 days and were admitted to ICU due to internal diseases not related to trauma or surgery. On the other hand the exclusion criteria were patients with renal failure, pancreatitis, short bowel syndrome and those that already have pressure ulcers and were HIV positive and also had bone marrow, lung, kidney and liver transplantation. Also all patients who were extubated within two days of establishment of mechanical ventilation or those died during the study period were excluded from this study.

The information of eligible patients consisting the age, gender, cause of hospitalization, diagnosis and the acute physiology and chronic health evaluation II (APACHE II) score was recorded on the day of their admission in the ICU. Moreover, in this study the ventilator associated pneumonia (VAP) was diagnosed based on Clinical Pulmonary Infection Score≥6 (11). In this experiment, patients were divided to two groups using block randomization technique (12) and assigned to receive selenium (group A) or placebo tablets (group B). Patients of group A, received one mg selenium as sodium selenite pentahydrate at the first day and 0.5 mg selenium daily for the following 13 days.

APACHE II score was calculated in all patients of both groups twice: one on the day of their ICU admission and, on the 14th day following selenium treatment, to define the influence of the selenium supplementation at APACHE II score and final prognosis. To calculate web based APACHE II score, age and 12 relevant physiological variables and 2 disease related variables used consisting: Glasgow Coma score, white blood cell count, hematocrit, heart and respiratory rate, mean arterial pressure (MAP), FiO_2 and PaO_2, body temperature, arterial pH, serum creatinine, serum potassium, serum sodium , the occurrence of acute renal failure or severe organ system insufficiency and immunocompromised state (13).

Pearson Chi-square test or Fisher's exact test was used to compare categorical data. In addition, Student's t test or Mann–Whitney U test was applied to compare continuous variables. A $P<0.05$ was considered statistically significant.

Results

Among 250 patients admitted in the ICU, 105 subjects were eligible to evaluation in this study. Here, 55 patients were male while 50 individuals were female which randomly divided in two experimental groups. One group treated with selenium (group A) and the other one received placebo (group B) while there was no significant difference between two groups based on the age and gender of patients. In this investigation, the underlying causes of hospitalization in ICU and mechanical ventilation evaluated and identified by the medical practitioners. In this regard, pulmonary diseases were the main reason of hospitalization in ICU in both groups that its incidence was about 70%. Sepsis was the second cause of these critically ill patients' condition with the prevalence of 14% and 16% group A and B, respectively. Also based on acquired data, 13% of subjects group A and 10% group B were admitted to ICU due to central nervous system (CNS) disorders (Table 1). Here, the severity of illness was defined using APACHE II scoring system at the time of their entrance to the ICU.

In this study statistical analysis of the acquired data from the point of interfering factors such as age, gender, the cause of hospitalization and illness severity revealed no significant difference between two experimental groups. According to obtained data the average APACHE II score of patients at the beginning of their admission to ICU was 20.6±7 and 21±8 in group A and B, respectively ($P= 0.1$). Following the employed nutritional treatment, the APACHE II score of group A reached to 18±3 while this score in group B was 19.1±4($P<0.05$), which shows a significant difference between two groups. Based on the APACHE II score, non-operation and post-operation predicted mortality percentage of patients in both groups were similar; however actual mortality in group A was 9 subjects (16.3%) and 12 subjects (24%) in group B which revealed the selenium supplemented nutrition resulted in a significant difference in the rate of death between groups ($P<0.05$). The incidence of VAP was another factor that has been evaluated between two groups that acquired data demonstrated 6 (10.9%) subjects in group A were infected while 5 (10%) patients in group B developed VAP which indicated no significant difference between groups ($P=0.3$). Also, there was a meaningful difference in duration of patients' stay in ICU among groups, as the number of days in ICU was 10.1±8 and 11.2±8.2 in group A and B, respectively ($P<0.05$) (Table 2).

Discussion

Incidence and cause of malnutrition in ICU are multifactorial (14) and loss of essential micronutrients is common among critically ill patients who admitted to critical care wards. This situation can be worse in patients who suffer from micronutrient deficiency prior to the illness. Selenium is one of these essential trace elements which becomes reduced remarkably following devastating conditions (6). Hence, in these patients selenium supplementation could be a valuable strategy to prevent multi organ dysfunction due to severe oxidative stress. The result of this prospective randomized and placebo-controlled, single-center trial revealed selenium supplementation is a critical adjuvant therapeutic approach to improve outcome of patients in ICU who were admitted due to pulmonary diseases, sepsis or CNS disorders. We found that selenium supplementation in mechanically ventilated, non-surgical/traumatic adult patients during the first days in the ICU was associated with better APACHE II score, shorter stay in the ICU and fewer rate of death.

This finding is in agreement with other single and multi-center trials which reported the important role of this essential trace element in nutrition plan of ICU admitted patients. In this regard, Heyland et al. in a systematic review on antioxidant supplementations reported that enhanced selenium (alone or in combination with other antioxidants) can be

Table 1: Patient characteristics on admission with detail of the diagnostic categories.

Variable	Group A (selenium)	Group B (placebo)	P value
Number	55	50	
Age (mean± SD)	47±9	49±8	P>0.05
Gender			P>0.05
Male	31	28	
female	24	22	
Illness causing hospitalization			
Pulmonary diseases	38 (69%)	36 (72%)	
Sepsis	8 (14%)	8 (16%)	
CNS disorders	7 (13%)	5 (10%)	
Others	2 (4%)	1 (2%)	

Table 2: The effects of selenium supplementation on clinical outcomes of critically ill patients.

Variable	Group A (selenium)	Group B (placebo)	P value
Admission APACHE II score	20.6±7	21±8	P<0.05
Predicted mortality	40/30 %	40/30 %	
Final APACHE II score	18±3	19.1±4	
Actual Mortality (%)	9 (16.3%)	12 (24%)	P<0.05
Length of ICU stay (Days)	10.1±8	11.2±8.2	P<0.05
VAP Incidence (%)	6 (10.9%)	5 (10%)	P>0.05

correlated with decreased rate of mortality (15, 16). Also a multiple-center study demonstrated that enhanced level of sodium-selenite reduced rate of mortality in patients with septic shock or severe sepsis (17). In addition, Andrews et al. found that daily selenium administration for at least five days, reduced new infections (18). On the other hand, Berger et al. reported that antioxidant supplements (mixture of selenium, zinc, vitamin C and vitamin B_1) for 5 days did not reduce infectious complications, length of hospital stay, early organ failure and mortality; however remarkably decreased the inflammatory responses in trauma patients or following cardiac surgery (19).

It has been assumed that antioxidant and anti-inflammatory properties of selenium are mediated through glutathione peroxidase and thioredoxin reductase which are crucial elements to maintain redox system in any types of cells in the body including the immune cells (20-22). These two enzymes reduce hydrogen peroxide, lipid, and phospholipid hydroperoxides and also diminish free radicals and ROS propagation (23). Following selenium supplementation the selenoprotein is rapidly generated which subsequently prevents endothelial cells from oxidative damage (24, 25).

To the best of our knowledge, although so many investigations reported the impact of selenium supplementation in clinically ill patients in other parts of the world, there is just one documented investigation in Iran about administration of this trace element and its influence on patients who admitted in the ICU due to trauma (26). Chelkeba et al. in 2015 reported the effects of parenteral selenium on outcomes of mechanically ventilated patients following sepsis, severe sepsis and septic shock and their study carried out in a center in Tehran, Iran; however, their findings and the target patients were different. This research group revealed selenium can reduce the occurrence of VAP in patients who mainly admitted in ICU due to trauma. Also their goal-directed therapy didn't change the mortality rate, significantly (26), while our supplementation resulted in reduction of mortality rate without significant effect on the incidence of VAP. Since VAP is the leading cause of death in the ICU, increases length of ICU and hospital stay and elevates mortality rate and costs, various treatments have been employed to reduce its incidence (27-29); however, in the present study, selenium supplementation did not affect VAP incidence.

Up until now there is no conclusive investigation to show where the balance should lie between therapeutic and toxic doses of selenium (6, 15). Therefore, the employed protocol of selenium administration can provide a useful insight about the required dose of this important trace element in the nutrition plan of patients with critical condition in our country. It is important to mention that our study was single-center trial that did not include patients from various geographical parts of Iran; therefore, it requires data of more centers to gain further validity. In addition, we did not measure selenium levels before and after the treatment, that is another limitation of the current investigation.

Conclusion

The obtained data of this single center clinical trial showed that selenium supplementation could improve clinical outcomes of critically ill patients.

Acknowledgment

The authors would like to thank the Clinical Research Development Center (CRDC) of Loghman Hakim Hospital, Shahid Beheshti University of Medical Sciences, Tehran, Iran for their support, cooperation and assistance throughout the period of study.

Conflicts of Interest

The authors declare that they have no conflict of interest.

References

1. Crimi E, Sica V, Williams-Ignarro S, et al. The role of oxidative stress in adult critical care. Free Radic. Biol. Med. 2006;40:398-406.
2. Schieber M, Chandel N S. ROS function in redox signaling and oxidative stress. Curr. Biol. 2014;24:R453-R62.
3. Goodyear-Bruch C, Pierce J D. Oxidative stress in critically ill patients. Am. J. Crit. Care. 2002;11:543-51.
4. Arthur J. The glutathione peroxidases. Cell. Mol. Life Sci. 2001;57:1825-35.
5. Allingstrup M, Afshari A. Selenium supplementation for critically ill adults. Cochrane Database Syst. Rev. 2015.
6. Andrews P J. Selenium and glutamine supplements: where are we heading? A critical care perspective. Curr. Opin. Clin. Nutr. Metab. Care. 2010;13:192-7.
7. Ehteshamfar S-M, Shapouri-Moghaddam A, Safarian M, Nematy M, Bahrami-Taghanaki H, Azizi H. Serum selenium concentration in Mashhad prisoners, Iran. Saudi Med. J. 2012;33:859-62.
8. Rafraf M, Mahdavi R, Rashidi M R. Serum selenium levels in healthy women in Tabriz, Iran. Food Nutr. Bull. 2008;29:83-6.
9. Safaralizadeh R, Sirjani M, Pourpak Z, et al. Serum selenium concentration in healthy children living in Tehran. Biofactors. 2007;31:127-31.
10. Nazemi L, Nazmara S, Eshraghyan M R, et al. Selenium status in soil, water and essential crops of Iran. Iranian journal of environmental health science & engineering. 2012;9:11.
11. Shan J, Chen H-L, Zhu J-H. Diagnostic accuracy of clinical pulmonary infection score for ventilator-associated pneumonia: a meta-analysis. Respir. Care. 2011;56:1087-94.
12. Efird J. Blocked randomization with randomly selected block sizes. Int. J. Environ. Res. Public Health. 2010;8:15-20.
13. Mahdaviazad H, Imanieh M, Masoompour S. Effectiveness of the APACHE II scoring system in an intensive care unit: results of a prospective study. Br. J. Med. Med. Res. 2015;8:1018-24.
14. Dock-Nascimento D B, Maeve Tavares V, de Aguilar-Nascimento J. Evolution of nutritional therapy prescription in critically ill patients. Nutr. Hosp. 2005;20:343-7.
15. Heyland D K. Selenium supplementation in critically ill patients: can too much of a good thing be a bad thing? Critical Care. 2007;11:153.
16. Heyland D K, Dhaliwal R, Suchner U, Berger M M.

Antioxidant nutrients: a systematic review of trace elements and vitamins in the critically ill patient. Intensive Care Med. 2005;31:327-37.

17. Angstwurm M W, Engelmann L, Zimmermann T, et al. Selenium in Intensive Care (SIC): results of a prospective randomized, placebo-controlled, multiple-center study in patients with severe systemic inflammatory response syndrome, sepsis, and septic shock. Crit. Care Med. 2007;35:118-26.

18. Andrews P J, Avenell A, Noble D W, et al. Randomised trial of glutamine, selenium, or both, to supplement parenteral nutrition for critically ill patients. BMJ. 2011;342:d1542.

19. Berger M M, Soguel L, Shenkin A, et al. Influence of early antioxidant supplements on clinical evolution and organ function in critically ill cardiac surgery, major trauma, and subarachnoid hemorrhage patients. Critical Care. 2008;12:R101.

20. de Vega J M A, Díaz J, Serrano E, Carbonell L F. Oxidative stress in critically ill patients with systemic inflammatory response syndrome. Crit. Care Med. 2002;30:1782-6.

21. Driscoll D M, Copeland P R. Mechanism and regulation of selenoprotein synthesis. Annu. Rev. Nutr. 2003;23:17-40.

22. Motoyama T, Okamoto K, Kukita I, Hamaguchi M, Kinoshita Y, Ogawa H. Possible role of increased oxidant stress in multiple organ failure after systemic inflammatory response syndrome. Crit. Care Med. 2003;31:1048-52.

23. Rayman M P. The importance of selenium to human health. The lancet. 2000;356:233-41.

24. Burk R F, Hill K E. Selenoprotein P: an extracellular protein with unique physical characteristics and a role in selenium homeostasis. Annu. Rev. Nutr. 2005;25:215-35.

25. Schomburg L, Schweizer U, Köhrle J. Selenium and selenoproteins in mammals: extraordinary, essential, enigmatic. Cell. Mol. Life Sci. 2004;61:1988-95.

26. Chelkeba L, Ahmadi A, Abdollahi M, et al. The effect of parenteral selenium on outcomes of mechanically ventilated patients following sepsis: a prospective randomized clinical trial. Ann. of Intensive Care. 2015;5.

27. Bashar F R, Manuchehrian N, Mahmoudabadi M, Hajiesmaeili M R, Torabian S. Effects of ranitidine and pantoprazole on ventilator-associated pneumonia: a randomized double-blind clinical trial. Tanaffos. 2013;12:16.

28. Hajiesmaeili M R, Moghadam O M, Sedaghat A, et al. Evaluation of ventilator-associated pneumonia according to stress related mucosal disease prophylaxis regimen in the intensive care unit. Archives of Anesthesiology and Critical Care. 2015;1:116-9.

29. Miroliaee A E, Salamzadeh J, Shokouhi S, et al. Effect of vitamin D supplementation on procalcitonin as prognostic biomarker in patients with ventilator associated pneumonia complicated with vitamin D deficiency. Iran J. Pharm. Res. 2017;16:1254.

21

Effects of Preemptive and Preventive Intravenous Paracetamol on Postoperative Pain and Opioid Consumption in Patients Undergoing Laparoscopic Nephrectomy

Alireza Jafari[1], Mohammadreza Kamranmanesh[1*], Homayoun Aghamohammadi[1], Babak Gharaei[1], Mehranoosh Noori Khorramabadian[1], Behzad Narouie[2], Payam Sarmadi[2], Reza Valipour[3], Abbas Vali[2]

Abstract

Background: Adequate pain control is a goal in postoperative recovery. Although opioids provide good analgesic effects, their side effects such as postoperative nausea and vomiting (PONV) limit their administration. Intravenous Paracetamol as a safe and well-tolerated drug with fewer side effects can be used instead of opioids for pain management. The aim of this study is to compare preemptive or preventive administration of paracetamol with placebo group to investigate its effects on pain control and opioid consumption in patients undergoing laparoscopic nephrectomy.

Materials and Methods: Ninety patients were randomly divided to three groups. Preemptive group received 1 gram Paracetamol in 100 milliliters of 0.9% saline 30 minutes before induction of anesthesia, the preventive group received 1 gram paracetamol in 100 milliliters of 0.9% saline before closure of the skin and placebo group just received 100 milliliters of 0.9% saline. Post-surgical pain was assessed using verbal rating scale (VRS). Pethidine 0.25 mg/kg was administered and repeated each 10 minutes to control pain as needed. Pain scores, total dose of opioid and symptoms like nausea and vomiting were recorded.

Results: Preemptive and preventive groups had lower pain scores than placebo group. Opioid consumption and PONV were significantly higher in placebo group. No significant differences were observed between Preemptive and preventive groups.

Conclusion: Intervenes Paracetamol can provide an adequate pain control with few side effects and may be an effective choice in management of postoperative pain in patients undergoing laparoscopic nephrectomy.

Keywords: Paracetamol, Preemptive analgesia, Preventive analgesia, PONV

1. Anesthesiology Research Center , Department of Anesthesia, Shahid Labbafinejad Medical Center, Shahid Beheshti University of Medical Sciences, Tehran, Iran
2. Urology and Nephrology Research Center; Department of Urology, Shahid Labbafinejad Medical Center, Shahid Beheshti University of Medical Sciences, Tehran, Iran
3. Department of Urology, Tehran Medical Sciences Branch, Islamic Azad University, Tehran, Iran

Corresponding Author:
Mohammadreza Kamranmanesh. MD, Anesthesiology Research Center, Department of Anesthesia, Shahid Labbafinejad Medical Center, Shahid Beheshti University of Medical Sciences, Boostan 9th Ave, Pasdaran St, Tehran, Iran;

Email:
mrz_kamranmanesh@yahoo.com

Introduction

One of the most important issues in postoperative recovery is pain management. Inadequate pain control increases the risk of postoperative complications such as deep vein thrombosis (DVT) and espiratory insufficiency (1). On the other hand, optimal post surgical pain control will lower duration and costs of hospital stay, reduces incidence of postoperative chronic pain and increases patients' outcome (2). For decades, opioids used to be the first line medications in post operative pain management (3). Because of greater analgesic efficacy and higher patient satisfaction, patient-controlled analgesia (PCA) is the method of choice in administration of opioids (4). During opioid PCA, adverse effects such as postoperative nausea and vomiting (PONV), drowsiness, respiratory depression, and gastrointestinal and bladder dysfunction are frequent (5). Methods such as adding non-opioid analgesics like nonsteroidal anti-inflammatory drugs (NSAIDs) (6) or utilizing other additives in the PCA pumps like ketamine (7), other modalities like oral Pregabalin, intravenous corticosteroid, Lidocaine and Nitroglycerine which were reported to decrease postoperative pain (8,10) are used to decrease these side effects.

One of the other approaches to achieve an optimal post surgical pain with minimal side effects is using of preemptive analgesia (11). Preemptive Analgesia is defined as an antinociceptive treatment starting before surgery that prevents establishment of altered central afferent input from injuries; this method was shown to be more effective than preventive Analgesia, which is the administration of intraoperative analgesic agents, in controlling pain-induced sensitization of the central nervous system (11, 12). Paracetamol is a safe, well-tolerated drug with proven efficacy as analgesic that rapidly passes the blood brain barrier (13, 14). Although Paracetamol has peripheral effects but its clinical manifestations arise most likely from central action (13, 14). Intravenous (IV) administration of Paracetamol is used to relief pain (13). Peak analgesic effect of IV Paracetamol is achieved in 1 hour and lasts for 4-6 hours (14). Since it is not sedative and has no major adverse effect like respiratory and circulatory depression, it is an ideal agent for day care procedures with mild to moderate pain (15). Recently, it is suggested to use intravenous Paracetamol in postoperative pain management (11, 13, 16).

The aim of this study was to compare two different protocols of postoperative pain management, using intravenous Paracetamol as preemptive or preventive analgesia in patients undergoing laparoscopic nephrectomy, and to investigate Paracetamol efficacy in reducing the postoperative opioid consumption and its related side effects.

Methods

In this Clinical Trial study, from February 2014 until March 2015, patients between the ages of 20 and 65 years, American society of anesthesiologists (the classification of the ASA) physical status I- II, who were referred for laparoscopic nephrectomy to Labbafinejad Hospital, Tehran, Iran, were included. Written informed consent was obtained from all participating patients and the Helsinki declaration and Labbafinejad ethics committee`s rules were respected all over the study course. Patients with a history of allergy to any of the study medications (opioid, general anesthetic agents or paracetamol), history of opioid or Paracetamol use during the last 48 hours before surgery, hepatic or renal disorders, coagulopathy, pregnancy, cancer, seizure and opioid or alcohol abuse were excluded from the study. Patients with severe hemorrhage (more than 1500 ml) and duration of surgery more than 4 hours were excluded from the study. In case of reoperation before 24 hours, the data was recorded but not included in analysis.

Patients were randomly divided to three groups based on computerized randomization. In preemptive paracetamol group, 1 gram (gr.) Paracetamol (one gr. ampule, authorized by Cobel Darou Co, Iran) in 100 ml 0.9% saline (normal saline) was given to patient 30 minutes before induction of anesthesia; they also received 100 ml of normal saline prior to skin closure during surgery. In preventive Paracetamol group, patients received 100 ml IV normal saline 30 minutes before induction and 1 gr. Paracetamol in 100 ml normal saline before closure of the skin in surgery. Placebo group received 100 ml normal saline 30 minutes before induction and 100 ml normal saline before closure of the skin. All patients received 2 μg/kg Fentanyl (ampule 10 mL, Fentanyl-Janssen™, Belgium) and 0.03 mg/kg Midazolam (ampule 5 mg, MIDAZOLEX®5, Exir-Iran) as premedication. They were oxygenated with 100% oxygen for 3 minutes and then went through induction by Sodium Thiopental (EXIPENTAL 1g, Exir-Iran) 5 mg/kg and Atracurium (ampule 10 mg., Mayne Pharma Plc™, UK) 0.6 mg/kg. After intubation, maintenance of anesthesia was continued by O_2/N_2O 50% and Isoflurane (AErrane; Baxter MFD, Puerto Rico) 1.2%. Patients were continuously monitored for blood pressure, O_2 saturation, heart rate and end-tidal CO_2. The anesthesiologist administered fentanyl (20% of first dose) as needed during the operation. 30 minutes before the end of the operation, Fentanyl was not administered anymore and all the patients received Morphine Sulfate (10 mg. ampule, Darou Pakhsh Co, Iran) 0.05 mg/kg.

Verbal Rating Scale (VRS) was used for assessment of post-surgical pain in all patients 30 minutes, 4, 8 and 24 hours after the operation. In VRS 0 represents "no pain" and 10 represents, "the worst pain possible". Patient`s first request for opioid, total dose of opioid and symptoms like nausea and vomiting were recorded. An anesthesiology resident collected data through provided questionnaire. In patients with scale 3 and higher, Pethidine (ampule 50 mg, Pethedine IPDIC, Caspian Tamin pharmaceutical co. Rasht-Iran) 0.25 mg/kg was administered intravenously and repeated each 10 minutes to control pain. Patients with pain greater than 3 despite two times Pethidine administration were excluded. In patients with history of allergy to Pethidine, Morphine 2.5 mg was administered. In case of vomiting, Metoclopramide (ampule 10 mg, PLADIC®, Caspian Tamin pharmaceutical co. Rasht-Iran) 0.1 mg/kg for the first time and Ondansetron (ampule 4mg, DEMITRON®,Tehran Chemie, Tehran-Iran) 4 mg for the second time were administered. A pilot study of pain reported by patients after nephrectomy revealed that the average VAS score for pain was 3.8 with a standard deviation of 1.5. Considering a power of 0.8, alpha error at 0.05 and maximum allowable difference of 1 in VAS score the sample size of 30 patients in each group was calculated.

Statistical analysis was performed by SPSS software version 19 using ANOVA and FISHER test. $P<0.05$ was considered significant in all tests.

Results

One hundred and four patients were observed for the study. However, ten of them were opioid abusers and four of them had metastatic cancer, they were excluded. Finally, ninety patients (n=30, for each group) met the inclusion criteria. No patients met severe hemorrhage and prolonged duration of surgery. We had no case of reoperation in the first 24 hours (Figure 1). There was no significant difference among the groups regarding patients' characteristics such as age, sex, weight and duration of surgery (Table 1).

Mean values of VRS scores, in recorded intervals show a lower pain severity in preemptive and preventive group in comparison to placebo group. This difference was statically significant. VRS scores

Table 1: Patients' Characteristics.

	Preemptive	Preventive	Placebo
Age(year)	49±10	51±8	50±8
Weight(kg)	73±8	71±4	70±5
Surgery duration(min)	229±14	236±16	233±10
Sex(male/female)	21/9	18/12	24/6
ASA Class(I/II)	18/12	21/9	21/9

ASA: American Societey of Anesthesiologist Class

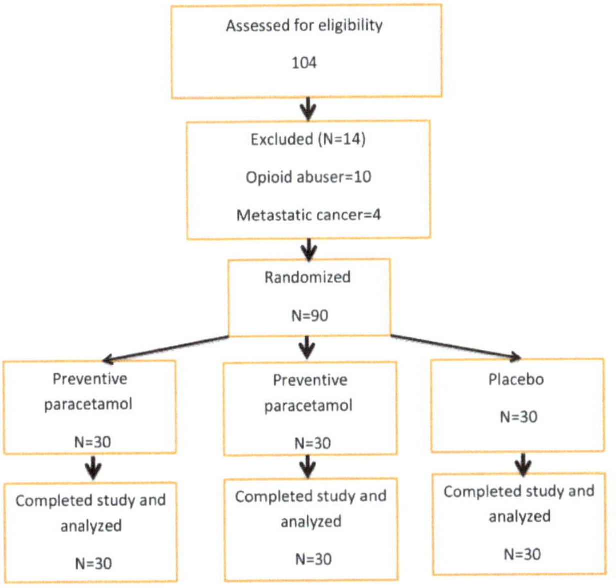

Figure 1. Consort flow diagram.

in preventive group were lower than preemptive group; however, this difference was not statically significant (Table 2). The time of first request for analgesia was also recorded. Due to our results, values of this variable in placebo group were significantly lower than preemptive and preventive group (6±2.0mins, 12±3 mins and 13±4mins respectively) (Table 2).

In all the recorded intervals, opioid consumption in placebo group was significantly higher than groups in which Paracetamol was used (P=0.001). This consumption was almost the same in preemptive and preventive group (Table 2).

Postoperative nausea and vomiting as one of the side effects of opioid, in 4 and 8 hours after operation was significantly lower in groups in which Paracetamol was used (Table 3).

Discussion

In November 2010, intravenous Paracetamol was approved by food and drug administration (FDA) for management of mild to moderate perioperative pain alone; management of moderate to severe pain with adjunctive opioid medication; and reduction of

Table 2: VRS Pain Scores and Opioid consumption in recorded intervals.

	preemptive	preventive	placebo	P-value
VRS 30	5.1±0.9	4.9±0.8	6.7±0.9	<0.0001
VRS 4	3.8±0.4	3.6±0.5	5.2±0.6	<0.0001
VRS 8	3.3±0.6	3.2±0.8	4±1.1	0.001
VRS 24	2.3±1.1	1.9±1.0	3.5±0.7	0.001
First analgesic request (minutes)	12±3	13±4	6±2.0	<0.0001
Recovery opioid consumption	52±14	50±16.0	72.5±18	0.01
Opioid consumption at 4h	40±17	45±15	72.5±14	0.001
Opioid consumption at 8h	32.5±12	27.5±8	50±10	0.001
Opioid consumption at 24h	15±10	17±10	27±8	0.001

Data presented as mean ± SD., VRS = Verbal Rating Scale (0-10)
H: hour

Table 3: The nausea and vomiting rate at 8 and 24 hours postoperative in groups.

		preemptive	preventive	Placebo	
PONV 8	**None**	18	12	9	P=0.02
	Nausea	9	12	8	
	vomiting	3	6	13	
PONV 24	**None**	18	21	17	P=0.04
	Nausea	9	6	3	
	vomiting	3	3	10	

fever. Before that, oral tablets, liquid and rectal suppository of Paracetamol were widely used for more than 4 decades (16). Administration of IV Paracetamol causes a rapid elevation in plasma concentration and higher peak levels when compared with its oral route (17). The mean peak concentration of intravenous rout is 70% higher than an equivalent oral dose. High plasma concentration causes diffusion of Paracetamol across the blood-brain barrier and results in rapid and high levels of drug in the cerebrospinal fluid (18, 19).

Intravenous Paracetamol has been shown to be effective in management of postoperative pains after several surgeries (11, 13, 15, 16). In our study, both preemptive and preventive Paracetamol lowered pain scores. Opioid consumption and side effects related to opioids like PONV were also reduced when Paracetamol was administered. Our results were consistent with Unal et al, who reported that use of preemptive or postoperative paracetamol reduces Fentanyl related nausea-vomiting in patients undergoing open nephrectomy; Although they did not observe significant decrease in total Fentanyl consumption in the early postoperative period (0-4 hours), but Paracetamol reduces total Fentanyl requirements in the first 24 hours postoperatively (13). Majumdar et al, also demonstrated that use of preemptive Paracetamol in palliative head and neck cancer surgery causes in Fentanyl requirements reduction and earlier discharge from hospital (20).

Hassan et al, compared post-surgical analgesic effects of preemptive and preventive Paracetamol in patients after cesarean section. They assessed postoperative pain by visual analog score (VAS). Their results show that preemptive Paracetamol and immediate postoperative opioid analgesia were more effective than preventive paracetamol (11). In our study, however, the differences between analgesic effects of preemptive and preventive were not significant.

Results of Khalili et al, were similar to our results, they compared analgesic effects of Paracetamol in preventive, preemptive and placebo groups on postoperative pain scores in patients undergoing lower extremity surgery. They used verbal rating scale (VRS) 5 minutes before anesthesia, and 6, 12, 18 and 24 hours after surgery. Due to their results, there were no significant differences in pain scores between the preemptive and preventive groups. However, in comparison with placebo group, Paracetamol lowered pain scores and total analgesic consumption (21).

Although paracetamol is a short acting analgesic, previous studies declared its effectiveness on postoperative side effects like PONV during the first 24 hours (22). It is proposed that decreasing the severity of pain during early postoperative period by Paracetamol could enhance its analgesic efficacy and may end up in opioid sparing until the late postoperative period.

Limitations of our study include a lack of proper method for blinding the investigators and the patients. While this may have a little disturbing effect on Data analysis, further observations with proper method for blinding are recommended.

Conclusion

We demonstrated that IV Paracetamol might be an effective choice in management of postoperative pain in patients undergoing laparoscopic nephrectomy. It lowers pain scores, opioid consumption and reduces side effects of opioid like PONV. Due to this study, there is no significant difference between Preemptive and Preventive protocols for Paracetamol administration.

Acknowledgment

Authors would like to thank members of operation rooms, urology and ICU wards of Labbafinejad hospital for their cooperation.

Conflicts of Interest

The authors declare that they have no conflict of interest.

References

1. Lawrence VA, Hilsenbeck SG, Mulrow CD, Dhanda R, Sapp J, Page CP. Incidence and hospital stay for cardiac and pulmonary complications after abdominal surgery. Journal of general internal medicine. 1995;10(12):671-8.

2. Imani F. Postoperative pain management. Anesth Pain. 2011;1(1):6-7.

3. Gianesello L, Pavoni V, Barboni E, Galeotti I, Nella A. Perioperative pregabalin for postoperative pain control and quality of life after major spinal surgery. Journal of neurosurgical anesthesiology. 2012;24(2):121-6.

4. Ballantyne JC, Carr DB, Chalmers TC, Dear KB, Angelillo IF, Mosteller F. Postoperative patient-controlled analgesia: meta-analyses of initial randomized control trials. Journal of clinical anesthesia. 1993;5(3):182-93.

5. Walder B, Schafer M, Henzi I, Tramer M. Efficacy and safety of patient- controlled opioid analgesia for acute postoperative pain. Acta Anaesthesiologica Scandinavica. 2001;45(7):795-804.

6. Marret E, Kurdi O, Zufferey P, Bonnet F. Effects of nonsteroidal antiinflammatory drugs on patient-controlled analgesia morphine side effectsMeta-analysis of randomized controlled trials. The Journal of the American Society of Anesthesiologists. 2005;102(6):1249-60--60.

7. Imani F, Faiz HR, M Sedaghat, Hajiashrafi M. Effects of Adding Ketamine to Fentanyl Plus Acetaminophen on Postoperative Pain by Patient Controlled Analgesia in Abdominal Surgery. Anesth Pain Med. 2014;4(1):e12162.

8. Alimian M, Imani F, Faiz SHR, Pournajafian A, Navadegi SF, Safari S. Effect of Oral Pregabalin Premedication on Post-Operative Pain in Laparoscopic Gastric Bypass Surgery. Anesth Pain Med. 2012;2(1):12-6.

9. Rahimzadeh P, Imani F, Faiz HR, Nikoubakht N, Sayarifard A. Effects of Intravenous Methylprenisolone on Pain after Intertrochanteric Femoral Fracture Surgery. J Clin Diagn Res. 2014;8(4):GC01-4.

10. Gharaei H, Imani F. Beneficial effect of intravenous nitroglycerin and lidocaine in severe pain due to acute arterial occlusion. Indian J Pain. 2014;28(1):42-3.

11. Hassan HIEA. Perioperative analgesic effects of intravenous paracetamol: Preemptive versus preventive analgesia in elective cesarean section. Anesthesia, Essays and Researches. 2014;8(3):339.

12. Shen X, Wang F, Xu S, Ma L, Liu Y, Feng S, et al. Comparison of the analgesic efficacy of preemptive and preventive tramadol after lumpectomy. Pharmacological Reports. 2008;60(3):415.

13. Unal S, Aksoy M, Ahiskalioglu A, Erdem A, Adanur S. The effect of intravenous preemptive paracetamol on postoperative fentanyl consumption in patients undergoing open nephrectomy: A prospective randomized study. Nigerian journal of clinical practice. 2015;18(1):68-74.

14. Arici S, Gurbet A, Türker G, Yavaşcaoğlu B, Sahin S. Preemptive analgesic effects of intravenous paracetamol in total abdominal hysterectomy. Agri. 2009;21(2):54-61.

15. Ali MA, Shamim F, Chughtai S. Comparison between intravenous paracetamol and fentanyl for intraoperative and postoperative pain relief in dilatation and evacuation: Prospective, randomized interventional trial. Journal of anaesthesiology, clinical pharmacology. 2015;31(1):54.

16. Lachiewicz PF. The role of intravenous acetaminophen in multimodal pain protocols for perioperative orthopedic patients. Orthopedics. 2013;36(2):15-9.

17. Schutz R, Fong L, Chang Y, Royal M, editors. Open-label, 4-period, randomized crossover study to determine the comparative pharmacokinetics of oral and intravenous acetaminophen administration in healthy male volunteers. Poster presentation at the 32nd Annual Meeting and Workshops American Society of Regional Anesthesia and Pain (ASRA); 2007.

18. Singla NK, Parulan C, Samson R, Hutchinson J, Bushnell R, Beja EG, et al. Plasma and cerebrospinal fluid pharmacokinetic parameters after single- dose administration of intravenous, oral, or rectal acetaminophen. Pain Practice. 2012;12(7):523-32.

19. Jensen L, Handberg G, Brøsen K, Schmedes A, Ørding H. Paracetamol concentrations in plasma and cerebrospinal fluid: A-785. European Journal of Anaesthesiology (EJA). 2004;21:193.

20. Majumdar S, Das A, Kundu R, Mukherjee D, Hazra B, Mitra T. Intravenous paracetamol infusion: Superior pain management and earlier discharge from hospital in patients undergoing palliative head-neck cancer surgery. Perspectives in clinical research. 2014;5(4):172.

21. Khalili G, Janghorbani M, Saryazdi H, Emaminejad A. Effect of

preemptive and preventive acetaminophen on postoperative pain score: a randomized, double-blind trial of patients undergoing lower extremity surgery. Journal of clinical anesthesia. 2013;25(3):188-92.

22. Cok OY, Eker HE, Pelit A, Canturk S, Akin S, Aribogan A, et al. The effect of paracetamol on postoperative nausea and vomiting during the first 24 h after strabismus surgery: A prospective, randomised, double- blind study. Eur J Anaesthesiol. 2011;28:836-41.

22

Rh-Incompatibility-Induced Delayed Hemolytic Transfusion Reaction: Role of Immunologic Reactions in RH-Incompatibility

Mohammadreza Moshari[1], Ronak Karbalaeifar[1], Maryam Vosoghian[1], Bahman Malek[1], Mastaneh Dahi-Taleghani[1]

Abstract

Blood transfusions cause to increase oxygen-carrying capacity and intravascular volume. Despite all the benefits of transfusion, it may have some complications. When mistransfusion occurs or when no other option is available, incompatible packed-cells may be infused, which puts the patient at risk of experiencing a hemolytic transfusion reaction (HTR). The HTRs are classified as acute or delayed reactions have wide spectrum of clinical presentations. In this report, we present a case of delayed hemolytic reaction due to rhesus factor (Rh) incompatibility in the operation room. Critical incident reporting and evaluation of adverse transfusion reactions may provide data for effective patient management and prevent the occurrence or repetition of these events.

1. Anesthesiology Research Center, Shahid Beheshti University of Medical Sciences, Tehran, Iran

Corresponding Author:
Ronak Karbalaeifar, MD,
Anesthesiology Research Center,
Shahid Beheshti University of Medical Sciences, Tehran, Iran;
e mail: ronak_k1990@yahoo.com

Keywords: Transfusion, hemolytic transfusion reaction, blood group incompatibility, antibody

Introduction

In general, incompatible transfusions should be strictly avoided, as hemolysis of the transfused red blood cells (RBCs) can happen with potentially fatal outcomes, known as hemolytic transfusion reactions (Figure 1) (1).

Clinical presentations of an incompatible transfusion cover a broad spectrum: in mild cases, the patients become immunized with alloantibodies bearing a potential risk for later transfusions or their pregnancies. Sometimes, serological tests become positive after the transfusion without any clinical presentations. In some other cases, the positive effect of the transfusion (e.g. rising of hemoglobin) is missing or too short lasting, but in a number of cases, severe or life-threatening events may occur (2).

According to published statistics (2011-2015), about 14% of all deaths due to blood transfusion were related to non-ABO-dependent types (3-4). In fact, by implementing this process, the serum IgM levels increase sharply. This causes intravascular hemolysis, which ultimately ends in renal dysfunction, shock and death. Although immunoglobulin M hemolytic transfusion reactions (IgM-HTRs) have lower prevalence rates than HTRs (IgG-HTRs), the severity of degradation due to increased IgM-HTRs is more than other types (5-7).

Antibody-induced hemolysis generally occurs by one of these two mechanisms; first, RBCs can be lysed intravascularly when complement is activated to form the Membrane Attack Complex (MAC). (8-11). This is usually due to IgM binding to the RBC membrane but can also occur with IgG (5-7).

Phagocytes can also opsonize the RBCs, a process called as extravascular hemolysis. If activation of complement does not lead to MAC formation to the extent that rapid intravascular hemolysis occurs, then C3 deposited on the RBC surface may convert to C3b and iC3b. In this case, Complement Receptors on phagocytes (i.e., CR1, CR2, and CR3) can consume C3b-coated RBCs. Second, antibody-induced opsonization can occur as a result of Fc domains of IgG bound to RBCs, which are recognized by Fcγ receptors (FcγRs) on phagocytes intravascularly (12-15). There is significant data mostly in animal models, which demonstrates the existence of each of these mechanisms of RBC clearance after binding to antibodies (8-11).

Regardless of the canonical pathways described, alternative mechanisms of IgG-mediated RBC clearance have been suggested, which involve neither complement nor FcγR pathways. These include destabilization of the RBC membrane by antibody binding which can induce eryptosis (programmed RBC death) (12-18).

Several in vitro investigations suggested that IgM and IgG antibodies interact with complement in different ways; it showed that one molecule of IgM on a cell surface is sufficient to initiate complement fixation, but a doublet (two molecules side by side) of the IgG in serum is required to form a complement-fixing site. Nevertheless, electron microscopic and molecular studies have suggested that IgG antibody, although inefficient at initiating fixation of complement, may produce more membrane damage in comparison to IgM. Meanwhile, a series of cell surface receptors have been described which improve the adherence of antibody and complement-coated erythrocytes to macrophages and lymphocytes. Receptors specific for IgM, IgG and complement on macrophages and for complement on lymphocytes; these cellular receptors play an important role in both sequestration and clearance (19-23).

Reporting the adverse transfusion reactions is not to find a guilty person but to reveal the cause of a transfusion reaction in order to treat the patient adequately and to prevent the occurrence or repetition of an adverse event (24).

Clinical Report

A 16-month old boy with left lateral neck mass (rhabdomyosarcoma) was brought to our operating room by the ear, nose, and throat (ENT) surgeons for palliative resection of the mass (Figure2). He had had the swelling of his left lateral neck for 9 months and underwent surgery in respect of the mass when he was 11-month old which was diagnosed as rhabdomyosarcoma in pathological studies. It started to grow again and became 62*31*52 millimeters involving facial muscles, candidate for palliative resection.

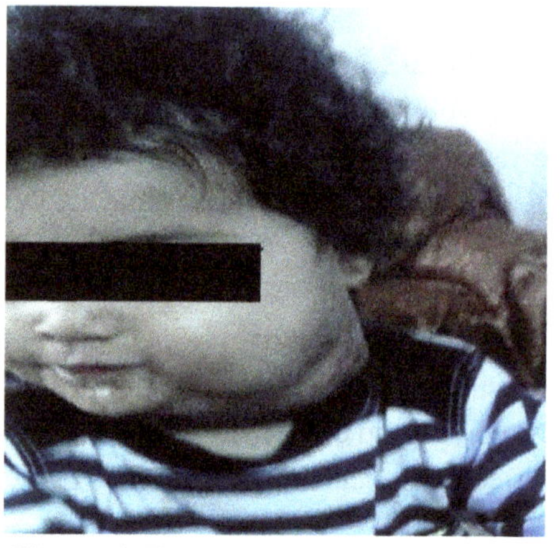

Figure 1. The patient with mandibular rhabdomyosarcoma.

On preoperative assessment, the patient weighed 12 kilograms. No other problem was found in history and physical examination except for being passive-smoker. The anteroposterior and lateral neck X-ray showed intact airway with small deviation of trachea to the right side (Figure 3). His blood group and Rh was B-negative and laboratory data was within normal range (hemoglobin = 11 gr/dL, hematocrit = 33.7%).

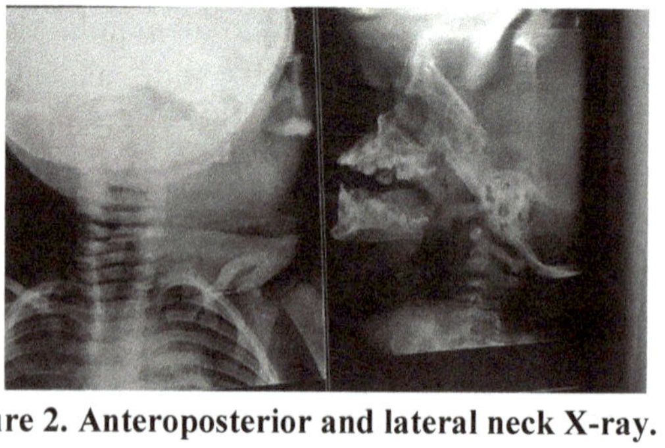

Figure 2. Anteroposterior and lateral neck X-ray.

Anesthesia induced using Sevoflurane 8% inhalation in oxygen; under basic monitoring (electrocardiogram, pulse oximetry, noninvasive blood pressure). Administering 0.25 mg atropine intravenously after about two minutes, the patient was successfully intubated in the first try by direct laryngoscopy using a #3.5 cuffed endotracheal tube. Then, 4 mg Atracurium and 25 microgram Fentanyl were infused through the intravascular (IV) line and maintenance of anesthesia was continued with Sevoflurane 2.5%.

After 30 minutes of surgery, according to estimated blood loss (140 cc), we prescribed 20 cc of packed-cell for the infant. Soon after blood transfusion, blood bank informed us about sending the wrong unit of O-negative blood to the operation room.

The transfusion was stopped. 200 mL of saline 0.9% was administered over 15 minutes; Foley catheter was inserted,10 gr of mannitol was infused over 15 minutes; 5 mg of Furosemide was injected; 10 mEq sodium bicarbonate was administered to alkalize the urine; the packed-cell and blood sample of patient was sent to the laboratory to repeat the crossmatch. Blood and urine samples were sent to the laboratory to check the blood cell count, partial thromboplastin time, fibrinogen level, direct coombs and urine analysis. Axillary temperature was 37.8°C.

Surgery lasted for about 90 minutes. He was extubated and taken to recovery when able to cry and according to lab results there was no hemoglobinuria, coagulation profile was normal and direct coombs was reported negative; but after six hours, the lab results were changed as below:

Hemoglobin: 6.3 g/dL, Platelet: 307000, Hematocrit: 20%, Reticulin count: 0.2% (corrected=1%), partial thromboplastin time: 30, prothrombin time: 12, International Normalized Ratio: 1.1, Urine Analysis: RBC: 3-5, pH 7.5, Hemoglobin: +, total Bilirubin: 0.6 mg/dL, direct Bilirubin direct: 0.2 mg/dL, Direct coombs: negative, Lactate Dehydrogenase: 870 U/L, Fibrinogen: 190 mg/dL.

Fifteen cc/Kg of iso-group and iso-Rh packed-cell was infused over 4 hours and 5 mg of furosemide was prescribed. Three hours after transfusion hemoglobin concentration was 9 gr/dL and no hemoglobinuria were found in urine sample. All other lab data was normal. He was discharged in a stable condition two days later, after removing the drain and hemovac. In a weekly follow-up of our patient during the next 2 months, no serum antibodies appeared.

Discussion

Human error is a substantial factor in iatrogenic injury (1). Fortunately, most of these errors do not result in patient injury, but a small number can have catastrophic effects and lengthen the hospital stay.

The reasons for mistransfusions may occur in the pre-analytical, laboratory and/or clinical periods of transfusion. Examples of pre-analytical errors are incorrect patient identification, donor mix-ups, and incorrect blood bag labelling. Laboratory errors may cause incorrect blood grouping or cross-matching. Clinical errors may happen at bedside testing or when the units are being transfused. Electronic data processing systems and various hemovigilance systems have been established during recent years to prevent these mistakes (25).

Chiaroni et al, found that during a 5-year period in France, the incidence of ABO discrepancies was 1 per 3,400 tests performed. In their experience, most discrepancies (58%) were secondary to phlebotomy errors in which the samples were obtained from the wrong patient, whereas the second common cause of discrepancy was error during patient registration (30%) (25). In comparison, in a study that Figueroa et al. have done, 90% of errors were due to patient identification at the time of phlebotomy, and only 10% were due to admission or registration errors (26).

MacDougall and co-workers have attempted to mitigate the risk of ABO mismatch associated with knowledge gap. Based on the findings, they found that the use of adaptive methods (for blood compatibility in ABO system) is helpful in blood donors and recipients. In fact, this can be done as a "forcing function" before the release of blood from the blood bank and before transfusion at the bedside to reduce transfusion mismatch associated with gaps in ABO compatibility knowledge especially in Fresh Frozen Plasma and Platelet transfusion (25).

Some options include easy access to standard operating procedure instructions in work areas (25), a blood-component lock system that will not allow the issuance of a component unless there is a patient wristband and blood component match (26), and computerized inventory control that will not permit issuance of a blood component that does not match the written request. Ultimately, automation may be the best solution. Handheld bar-code devices that may be used at the bedside can prevent the need for visual matching of data (26-28).

Ahrens et al. reported that of 21 transfusion-related errors, one (4.8%) was a pre-analytical error, 4 (19.0%) were laboratory errors and 16 (76.2%) were clinical errors (28). Their results confirm that bedside testing is the weakest link in the safety chain of transfusion in medical practice (26-29).

Delayed hemolytic transfusion reactions have been studied widely in the setting of sickle cell disease and beta-thalassemia, emphasizing the risk of adverse events in patients with baseline hematologic deficiencies (26-29). Chadebech et al, reported two cases of sickle cell disease with delayed hemolytic transfusion reaction in the absence of detectable antibody. Even in monthly follow-up of the serum of these patients in 6 months, no antibodies appeared (26).

Within the pediatric population, allergic reactions to platelets and RBCs were the most common reported reaction types. As said by Vossoughi et al. the rate of allergic reactions to platelets was more than three times, and the rate of allergic reactions to RBCs was more than seven times the adult rate (26).

Irani et al, reported a case of a delayed hemolytic transfusion reaction due to anti-e, an antigen in the Rh blood group system, after a liver transplant that was a consequence of receiving emergent incompatible RBC transfused during surgery that was treated successfully using an automated red cell exchange. According to this study, they stated that how a red cell exchange can reduce the potentially harmful effects of a delayed hemolytic transfusion reaction caused by anti-e or any clinically significant red blood cell antibody (26).

Werch et al, reported two women in child bearing age who had D2 blood type and received two units of D1 RBCs. Prompt delivery of intravenous RHIG (Rh Immunoglobulin) prophylaxis could prevent alloimmunization and associated complications in those two patients (27).

Arneja et al, have combined a recently developed mouse model for transfusion mediated RBC alloimmunization with mice genetically deficient in interleukin-6 receptor (IL-6Rα) to determine the role of IL-6Rα signaling in regulating RBC alloimmunization. The findings indicated that IL-6Rα signaling plays a key role in the generation of anti-RBC alloantibodies in response to transfused RBCs. Based on these results, available biologics targeting IL-6Rα can be a therapeutic option for the prevention of RBC alloimmunization (27).

While much remains to be learned, better concept of the cellular and molecular mechanisms that govern the course of HTRs, will undoubtedly lead to better therapy and improved survival for patients suffering this life-threatening complication of transfusion and shorten the duration of their hospital stay.

Conclusion

By decreasing the incidence of human errors we can prevent complications of mistransfusion. There are so many unknown aspects of cellular and molecular pathophysiology of mistransfusion which could be a good target for future researches. By preventing human errors and improving our knowledge and skill to face these kind of complications, we can hopefully improve survival of our patients.

Acknowledgment

The authors want to thank Dr Hengameh Asadi for her kind cooperation.

Conflicts of Interest

The authors declare that there are no conflicts of interest.

References

1. Vamvakas EC, Blajchman MA. Transfusion-related mortality: the ongoing risks of allogeneic blood transfusion and the available strategies for their prevention. Blood. 2009;113(15):3406-17.
2. Zimring JC, Spitalnik SL. Pathobiology of transfusion reactions. Annual review of pathology. 2015;10:83-110.
3. Mollison PL, Engelfriet P. Blood transfusion. Seminars in hematology. 1999;36(4 Suppl 7):48-58.
4. Mollison PL. The genetic basis of the Rh blood group system. Transfusion. 1994;34(6):539-41.
5. Kolins J. Fatalities from blood transfusion. Jama. 1981;245(11):1120.
6. Holness L, Knippen MA, Simmons L, Lachenbruch PA. Fatalities

caused by TRALI. Transfusion medicine reviews. 2004;18(3):184-8.
7. Gaines AR. Disseminated intravascular coagulation associated with acute hemoglobinemia or hemoglobinuria following Rh(0)(D) immune globulin intravenous administration for immune thrombocytopenic purpura. Blood. 2005;106(5):1532-7.
8. van der Schoot CE, de Haas M, Clausen FB. Genotyping to prevent Rh disease: has the time come? Current opinion in hematology. 2017;24(6):544-50.
9. Sandler SG, Chen LN, Flegel WA. Serological weak D phenotypes: a review and guidance for interpreting the RhD blood type using the RHD genotype. British journal of haematology. 2017;179(1):10-9.
10. Quraishy N, Sapatnekar S. Advances in Blood Typing. Advances in clinical chemistry. 2016; 77:221-69.
11. Belsito A, Magnussen K, Napoli C. Emerging strategies of blood group genotyping for patients with hemoglobinopathies. Transfusion and apheresis science: official journal of the World Apheresis Association: official journal of the European Society for Haemapheresis. 2017;56(2):206-13.
12. Garratty G. Advances in red blood cell immunology 1960 to 2009. Transfusion. 2010;50(3):526-35.
13. Daniels G. A century of human blood groups. Wiener klinische Wochenschrift. 2001;113(20-21):781-6.
14. Daniels G. Functional aspects of red cell antigens. Blood reviews. 1999;13(1):14-35.
15. Agarwal B. Autoimmune hemolytic anemia. Indian journal of pediatrics. 1998;65(5):663-8.
16. Repsold L, Joubert AM. Eryptosis: An Erythrocyte's Suicidal Type of Cell Death. Biomed Res Int. 2018; 2018:9405617.
17. Jemaa M, Fezai M, Bissinger R, Lang F. Methods Employed in Cytofluorometric Assessment of Eryptosis, the Suicidal Erythrocyte Death. BioMed research international. 2017;43(2):431-44.
18. Farag MR, Alagawany M. Erythrocytes as a biological model for screening of xenobiotics toxicity. Chemico-biological interactions. 2018;279:73-83.
19. Wouters D, Zeerleder S. Complement inhibitors to treat IgM-mediated autoimmune hemolysis. Haematologica. 2015;100(11):1388-95.
20. Lunn MP, Nobile-Orazio E. Immunotherapy for IgM anti-myelin-associated glycoprotein paraprotein-associated peripheral neuropathies. Cochrane Database Syst Rev. 2016;10: Cd002827.
21. Bakchoul T, Jouni R, Warkentin TE. Protamine (heparin)-induced thrombocytopenia: a review of the serological and clinical features associated with anti-protamine/heparin antibodies. Journal of thrombosis and haemostasis : JTH. 2016;14(9):1685-95.
22. Mousavi Hosseini K, Ghasemzadeh M. Implementation of Plasma Fractionation in Biological Medicines Production. Iranian journal of biotechnology. 2016;14(4):213-20.
23. Greinacher A, Selleng K, Warkentin TE. Autoimmune heparin-induced thrombocytopenia. Journal of thrombosis and haemostasis : JTH. 2017;15(11):2099-114.
24. Leape LL. Error in medicine. JAMA 1994; 272:1851-7.
25. Faber JC. Worldwide overview of existing haemovigilance systems. Transfus Apheresis Sci. 2004; 31:99–110.
26. Chiaroni J, Legrand D, Dettori I. Analysis of ABO discrepancies occurring in 35 French hospitals. Transfusion. 2004; 44:860-864.
27. Figueroa F, Priscilla I. "Nearly two decades using the check-type to prevent ABO-incompatible transfusions: one institution's experience." American journal of clinical pathology. 2006;422-6.
28. MacDougall, Nickolas, et al. "Preventing Mistransfusions: An Evaluation of Institutional Knowledge and a Response." Anesthesia & Analgesia. 2018.1;247-251.
29. Newton JM, DeVeaux J, Brendel J, et al. Job aides, a novel approach to standardized blood collection (abstract). Transfusion. 1999;39(Suppl):129S.

Epidural Anesthesia with Lidocaine and Dexmedetomidine, Versus Lidocaine Alone on Plasma Levels of IL-6 in Patients with Proximal Femoral Fracture

Mohammadreza Moshari[1], Bahman Malek[1], Adel Ebrahimpour[2], Maryam Vosoughian[1], Mastane Dahi-Taleghani[1], Ehsan Ghorbani[1], Seyed Mohammad Seyed-Alshohadaei[1]

Abstract

Background: Interleukin-6 (IL-6) plays an important role in inflammatory. Epidural anesthesia is an appropriate method for controlling pain in lower limb surgeries. The aim of this study was to evaluate the effect of Dexmedetomidine and Lidocaine in the epidural injection by measuring IL-6 plasma levels.

Materials and Methods: Fifty-two patients with lower limb fractures in two groups receiving Dexmedetomidine doses and controls for the quality of epidural anesthesia and IL-6 index. After explaining the design and obtaining informed written consent, patients were randomly divided into two groups. After 4–6 minutes of administering the test dose, patients in group RC received 5 ml of 1.5% Lidocaine solution via epidural catheter. Patients in group RD were administered 15 ml solution of 1.5% ropivacaine and 0.6 µg/kg of Dexmedetomidine. The levels of IL-6 were evaluated before surgery and 6 hours after surgery.

Results: The two groups did not show a significant difference in age and level of interleukin prior to the operation. There was a significant difference in the second injection time and total drug volume between the control and intervention groups. Dexmedetomidine reduced the volume of total drug needed and increased the time interval from the first injection to the second one (p <0.001).There was also lower levels of interleukin 6 in the Dexmedetomidine group at the 6th hour-after the operation.

Conclusion: Dexmedetomidine does not only reduce the need for patients on the amount and frequency of analgesic drugs, but also reduces stress and cellular damage.

Keywords: Interleukin-6, Dexmedetomidine, Lidocaine, Anesthesia

1. Anesthesiology Research Center, Shahid Beheshti University of Medical Sciences, Tehran, Iran
2. Department of Orthopedic Surgery, Taleghani Hospital, Shahid Beheshti University of Medical Sciences, Tehran, Iran

Corresponding Author:
Mohammadreza Moshari, MD, Assistant Professor, Anesthesiology Research Center, Shahid Beheshti University of Medical Sciences, Tehran, Iran;

Email: rmoshari@sbmu.ac.ir

Introduction

The increasing use of topical anesthetic, major and minor neural blocks has led to the selective use of general anesthesia. This is because avoiding general anesthesia risks, better postoperative pain control, and some other factors in long-term surgery and long-term postoperative pain control, local anesthetic drugs with a long-lasting effect are common. Meanwhile, auxiliary drugs are also used to maximize the length of the base drug (1).

Considering the history of local anesthesia and

many studies in this field, today, the tendency of anesthesiologists to perform local block has increased and this may reduce the need for general anesthesia (1). This method is used to carry out surgical procedures or control postoperative pain in order to remove pain and to create anesthesia (2), creating favorable conditions during surgery and faster postoperative patient mobility, and decreasing the risks of general anesthesia and hospital costs (3).

Lidocaine reduces inflammatory processes. The substance acts by lowers the release of cytokines from epithelial cells and neutrophils and reducing the production of cytokines caused by damage to endothelial cells (4). These cytokines are of the pro-inflammatory type (5).

Dexmedetomidine is an α-agonist (11). Some studies have shown that the use of this drug (due to its low toxicity) can reduce cell death. (6). This drug lowers the concentration of tumor necrosis alpha (TNF-α) (7,8). On the other hand, in various studies on apoptosis of the epithelial cells of the intestine, it has reduced the inflammatory response and accelerated the intestinal improvement after trauma (9,10). In several studies, the positive effect of intravenous Dexmedetomidine on the control of inflammatory responses and the reduction of levels of inflammatory mediators such as IL-6 has been confirmed (12-15).

The purpose of this study was to learn whether the use of this drug as an adjuvant in epidural injection has meaningful effects. Confirmation of this positive effect can provide a low cost and easy method to reduce the complications of inflammatory response after lower limb surgery.

Methods

In this study, all patients were referred to Taleghani Hospital (affiliated to Shahid Beheshti University of Medical Sciences, Tehran, Iran) in 2017, who suffered from lower limb fractures and who needed surgery were evaluated. The inclusion criteria were: 18-75 years old, lower limb fractures, ASA Class I & II, and no history of allergy. However, the following patients were not included in the study: absolute contraindication for using local anesthetics, and the presence of these comorbidities: diabetes mellitus, myocardial infarction, major cardiovascular events, cerebrovascular accidents, hypertension, malignancy, renal failure, liver dysfunction and coagulation disorders.

After explaining the design and obtaining informed written consent, patients were randomly divided into two groups. Patients were administered epidural block with 18-gauge Tuohy needle and catheter was secured 3–4 cm into epidural space and a test dose of 3 ml of 2% Lidocaine solution containing adrenaline 1:200,000 was injected. After 4–6 minutes of administering the test dose, patients in group RC received 5 ml of 1.5% Lidocaine solution. Patients in group RD were administered 15 ml solution of 1.5% ropivacaine and 0.6 μg/kg of Dexmedetomidine. The bilateral pin-prick method was used to evaluate and check the sensory level while a modified Bromage scale (0 = no block, 1 = inability to raise extended leg, 2 = inability to flex knee and 3 = inability to flex ankle and foot) was used to measure the motor blockade effect at 5, 10, 15, 20, 25 and 30 minutes intervals after the epidural administration of the drugs.

The second dose was injected every 45-60 minutes based on need (VAS> 3; Visual Analog Scale: VAS), then 8 mL of 1.5%, Lidocaine and the final dose of the received drug was recorded at the end of the operation. Blood samples were taken from all patients before entering the operating room to determine the level of the interleukin-6. During surgery, the onset of anesthesia, time to second injection, duration of operation and volume of blood loss, the volume of intake and output, and the amount of injected drug by the epidural catheter were recorded. In order to control the pain in all patients, intravenous morphine infusion pump was given at a dose of 3 to 5 mg/hr. Additional drug doses were prescribed if necessary to maintain VAS <3 in the first 24 hours. Blood samples were taken at 6 hours after surgery to measure the level of interleukin-6 in all patients.

IL-6 detection method

5 cc blood samples were taken from the patient and placed in a simple test tube. After blood clotting at room temperature (15-30 minutes), it was centrifuged (3000 to 3500) at room temperature for 15 minutes. The yielding plasma was poured into the microtube and stored in -70°C. Collected samples evaluated by Bio-Science ELISA Kits.

The obtained data was collected and using descriptive statistics, the results of IL-6 were reported according to the variables in question. In addition, to compare the IL-6 level among the patients in both groups, independent t-test was used.

Results

Table 1: Descriptive statistics of variables

	N	Minimum	Maximum	Mean	Std. Deviation
Age (years)	52	24.00	75.00	53.4038	15.8439
Onset time (min)	52	10.00	22.00	15.8846	3.12268
Second injection(min)	51	35.00	165.00	60.7647	21.71690
LA Final Vol (ml)	52	20.00	65.00	42.0385	9.48469
Received fluid (L)	52	1.50	28.00	3.0808	3.55500
Blooding volume (ml)	52	50.00	600.00	257.3077	122.60434
Urine volume (ml)	52	50.00	1000.00	595.1923	173.56120
Base Serum IL (pg/ml)	52	0.20	23.50	4.1892	5.70042
Six hours IL_6 (pg/ml)	52	1.1	120	20.07	19.93
Surgery time (min)	52	75.00	300.00	177.2115	43.81796
Valid Number of cases	51				

In this study, 52 patients, 19 women (36.5%) and 33 men (63.5%), were divided into two groups of 26 patients. The mean age of the patients was 15.8±53.4 years (Table 1).

Based on the results, the mean of the second injection requirement (51 out of 52) was 60.7 ± 21.7. Duration of surgery was same between the two groups. Also no significant difference in volume of received fluid during surgery and the level of baseline interleukin was seen. On the other hand, based on independent t-test, there was a significant difference between the two groups regarding the bleeding and urine volumes ($p < 0.05$) (Table 2).According to the U Mann Whitney test, the second injection and drug levels were significantly different between the control and intervention groups. Dexmedetomidine reduced the need for a second injection ($p < 0.001$) (Table 3).

There was a significant difference between the two groups in terms of IL-6 after 6 hours of operation, and this was lower in the Dexmedetomidine group (Table 4).

Discussion

Today, use of regional anesthesia is superior to general anesthesia in many procedures, because it has fewer side effects and makes it easier for the patient to have mobility and daily activities. In recent years, however, stress and cellular damage have become a problem that attracts the attention of experts and researchers and has attracted efforts to reduce it. This study also considers the importance of the present method using two different drugs.

Lidocaine and relevant drugs, which are used primarily as positional anesthetics and antiarrhythmic factors. Lidocaine exerts immunoregulatory effects on a variety of cell types. For example, lidocaine-related local anesthetics were shown to inhibit lymphocyte maturation and proliferation, the migration of macrophages into tissues (16), the expression of CD11b/CD18 by polymorphonuclear cells (19), the adhesion of leucocytes to injured venules (17–19) and the LPS-stimulated secretion of LTB4 and IL-1a from peripheral blood mononuclear cells (20). Moreover, the anti-inflammatory effects of lidocaine were shown by in vivo studies as well. Taniguchi *et al.*, have shown that lidocaine treatment of rabbits injected with endotoxin reduced the serum concentrations of IL-8 and IL-6 (21).

Previous studies have shown DEX has a low cytotoxic effect, which in some studies reduces cell death (6). On the other hand, this drug lowers the concentration of tumor necrosis alpha (TNF-α) (7,8). In various studies on apoptosis of the epithelial cells of the intestine, it reduces the inflammatory response and accelerates the intestinal improvement after trauma (9,10). In several studies, the positive effect of intravenous Dexmedetomidine on the control of inflammatory responses and the decrease, of levels of inflammatory mediators such as IL-6 has been confirmed (12-15).

Accordingly, based on these results, dexmedetomidine not only reduces the amount and frequency of analgesic drug administration, but also reduces stress and cellular damage. So, dexmedetomidine is suggested as a good option for similar surgeries. Of course, further studies are needed in order to evaluate the best application and other effects of the drugs used in this study can lead to better anesthesia plans.

Conclusion

Not only does dexmedetomidine reduce the need for patients on the amount and frequency of analgesic drugs, but also it lowers stress and cellular damage.

Acknowledgment

The authors would like to acknowledge the kind help of all physicians and nurses of Taleghani Hospital, SBMU, Tehran, Iran for their kind assistance.

Conflicts of Interest

The authors declare that they have no conflict of interest.

References

1. Charles B, Strichantz B&GR. Local anesthetics: In Miller, RD, editor. Anesthesia. Vol 1, 5th ed.Philadelphia: Churchill Livingstone; 2000, P. 491-517.

2. Turkan H, Baykal B, Ozisik T. Axillary brachial plexus blockade: an evaluation of three techniques. Mil Med. 2002;167(9):723-5.

3. Bergendahl H, Lönnqvist PA, Eksborg S. Clonidine: an alternative to benzodiazepines for premedication in children. Current opinion in anesthesiology. 2005;18(6):608-13.

4. Hollmann MW, Durieux ME. Local anesthetics and the inflammatory response: a new therapeutic indication. Anesthesiology. 2000;93:858–75.

5. Lahav M, Levite M, Bassani L. Lidocaine inhibits secretion of IL-8 and IL-1beta and stimulates secretion receptor antagonist by epithelial cells. ClinExpImmunol. 2002;127:226–33.

6. Sinclair R, Eriksson AS, Gretzer C, et al. Inhibitory effects of amide local anesthetics on stimulus-induced human leukocyte metabolic activation, LTB4 release and IL-1 secretion in vitro. Acta Anaesthesiol Scand. 1993;37:159–65.

7. Sanders RD, Xu J, Shu Y, Januszewski A, Halder S, Fidalgo A, Sun P, Hossain M, Ma D, Maze M. Dexmedetomidine attenuates isoflurane-induced neurocognitive impairment in neonatal rats. Anesthesiology. 2009;110:1077–85.

8. Li B, Li Y, Tian S, Wang H, Wu H, Zhang A, et al. Anti-inflammatory effects of perioperative dexmedetomidine administered as an adjunct to general anesthesia: a meta-analysis, Sci. Rep. 5(2015):12342.

9. Kuru S, Bozkirli OB, Barlas AM, Duymus ME, Senes M, Yumusak N, et al. The preventive effect of dexmedetomidine against postoperative intra-abdominal adhesions in rats, Int. Surg. 2015;100(1):87–95.

10. Liu YE, Tong CC, Zhang YB, Jin HX, Gao Y, Hou MX. Effect of dexmedetomidine on rats with renal ischemia-reperfusion injury and the expression of tight junction protein in kidney, Int. J. Clin. Exp. Med. 2015;8(10):18751–7.

11. Riquelme JA, Westermeier F, Hall AR, Vicencio JM, Pedrozo Z, Ibacache B, et al. Dexmedetomidine protects the heart against ischemia-reperfusion injury by an endothelial eNOS/NO-dependent mechanism, Pharmacol. Res. 2016;103:318–27.

12. Xin Y, Xie K, Xie H. Effects of Dexmedetomidine on Survival Rate, IL-6, and IL-10 of Rats with Sepsis. Sepsis. 2012;5:020.

13. Yun SH, Park JC, Kim SR, Choi YS. Effects of Dexmedetomidine on Serum Interleukin-6, Hemodynamic Stability, and Postoperative Pain Relief in Elderly Patients under Spinal Anesthesia. ActaMedica Okayama. 2016;70(1):37-43.

14. Farghaly HS, Mahmoud AM, Abdel-Sater KA. Effect of dexmedetomidine and cold stress in a rat model of neuropathic pain: Role of interleukin-6 and tumor necrosis factor-α. European journal of pharmacology. 2016;776:139-45

15. Ebrahimpour A, Okhovatpour MA, Sadighi M, Sarejloo AH, Sajjadi MR. Comparative investigation of percutaneous plating and intramedullary nailing effects on IL-6 production in patients with tibia shaft fracture. Acta orthopaedica et traumatologica turcica. 2017;51(6):478-81.

16. Dickstein R, Kiremidjian-Schumacher L, Stotzky G. Effects of lidocaine on the function of immunocompetent cells. I. In vitro exposure of mouse spleen lymphocytes and peritoneal macrophages. Immunopharmacology. 1985;9(3):117-25.

17. Giddon DB, Lindhe J. In vivo quantitation of local anesthetic suppression of leukocyte adherence. The American journal of pathology. 1972;68(2):327.

18. MacGregor RR, Thorner RE, Wright DM. Lidocaine inhibits granulocyte adherence and prevents granulocyte delivery to inflammatory sites. Blood. 1980;56(2):203-9.

19. Martinsson T, Oda T, Fernvik E, Roempke K, Dalsgaard CJ, Svensjö E. Ropivacaine inhibits leukocyte rolling, adhesion and CD11b/CD18 expression. Journal of Pharmacology and Experimental Therapeutics. 1997;283(1):59-65.

20. Sinclair R, Eriksson AS, Gretzer C, Cassuto J, Thomsen P. Inhibitory effects of amide local anaesthetics on stimulus-induced human leukocyte metabolic activation, LTB4 release and IL-1 secretion in vitro. Acta anaesthesiologica scandinavica. 1993;37(2):159-65.

21. Taniguchi T, Shibata K, Yamamoto K et al. Effects of lidocaine administration on hemodynamics and cytokine responses to endotoxemia in rabbits. Crit Care Med 2000; 28:755–9

Table 2- Based on independent t-test, among the variables studied in this study, the mean volume of bleeding and volume of urine show a significant difference between the control and intervention groups.

		Leven's Test for Equality of Variances		t-test for Equality of Means						
		F	Sig.	t	d.f	Sig.(2-tailed)	Mean Difference	Std. Error Difference	95% Confidence interval of the Difference	
									Lower	Upper
Blooding volume	Equal variances assumed	0.205	0.653	3.315	50	0.02	103.07692	31.09539	40.62000	165.53385
	Equal variances not assumed			3.315	49.843	0.02	103.07692	31.09539	40.61514	165.53871
Urine volume	Equal variances assumed	2.370	0.130	2.472	50	0.017	113.46154	45.89188	21.28498	205.63810
	Equal variances not assumed			2.472	46.173	0.017	113.46154	45.89188	21.09528	205.82779
Surgery time	Equal variances assumed	1.405	0.241	0.424	50	0.674	5.19231	12.25186	-19.41627	29.80089
	Equal variances not assumed			0.424	46.215	0.674	5.19231	12.25186	-19.46630	29.85092

Table 3- According to the U Mann Whitney test, the second injection and drug levels had a significant difference between the control and intervention groups

	Group	N	Mean Rank	Sum of Ranks
Drug rate	Normal saline	26	14.00	364.00
	Dexmedetomidine	26	39.00	1014.00
	Total	52		
Second injection	Normal saline	26	18.58	483.00
	Dexmedetomidine	25	33.72	843.00
	Total	51		
Received fluid	Normal saline	26	27.71	720.50
	Dexmedetomidine	26	25.29	657.50
	Total	52		
Base serum IL-6 level	Normal saline	26	26.15	680.00
	Dexmedetomidine	26	26.85	698.00
	Total	52		

Table 4: The mean level of interleukin six hours after surgery, which was the main presumption in this study, is also $p < 0.05$, which shows a significant difference between the two groups.

	Group	N	Mean	Std. Deviation	Std. Error Mean
Six hours IL-6 level	Normal saline	27	26.6333	24.44054	4.70358
	Dexmedetomidine	25	12.9800	9.81411	1.96282

The Preconditioning Effect of Sevoflurane on Coronary Artery Bypass Surgery Patients

Abdorasoul Anvaripour[1], Houshang Shahryari[1], Sayed Mehran Marashian[2], Alireza Jahangirifard[3]*

Abstract

Background: One of the most important issues in the field of surgery is ischemic preconditioning (IPC) of the myocardium during the coronary artery bypass grafting (CABG). The current study attempted to reevaluate the issue to find a potential approach to diminish morbidity, inotrope administration, ischemia and possibly intensive care unit stay after CABG in adult patients.

Materials and Methods: Through randomized single-blind clinical trial, all elective coronary bypass surgeries in 40 to 80 years-old patients enrolled the study. Atrioventricular (AV) block (mobitz2); complete heart block; left bundle branch block (LBBB); acute heart failure (ejection fraction (EF) <30%); re-exploration due to surgical complications and MI cases in the last 7 days were excluded. In all patients, induction (sufentanil, cis-atracurium and etomidate) and maintenance phase (sufentanil, midazolam, cis-atracurium) of anesthesia were done following the same protocol. After cross-clamp of aorta in intervention group, the patients received oxygen (2Lit/min) and sevoflurane (4%) during coronary bypass surgery. After rewarming of the patients, sevoflurane was discontinued. Main outcome measures were troponin 4, 8, 24, 48 hours after surgery with charting the electrocardiogram (ECG) changes, need for inotrope agents and hemodynamic indices during and after CABG in ICU.

Results: 58 CABG candidates enrolled the current study: 29 in intervention group and 29 in control group. There were no statistical differences between the groups concerning hemodynamic issues, Central Venous Pressure (CVP), hematocrit (HCT), ECG changes, demands for inotrope, or ICU stay between the groups.

Conclusion: No significant relationship between application of 4% sevoflurane and IPC was found in adult CABG patients. However, the effect of Sevoflurane on IPC might be dose-related.

Keywords: Ischemic preconditioning (IPC); Sevoflurane; Coronary Artery Bypass Surgery (CABG)

Bushehr, Iran

2. Chronic Respiratory Diseases Research Center, National Research Institute of Tuberculosis and Lung Diseases (NRITLD), Shahid Beheshti University of Medical Sciences, Tehran, Iran

3. Lung Transplantation Research Center, National Research Institute of Tuberculosis and Lung Diseases (NRITLD), Shahid Beheshti University of Medical Sciences, Tehran, Iran

Corresponding Author: Alireza Jahangirifard, MD, Masih Daneshvari Hospital, Darabad, Tehran, Iran.

Email: alirezajahangiri@sbmu.ac.ir

Introduction

Ischemic preconditioning (IPC) is a protective way to lessen the ischemia of myocardium. IPC is a natural defensive mechanism that helps the heart tolerate ischemic condition that firstly raised by Murry et al, in the 1986 (1, 2). In this process, many mechanisms are involved such as myocardial G-protein paired receptors, adenosine A1 receptors and α_1 adrenergic receptors. Protein Kinase-C is another mediator involved as a cardiac potassium channel activator (1).

Sevoflurane is one of the liquid general anesthetic medications affecting on ion channels, especially on receptors of acetylcholine, gamma-aminobutyric acid (GABA) and glutamate. This anesthetic has several side effects such as malignant hyperthermia, dose-dependent hypotension, bradycardia, tachycardia, nausea and vomiting (3). Sevoflurane role has been shown as an inhaled anesthetic medication in protection through ischemic preconditioning (IPC) as well. Adenosine administration may induct IPC through previous experiences either before Coronary Artery Bypass Graft (CABG) or before being used along with cardioplegic solutions. IPC facilitates myocardial recovery after surgery via lower myocardial damage and decreased inotrope administration need.

Through a meta-analysis in 2007, clinical trials to compare Sevoflurane and Desflurane were studied concerning mortality and morbidity after CABG to conclude protective effects of halogen-containing anesthetic medicinal diet on heart (4). In addition, a drop in hemodynamic side effects was shown by Annecke et al, using sevoflurane in pigs through general anesthesia compared to propofol as well as a decrease in cellular markers regularly released because of myocardial damage (5).

Measuring Troponin-I four hours after surgery, as a marker of myocardial tissue damage, Frabdorf et al, found that two 5-min cycles of minimum dose of sevoflurane, 10-minute before external blood flow, obviously resulted in less myocardial damage comparing to intravenous Sufentanil and Propofol (6). They confirmed that Sevoflurane inducted strongly dose-dependent IPC.

A comparison between interrupted and continuous administration of Sevoflurane and Propofol was carried out in 2008 by Bein et al, through CABG to realize that interrupted sevoflurane could prominently reduce myocardial damage based on a drop in Troponin-I and creatine phosphokinase-MB (CK-MB) (7). Later in 2014, Kortekaas et al, observed that cardio-specific Sevoflurane administration strongly reduced systemic inflammation without attenuating cell damage markers when used during mitral value repair surgery (8).

Kawamura et al, in 2006 had assessed the effects of sevoflurane and Propofol on interleukin (IL)-10, IL-8, IL-6 and IL-1 receptor antagonist (IL-1ra) in 23 patients to know that Sevoflurane suppressed IL-6 and IL-8 release but had no obvious effect on IL-10 and IL-1ra. They also raised the doubt that its protective role for myocardium may be resulted by a change in the balance between pre-inflammatory and anti-inflammatory cytokines (9).

Finally, two separate studies by Bouwman et al, and Lorsonradee et al, showed the key protective role of sevoflurane on cardiac contracture, kidney, and liver to get better recovery results (10, 11).

In detail, Sevoflurane involves ca-dependent PKC-α channel to protect myocardium during IPC in addition to keeping serum glutamic-oxaloacetic transaminase (SGOT), serum glutamic pyruvic transaminase (SGPT), lactate dehydrogenase (LDH) and serum creatinine better than Propofol.

Few studies have focused on the effects of Sevoflurane on cardiac preconditioning through CABG among which the optimal administration dose to get optimal protection was not precisely available. Therefore, the current study attempted to reevaluate the issue to find better way of diminish in morbidity, inotrope administration, and ischemia and consequently ICU stay after CABG.

Methods

Patients and sample size

Through a randomized clinical trial, 58 patients of CABG were participated to be divided to two groups of intervention and control each containing 29 regarding inclusion criteria. The participants were 40-80 years of age who were candidates for elective CABG referred to a university hospital in Bushehr, Iran, between 2016 and 2017. Background information such as age, sex, ejection fraction, history of myocardial infarction, cardiomegaly, angiotensin-converting enzyme (ACE) inhibitors administration an also diabetes mellitus types I and II were basically recorded for all the participants.

Simple randomization was done using random numbers to enter the patients into the named groups of this study. The sample size was calculated 30 patients based on previous studies and the following formula:

$$n = \frac{2\left(z1 - \frac{\alpha}{2} + z1 - \beta\right)^2 s}{d2}$$

α=0.05 β=0.8 d=0.04 Tn-I plasma level SD=4.5ng/ml

Two patients had some lost information and were excluded from the study.

Procedure process

Premedication was done night before surgery as well as early morning at surgery date with Lorazepam and intramuscular injection of morphine regarding systolic blood pressure more than 100 mmHg, 30 minutes before entering operation room. All cardiac medications except ACE inhibitors and anticoagulants (like Plavix®) continued until procedure date. Arterial line was inserted left radial or brachial arteries under local anesthesia with lidocaine immediately after entering the operation room. Tracheal intubation, pulse-oximetry, V_2 and V_5-lead ECG and capnography were carried out. All the participants experienced similar protocol of general anesthesia with 1-1.5 µg/kg Sufentanil , 0.1 mg/kg Midazolam, 0.15-0.2 mg/kg Cis-atracurium and 0.2 mg/kg Etomidate followed by maintenance with 2µg/kg/hour Sufentanil+ 1µg/kg/min Midazolam+2µg/kg/min Cis-atracurium. Revascularization was done via left internal mammary artery (LIMA) and saphenous vein. Cannulation of aorta and right atrium was then conducted after 300 U/kg Heparin administration via central venous catheter while activated clotting time (ACT)>400 seconds. Cardioplegic solution was cold liquid plasmalight (6°C) containing 165 mEq sodium chloride, 25 mEq sodium bicarbonate, 45 mEq potassium, 138 mEq chloride with 1800 cc prime volume.

For the group of intervention, participants were administered sevoflurane 4% via vaporizer along with 2 liters oxygen during bypass pump while oxygen was the only thing administered in the control group. Sevoflurane was withdrawn after rewarming. The patients were admitted in ICU after the procedure ended by closing sternum. Analgesia was done using an intravenous pump containing a mixture of 10 mg morphine 2 g Apotel, and 4 mg Ondansetron.

Any changes in ECG showing ischemia as well as any ventricular arrhythmia, which needed medications (such as ventricular fibrillation (VF), ventricular tachycardia verotoxin (VT), or premature ventricular contractions (PVC)) beside atrial fibrillation atrial flutter amniotic fluid (AF) or atrial flutter, were recorded carefully. Ischemic changes of ECG follows:

1- Q-wave myocardial infarction (MI) evidenced by the appearance of new persistent (<24 hours) Q waves >0.04 seconds in greater than or equal to 2 contiguous leads of the same vascular territory or equivalent R-wave increments (R/S ratio >1 in leads V1and V2).

2- A non–Q-wave MI was diagnosed by ST-segment elevation or depression >1 mV 0.08 seconds after the J-point or T-wave inversion of 1 to 2 mV 0.08 seconds after the J-point in 2 contiguous leads of the same vascular territory.

Needed inotropes including Epinephrine, Norepinephrine, Milrinone and Vasopressin at the time of cardiopulmonary bypass (CPB) emerging was recorded as well. ECG changes were recorded at ICU admission time, 24 and 48 hours later. Serum troponin level was also recorded at 4, 8, 24 and 48 hours following operation. Systolic and diastolic blood pressure in addition to mean arterial pressure and heart rate were other parameters to record before anesthesia induction as well as 10 minutes, 60 minutes and 8 and 24 hours after end of CPB.

The current study was approved by the local ethics committee under the code: IR.BPUMS.REC1395.23 and finally by the ministry of health of Iran through approval number: IRCT2016061528477N1.

Regarding 95% confidence interval and significance of 0.05, frequency, mean, standard deviation and range of changes were analyzed using Chi-Square test, Mann-Whitney U test, ANCOVA and Friedman by SPSS 24 for windows.

The current study chiefly faced challenges such

as shortness in Sevoflurane stock as well as patient exclusion due to postoperative uncontrolled bleeding.

Results

Totally, 58 CABG candidates enrolled the current study including 29 in intervention group and 29 in control group. The mean age was 56.24 ± 8.80 (45-70 years) in the former group and 59.59±10.76 (31-81 years) in the latter with no significant difference (Mann-Whitney U: P value=0.348).

Sex wise, no difference was found between the groups as can be seen in table 1 ($X^2_{(1)}$ = 0.672; P value=0.585 by Fisher Exact test). There was no statistical difference between the groups concerning ejection fraction as checked with Mann-Whitney U (P value=0.177).

Table 1 summarizes some key demographic as well as medical history of the participants regarding their groups. History of cardiomegaly (P =0.431), ACE-inhibitors (P =0.065) and diabetes mellitus type Iand II (P =0.248) was not statistically different at all.

The serum level of troponin was the first concern, which showed similar results in intervention and control groups 4, 8, 24 and 48 hours after the surgery (Table 2).

Another factor to be assessed was ECG changes after surgery including Q and non-Q-wave-MI which were similar in the studied groups as observed in table 3.

Similar results were found for the need of Inotropes during on-pump process (P>0.089) and continued during off-pump (P=0.412) (Table3).

Inotropes were similarly needed through postoperative ICU stay as can be checked in table 3. (P=0.506) Inotrope need during intra-aortic balloon pump (IABP) did not differ between the groups (P=0.492).

Concerning hemodynamic factors, no item but systolic blood pressure (P=0.020) and the mean arterial blood pressure (P=0.002) differed statistically when compared the groups preoperatively. After 60 minutes of pump phase, like what happened 7 hours later, statistically similar hemodynamic parameters were obviously found between the groups as can be seen in table 4 as well. This similarity was showed 24 hours after the pump phase (Table 4).

In terms of hematocrit, findings shown no

Table 1: Demographics and some histories of diseases and medications.

		Group	Number	Frequency
Sex	**Male**	Intervention	17	58.6
		Control	20	69
	Female	Intervention	12	41.4
		Control	9	31
Recent MI	**Yes**	Intervention	5	17.2
		Control	5	82.8
	No	Intervention	24	17.2
		Control	24	82.8
Cardiomegaly	**Yes**	Intervention	16	55.2
		Control	12	41.4
	No	Intervention	13	44.8
		Control	17	58.6
ACE-I	**Yes**	Intervention	10	34.5
		Control	18	62.1
	No	Intervention	19	65.5
		Control	11	37.9
History of type 1 Diabetes Mellitus	**Yes**	Intervention	3	10.3
		Control	26	97.7
	No	Intervention	3	10.3
		Control	26	97.7
History of type 2 Diabetes Mellitus	**Yes**	Intervention	11	37.9
		Control	6	20/7
	No	Intervention	18	62.1
		Control	23	97.3

Table 2: Serum troponin levels at evaluating times.

Troponin	Group	Mean	SD	Min	Max	P-value
4 hours afterwards	Intervention	3.56	2.73	0.50	12.12	0.859
	Control	3.81	3.27	0.06	15.55	
8 hours afterwards	Intervention	5.58	7.28	0.43	32.00	0.446
	Control	5.17	5.28	0.62	50.25	
24 hours afterwards	Intervention	3.72	4.21	0.15	18.00	0.525
	Control	5.24	10.12	0.30	56.00	
48 hours afterwards	Intervention	2.15	2.63	0.00	8.80	0.294
	Control	3.74	8.79	0.12	48.70	

Table 3: ECG changes at different times of the study.

MI	Group	N (%)	P-value
Q wave MI	Intervention	0(0.00)	>0.05
	Control	1(3.30)	
Non-Q wave MI	Intervention	6(20.00)	0.761
	Control	8(26.70)	
On-Pump Inotrope Need	Intervention	7(23.3)	>0.05
	Control	8(26.7)	
Off-Pump Inotrope Need	Intervention	18(60.0)	0.412
	Control	22(73.3)	
ICU Inotrope Need	Intervention	4(13.3)	0.506
	Control	7(23.3)	

statistical discrepancy between the studied groups at basic time and 15 mins and 30 mins later like at the end point of pump phase (Table 5). Likely, basic CVP (central vein pressure) and post-pump CVP were statistically similar in the groups (Table 6).

Graft number showed the means of 3±0.13 (±SE) and 3±0.18 in the groups of intervention and control respectively with no statistical difference reported by Mann-Whitney U (P value=0.950).

Two complications including ventricular fibrillation (VF) and ventricular tachycardia (VT) were assessed for occurrence to find similar frequency in the groups (P value>0.05).

Discussion

The current study attempted to find positive effect of Sevoflurane on general anesthesia among 58 CABG surgeries with less hemodynamic and ECG changes finally to confirm similar responses compared to regular techniques of intravenous anesthesia.

Lemoine et al, in 2017 investigated cardio protective effects of sevoflurane through elective on-pump CABG surgery compared with no halogenated volatile anesthesia to conclude that sevoflurane could half the cardiac troponin I in serum of what seen in controls as well as less need to inotropic support (12). At the same time, Wang et al, tried to reveal the biological mechanism involving in sevoflurane-induced anesthesia in CABG surgery based on gene expression features to realize that neuroactive ligand-receptor interaction may play the main role in cardio protective effects of sevoflurane through regulating the pathway (13).

Zhang et al, in 2016 tried to compare the effects of Sevoflurane and regular method of general anesthesia only with inhaled oxygen regarding cardiac enzymes and hemodynamic features to find that Sevoflurane provided lower mean of arterial pressure, heart rate and left ventricle ejection fraction (LVEF) as well as significantly lower plasma level of CK-MB. Additionally, they studied respiratory parameters like tidal volume and vital capacity, respiratory rate and P_aO_2/Fio_2 to get fluctuated data not enough to assess sevoflurane-related improvements. However they realized that Sevoflurane, despite lower LVEF, may contribute to Stabilization of cardiopulmonary function and prevention of myocardial injury (14).

Table 4: Hemodynamics at different points of the study regarding the groups*

Hemodynamics	Group	Mean	SD	Min	Max	P-value
SBP	**Intervention**	152.71	26.53	100.00	200.00	0.020
	Control	169.54	23.08	120.00	220.00	
DBP	**Intervention**	73.27	11.41	50.00	100.00	0.620
	Control	74.61	10.56	50.00	100.00	
MAP	**Intervention**	96.27	13.42	72.00	115.00	0.002
	Control	110.24	16.25	80.00	153.00	
HR	**Intervention**	79.84	15.67	47.00	115.00	0.982
	Control	80.74	15.89	50.00	113.00	
MAP15	**Intervention**	60.74	9.13	45.00	76.00	0.849
	Control	62.04	9.25	40.00	76.00	
MAP30	**Intervention**	65.17	7.75	52.00	81.00	0.812
	Control	66.00	9.53	48.00	85.00	
End-Pump	**Intervention**	54.94	10.74	36.00	72.00	0.538
	Control	58.14	11.21	40.00	85.00	
SBP after 10 min	**Intervention**	119.31	11.21	99.00	141.00	0.140
	Control	114.27	9.96	90.00	133.00	
DBP after 10 min	**Intervention**	56.81	6.08	45.00	70.00	0.941
	Control	56.81	6.39	45.00	70.00	
MAP after 10 min	**Intervention**	73.07	6.32	65.00	85.00	0.486
	Control	74.14	6.65	58.00	86.00	
HR after 10 min	**Intervention**	100.27	8.31	80.00	116.00	0.554
	Control	98.44	9.77	78.00	116.00	
SBP60min	**Intervention**	127.91	13.49	100.00	160.00	0.351
	Control	124.34	13.41	100.00	145.00	
DBP60min	**Intervention**	62.74	9.09	46.00	80.00	0.599
	Control	63.81	8.85	48.00	80.00	
MAP60min	**Intervention**	81.77	11.98	67.00	111.00	0.545
	Control	109.27	153.65	65.00	921.00	
HR60min	**Intervention**	94.27	9.87	75.00	117.00	0.841
	Control	92.54	18.57	10.00	115.00	
SBP8hrs	**Intervention**	138.57	19.56	90.00	180.00	0.116
	Control	140.11	18.94	101.00	190.00	
DBP8hrs	**Intervention**	75.71	12.02	54.00	105.00	0.491
	Control	72.91	10.18	50.00	89.00	
MAP8hrs	**Intervention**	95.24	16.72	68.00	138.00	0.637
	Control	91.21	16.51	62.00	128.00	
HR8hrs	**Intervention**	95.07	14.22	67.00	121.00	0.894
	Control	96.17	10.66	75.00	118.00	
SBP24hrs	**Intervention**	133.91	16.93	103.00	167.00	0.220
	Control	137.84	17.86	107.00	170.00	
DBP24hrs	**Intervention**	72.17	11.32	53.00	100.00	0.801
	Control	72.54	11.21	51.00	91.00	
MAP24hrs	**Intervention**	88.51	17.33	58.00	132.00	0.674
	Control	89.34	14.19	60.00	129.00	
HR24hrs	**Intervention**	91.47	11.13	73.00	110.00	0.599
	Control	90.11	12.17	69.00	117.00	

*SBP: Systolic Blood Pressure; DBP: Diastolic Blood Pressure; MAP: Mean Arterial Pressure

A meta-analysis showed in 2016 demonstrated no statistical difference between data about postoperative CK-MB levels among total 384 patients undergoing on-pump CABG with Sevoflurane; though postoperative myocardial troponin levels were significantly lower in sevoflurane group (15).

Table 5: Hematocrit at on-pump and off-pump phases (HCT: Hematocrit)

	Group	Mean	SD	Min	Max	P-value
Base HCT	**Intervention**	39.31	5.21	25.00	48.00	0.563
	Control	38.74	5.15	28.00	54.00	
HCT pump1	**Intervention**	24.64	4.23	17.00	32.00	0.108
	Control	22.74	4.21	16.00	32.00	
HCT pump2	**Intervention**	26.04	4.38	19.00	36.00	0.238
	Control	24.24	4.65	16.00	32.00	
HCT: off-pump	**Intervention**	28.37	6.34	5.00	36.00	0.232
	Control	27.67	3.81	21.00	35.00	

Table 6: Central Venous Pressure (CVP) in two groups at the times of on- and off-pump (SD: Standard Deviation).

	Group	Mean	SD	Min	Max	P-value
CVP: base value	**Intervention**	9.64	2.36	5.00	15.00	0.549
	Control	9.94	2.41	4.00	15.00	
CVP: off-pump	**Intervention**	9.74	3.28	2.00	17.00	0.153
	Control	11.10	2.73	6.00	16.00	

The current study showed reduced length of ICU stay among patients who took Sevoflurane during surgery which was previously pointed out by Likhrantsev et al, in 2016 (16). The named study also confirmed reduced serum levels of cardiac biomarkers like troponin T and N- terminal pro-brain natriuretic peptide as well as mortality.

Sirvinskas et al, raised mitochondrial function involvement in 2015 to explain the effects of Sevoflurane on clinical parameters in CABG surgery to believe that Sevoflurane could slightly protect the mitochondrial outer membrane from ischemia-reperfusion injury and the loss of cytochrome C in addition to its significantly lower postoperative serum troponin levels when compared to Propofol. (17) However, little changes in hemodynamics through the current study were probably due to low dose of Sevoflurane to use; and higher doses may strengthen the protective features.

Regarding clinical and basic studies on the effects of harm reduction of CABG surgery, there are many aspects of studies to perform to get enough reliable documents about protective role of sevoflurane in cardiac safety during and after the named surgery.

Conclusion

The current study could not find significant clinical effect and additional benefit of sevoflurane on ischemic preconditioning with the used dosage in on-pump CABG surgeries. The effect of sevoflurane is probably dose-dependent which would be, in turn, a hypothesis to assess through more future trials as we believe.

Acknowledgment

The authors would like to acknowledge the kind efforts of all physicians and nurses in the operating room that was the research location.

Conflicts of Interest

The authors declare that they have no conflict of interest.

References

1. Shvedova M, Anfinogenova Y, Popov SV, Atochin DN. Connexins and Nitric Oxide Inside and Outside Mitochondria: Significance for Cardiac Protection and Adaptation. Front Physiol. 2018;9:479.

2. Murry CE, Jennings RB, Reimer KA. Preconditioning with ischemia: a delay of lethal cell injury in ischemic myocardium. Circulation. 1986;74(5):1124-36.

3. Miller RD. Miller's anesthesia. 8th ed, 2014, Saunders, Philadelphia.ISBN: 9780702052835.

4. El Dib R, Guimarães Pereira JE, Agarwal A, Gomaa H, Ayala AP, Botan AG, Braz LG, de Oliveira LD, Lopes LC, Mathew PJ. Inhalation versus intravenous anaesthesia for adults undergoing on-pump or off-pump coronary artery bypass grafting: A systematic review and meta-analysis of randomized controlled trials. J Clin Anesth. 2017;40:127-138.

5. Annecke T, Kubitz JC, Kahr S, et al. Effects of sevoflurane and

propofol on ischaemia–reperfusion,injury after thoracic-aortic occlusion in pigs. Br J Anaesth. 2007;98(5):581-90.
6. Fräßdorf J, Borowski A, Ebel D, et al. Impact of preconditioning protocol on anesthetic-induced cardioprotection in patients having coronary artery bypass surgery. J ThoracCardiovasc Surg. 2009;137(6):1436-42.
7. Bein B, Renner J, Caliebe D, et al. The effects of interrupted or continuous administration of sevoflurane on preconditioning before cardio-pulmonary bypass in coronary artery surgery: comparison with continuous propofol. Anaesthesia. 2008;63(10):1046-55
8. Kortekaas KA, van der Baan A, Aarts LP, et al. Cardiospecific sevoflurane treatment quenches inflammation but does not attenuate myocardial cell damage markers: a proof-of-concept study in patients undergoing mitral valve repair. British Journal of Anaesthesia. 2014;112(6):1005-14.
9. Kawamura T, Kadosaki M, Nara N, et al. Effects of sevoflurane on cytokine balance in patients undergoing coronary artery bypass graft surgery. J CardiothoracVascAnesth. 2006;20(4):503-8
10. Bouwman R A, Musters R J P, van Beek-Harmsen B J, et al. Sevoflurane-induced cardioprotection depends on PKC-α activation via production of reactive oxygen species. British Journal of Anaesthesia. 2007;99(5):639-45.
11. Lorsomradee S, Cromheecke S, Lorsomradee S, De Hert SG. Effects of sevoflurane on biomechanical markers of hepatic and renal dysfunction after coronary artery surgery. J CardiothoracVascAnesth. 2006; 20(5):684-90
12. Lemoine S, Zhu L, Gérard JL, Hanouz JL. Sevoflurane-induced cardioprotection in coronary artery bypass graft surgery: Randomised trial with clinical and ex-vivo endpoints. Anaesth Crit Care Pain Med. 2018;37(3):217-23.
13. Wang J, Cheng J, Zhang C, Li X. Cardioprotection Effects of Sevoflurane by Regulating the Pathway of Neuroactive Ligand-Receptor Interaction in Patients Undergoing Coronary Artery Bypass Graft Surgery.Computational and Mathematical Methods in Medicine. 2017:7.
14. Zhang J, Wang S. Effects of sevoflurane on cardiopulmonary function in patients undergoing coronary artery bypass.J BiolRegulHomeost Agents. 2016;30(4):1079-83
15. Lu Y, Wang L, Liu N, Dong T, Li R. Sevoflurane preconditioning in on-pump coronary artery bypass grafting: a meta-analysis of randomized controlled trials.J Anesth. 2016;30(6):977-86.
16. Likhvantsev VV, Landoni G, Levikov DI, Grebenchikov OA, Skripkin YV, Cherpakov RA. Sevoflurane Versus Total Intravenous Anesthesia for Isolated Coronary Artery Bypass Surgery With Cardiopulmonary Bypass: A Randomized Trial.J CardiothoracVascAnesth. 2016;30(5):1221-7.
17. Sirvinskas E, Kinderyte A, Trumbeckaite S. Effects of sevoflurane vs. propofol on mitochondrial functional activity after ischemia-reperfusion injury and the influence on clinical parameters in patients undergoing CABG surgery with cardiopulmonary bypass.Perfusion. 2015;30(7):590-5.

Effect of Spinal and General Anesthesia on Serum Cytokine Levels Following Cesarean Section in Preeclampsia

Maryam Vosoughian[1], Mastaneh Dahi-Taleghani[1], Mohammadreza Moshari[1], Samira Rajaei[2], Shima Rajabi[1], Farinaz Taheri[1]

1. Anesthesiology Research Center, Shahid Beheshti University of Medical Sciences, Tehran, Iran
2. Department of Immunology, School of Medicine, Tehran University of Medical Sciences, Tehran, Iran

Corresponding Author: Mastaneh Dahi-Taleghani
Email: ma_dahi@yahoo.com

Abstract

Background: The purpose of this study is to investigate the impact of different anesthetic techniques on the release of cytokines interleukin IL-6, IL-10 and tumor necrosis factor (TNF)-α in preeclampsia patients who undergo cesarean section.
Materials and Methods: In the study 40 patients were enrolled with preeclampsia undergoing cesarean section, allocated into two equal groups to receive either general anesthesia ($n = 20$) or spinal anesthesia ($n = 20$). Non-invasive hemodynamic monitoring was used. Serum levels of IL-6, IL-10 and TNF-α were measured before and at the end of surgery.
Results: There was no significant rise in serum levels of TNF-α in general anesthesia while IL-6 and IL-10 serum levels increased significantly. Also, compared with patients anaesthetized with general anesthesia patients who received regional anesthesia notably had lower levels of IL-6 and IL-10 after surgery ($p < 0.05$).
Conclusion: Spinal anesthesia causes significant difference in post-operation IL-6 and IL-10 serum levels in preeclampsia patients undergoing cesarean section. Nevertheless, neither general nor spinal anesthesia made such effect on serum level of TNF-α. Further studies with higher sample size and comparing preeclamptic patients to healthy mothers undergoing cesarean section are required.
Keywords: Spinal Anesthesia, Preeclampsia, General anesthesia, Interleukin-10, Interleukin-6, TNF-α, Cesarean Section

Introduction

Preeclampsia (PE) is a syndrome that affects 2% to 8% of human pregnancies and constitutes a major cause of maternal and perinatal morbidity and mortality (1). It is a systemic disease characterized by an inflammatory response and endothelial disorder, and is clinically identified by a combination of hypertension and proteinuria, presenting after 20 weeks of gestation in a previously normotensive pregnant woman (2, 3). Previous studies suggested that an abnormality in immunologic balance has been implicated in the pathology of preeclampsia (4). The ischemia and hypoxia resulting from the inappropriate trophoblast invasion lead to an increased production of pro-inflammatory cytokines in the placenta (5).

The roles of the various cytokines in the pathology of preeclampsia have been studied by several authors, with conflicting reports on the serum concentrations of interleukins in preeclampsia (6-8). These studies showed high levels of interleukin (IL)-1, IL-6 and tumor necrosis factor alpha (TNF-α), IL-2 and interferon gamma (IFN-γ), are overexpressed and secreted in placentas of preeclamptic women likely due to hypoxia-reoxygenation caused by intermittent placental perfusion (9). All these inflammatory cytokines seem to have deleterious effects on pregnancy development (10-12).

Prompt control of hypertension, fluid restriction, seizure prophylaxis in high-risk groups, and expedited delivery in the presence of severe maternal disease features or fetal compromise, are the core principles during preeclampsia management (13, 14).

As with other surgical procedures cesarean section provokes further increases in serum cytokine levels with consequences on host immunomodulation and recovery of the parturient (15).

The establishment of safe regional anesthesia (RA) for labor and caesarean delivery in preeclampsia is one of the most important developments in the past 25 years in obstetric anesthesia. Spinal anesthesia offers advantages in preeclampsia in terms of hypertension control and simplicity of airway management (16, 17). The advantages of regional anesthesia over general anesthesia are documented in many studies (e.g., inhibition of metabolic and hormonal responses to stress, reducing the incidence of post-operative pain, speeding peristalsis after abdominal operations, reducing the incidence of deep vein thrombosis, and shorter hospital stay). Unfortunately, it cannot always be applied. The potential disadvantage of regional anesthesia is its limited duration (18).

The indications for general anesthesia (GA) for caesarean section in preeclamptic women with preserved ejection fraction are eclampsia with altered mentation, coagulopathy, and thrombocytopenia. Although new evidence is sparse, in hemolysis, elevated liver enzyme levels, and low platelet levels (HELLP) syndrome most anesthesiologists adhere to an early report, which showed that thromboelastographic maximum amplitude, decreased once platelet numbers dropped below 75x109.L-1. Abruptio placentae without maternal hemodynamic compromise or cardiotocography abnormality are not a contraindication to RA (19). General anesthesia introduces problems of difficult tracheal intubation, and the hypertensive response. Therefore, ideal modern management for preeclamptics is early establishment of epidural analgesia in labor and spinal anesthesia for caesarean delivery in cases in whom an epidural catheter has not been inserted. However, many units around the world still provide routine general anesthesia (20-23). The advantages of general anesthesia are its simple and easy method of application, rapid sedation of the patient, and increased comfort of surgeons and anesthesiologists when the surgery has to last longer. The disadvantages of general anesthesia are airway management during intubation, challenges in controlling hypertension caused by intubation and extubation, and postoperative adverse effects (e.g. nausea, vomiting, and pain) (24). Although several studies have been conducted on the effects of different anesthetic methods on activity of inflammatory cells and serum levels of interleukins, but so far, no studies have been established to compare both general and regional anesthesia on the interleukin levels in pregnant women with preeclampsia. The aim of the study was to determine the significance of spinal anesthesia in suppressing levels of immune-associated compounds found in the plasma of patients suffering from preeclampsia comparing to general anesthesia.

Methods

Patients

The study included 48 patients, 24 in the general anesthesia group and 24 in the spinal anesthesia group (Fig. 1). In the general anesthesia group (group I), four patients were excluded due to technical issues in sample collecting. In the spinal anesthesia group (group II), two patients were excluded due to conversion from spinal anesthesia to general anesthesia during surgery, and another two patients were dismissed from the study due to technical laboratory problems. A total of 40 preeclampsia patients undergoing Cesarean Section (C/S), with an American Society of Anesthesiologists (ASA) physical status of I or II were included in the current study. The Ethics Committee of Shahid Beheshti University of Medical Sciences approved the study protocol and all the patients provided written informed consent prior to inclusion. The exclusion criteria included eclampsia, coagulation disorders of any type, history of anti-phospholipid syndrome and history of any allergy to the drugs used in the study.

The lead physician independently conducted patient assessments for inclusion based on the patient's medical history. Subsequently, the patients were randomly assigned in two groups (n=20 per group) using a computer-generated table of random numbers. The lead physician was also primarily responsible for drug preparation in order to ensure consistency of drug administration throughout the study.

Types of anesthesia

Group I received general anesthesia and group II received spinal anesthesia. During the operation, patients were continuously monitored using a combination of electrocardiography, noninvasive blood pressure recordings and pulse oximetry techniques.

Group I patients received intravenous anesthesia induction with 4-6 mg/kg Thiopental and 1-1.5 mg/kg Succinylcholine following 0.8% Isoflurane for anesthesia maintenance. Spinal anesthesia performed by injection of single dose of 2.8 cc Bupivacaine 0.5% at the L3–L4 interspace using a 25-gauge Quincke point needle in groups II.

Clinical Diagnosis of PE

Preeclampsia was diagnosed by new-onset blood pressure ≥140/90 mmHg and significant proteinuria (urinary total protein/creatinine ratio >30 or +1 on urine dipstick). All cases were diagnosed after 34 weeks' gestation (late-onset PE).

Blood samples

Peripheral blood samples for the detection of IL-6, IL-10 and TNF-α levels were collected prior to the induction of anesthesia (T0), and postoperatively, 30 minutes after transferring the patient to recovery room and before discharge (T1). The sampled blood was collected into EDTA tubes and centrifuged at 2000 rpm for 3 min at 4˚C immediately after sampling. Thereafter, the plasma samples were stored at -20˚C until all the samples were collected. The samples with the temperature of 0°C were transferred to laboratory at Department of Immunology to assess with an ELISA assay (Mabtech, Nacka Strand, Sweden).

Detection of plasma IL-6, IL-10 and TNF-α levels

Interleukin-6, IL-10 and TNF-α levels in the plasma were assessed using commercial quantitative ELISA assay kits (Mabtech, Nacka Strand, Sweden) according to the manufacturer's instructions. Standards were prepared and the appropriate volume of sample or standard was added to a 96-well polystyrene microtiter plate pre-coated with monoclonal antibodies either to the appropriate cytokine or to the related antigen. All samples and standards were run in duplicate and the plates were incubated for the recommended time. Each well was subsequently aspirated and the plates were washed with the provided buffered surfactant. An enzyme-linked polyclonal antibody against the cytokine was then added and the plates were incubated a second time prior to final washing. After addition of the substrate solution to each well, the optical density was read at the appropriate wavelength for each assay period. All the values were reported as picograms/milliliter. Interleukins were measured (with a sensitivity of 0.5 to 1 micrograms/liter. Cross-reactivity with other factors was considered negligible in all the cytokine assays.

Statistical analysis

All quantitative data are expressed as mean ± SD. Patients characteristics such as age and sera interleukin levels were calculated by student t-test. Categorical data were described as absolute frequencies and analyzed using the Pearson's $\chi 2$ and Fisher's exact tests. $P<0.05$ was considered to indicate a statistically significant difference. All the data were analyzed using the SPSS statistical software, version 22.0 (SPSS Inc., Chicago, IL, USA).

Results

Data from 40 patients, 20 in the general anesthesia group and 20 in the spinal anesthesia group, were included in the final analysis. None of the patients

Table 1: Baseline demographics and surgical procedure

	I	II	P value
Age	32.63±1.4	32.73±4.3	0.94
Mean number of previous pregnancies	1.75±1.0	2.10±1.1	0.29
Number of previous abortion	2 (10%)	4 (20%)	0.50

The results are expressed as mean ± SD or number of patients

The differences between groups were not significant (p > 0.05)

Table 2: Prevalence of intraoperative methyldopa, labetalol and magnesium sulfate

	I (%) N	II (%) N	P value
Methyldopa	(65%) 13	(35%) 7	0.113
Labetalol	(70%) 14	(40%) 8	0.111
Magnesium sulfate	(80%) 16	(65%) 13	0.480

The differences between groups were not significant (p > 0.05)

Table 3: Comparison of IL-6, IL-10 and TNF-α serum levels before and after surgery in each group.

	T0		T1		P value
	I	II	I	II	
IL-6 (pg/mL)	2.81±1.5	2.52±0.9	10.44±7.4	5.80±4.2	0.04*
IL-10 (pg/mL)	3.72±3.5	5.44±4.1	8.14±6.3	5.41±4.4	0.02*
TNF-α (pg/mL)	3.59±0.3	3.25±0.2	3.69±0.3	3.67±0.6	>0.05

The results are expressed as mean ± SD or number of patients, T0=before surgery, T1=after surgery.

*between two groups in T1

had signs of preoperative infection. All patients underwent C/S because of preeclampsia. No significant differences were found between the groups regarding their demographics (Table 1).

Neither were there any significant differences in the use of intraoperative methyldopa, labetalol and magnesium sulfate that could have influenced the inflammatory response (Table 2). Patients in spinal

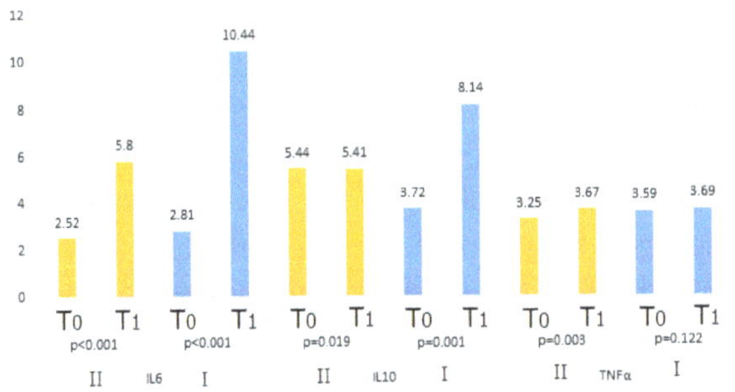

Figure 1. Comparison of changes in IL-6, IL-10 and TNF-α levels before surgery and 30 min after arrival in the recovery room in each group. Values are in pg/mL
I=general anesthesia, II= spinal anesthesia
T0=before surgery, T1=after surgery
P-value<0.05 was considered statically significant

anesthesia group had significant lower IL-6 serum level in comparison with general anesthesia in T1 (p=0.04) (Table 3).

Discussion

We hypothesized spinal analgesia in compare with general anesthesia could dampen release of inflammatory cytokines response to C/S in pregnant women with PE. Results of this study demonstrated a statistically significant increase in post-operation levels of the inflammatory cytokines (IL-6, IL-10 and TNF-α). In addition, there were significantly higher serum levels of the IL-6 and IL-10, in the pregnant women with preeclampsia in general anesthesia group compared with those in spinal anesthesia after C/S.

Naturally, there is a balance between the release of pro and anti-inflammatory cytokines. But inflammatory reactions induced by immune cells can exacerbate the pro-inflammatory response and increase the incidence of postoperative complications, including infections, delayed surgical wound healing, cognitive impairment and even progression of malignancies, systemic inflammatory response syndrome (SIRS), and lead to severe hemodynamic disorders and multiple organ failure (25-28).

There is a consensus about the role of surgical incision and any tissue damage in increasing the serum levels of pre-inflammatory cytokines such as interleukin-1, interleukin-6 and TNFα, in turn enhancing the activity of the hypothalamic-pituitary-adrenal axis and the secretion of glucocorticoids (29, 30)

On the other hand, recent studies showed that although normal pregnancy is associated with a controlled inflammatory process, but pathological conditions like PE associated with higher levels of IL-1, IL-6, IL-10 and tumor necrosis factor alpha (TNF-α), as well as IL-2 and interferon gamma (IFN-γ), in plasma and amniotic fluid of PE women. All these inflammatory cytokines seem to have deleterious effects on pregnancy development (4, 31, 32).

Taylor *et al.*, examined IL-6 levels during the second trimester and found that elevated levels of this cytokine predicted term PE (33). In other case–control studies during the third trimesters, researchers reported a significant increase in levels of IL-6 in pregnancies complicated by PE compared to normal pregnancies (34-38). In the same way, other researchers showed significant increased levels of IL-10 and TNF-α in pregnancies with PE when compared to normal pregnancies in the third trimester (38-42).

It is also demonstrated that anesthetic agents, anesthesia type, and anesthesia duration might affect the neuro-immuno-endocrine systems during surgery and influence this response (43-46).

The effects of different anesthetic techniques on perioperative changes in cytokine serum levels have been studied in surgical patients. When compared to general anesthesia alone, general anesthesia combined with continuous epidural anesthesia has not been shown to attenuate increases in IL-6 levels following radical esophagostomy, while TNF-α levels did not change in either group (47).

Circulating IL-6 levels have been found to increase in patients undergoing total hip replacement under both general and spinal anesthesia, while no significant changes were observed in TNF-α levels in either group (48). Similarly, 24 hours after hemorrhoidectomy under general or spinal anesthesia IL-6 increased with both anesthetic techniques while TNF-α levels remained the same (49).

In another study, IL-6 levels have been shown not to differ between patients undergoing abdominal hysterectomy under general or combined epidural and general anesthesia (50).

In liver cancer resection surgery, serum level of IL-10 of patients who underwent general anesthesia combined with epidural block showed a non-significant decrease immediately after surgery, but increased 24 hours after surgery, and the increase was greater than that of the general anesthesia group (51). Sun *et al.*, reported significant differences in IL- 6, and IL- 10 serum levels between the combined intravenous and inhalation anesthesia and the combined general and epidural anesthesia groups 72 hours after surgery (52).

Different general anesthesia techniques for hysterectomy have been shown to influence cytokine levels, with Propofol and Alfentanil associated with lower serum IL-6 levels than isoflurane anesthesia (53). However, it has been reported, again with abdominal hysterectomy, that IL-6 levels increased in a similar fashion after fentanyl administration (54). In patients undergoing pancreatoduodenectomy both IL-6 and TNF-α levels increased, an effect that was not influenced by supplemental epidural analgesia (55). However, all these studies included only small numbers of patients and may therefore have been underpowered.

Karadeniz *et al.*, showed that, there was no statistically significant difference in serum TNF-α levels between groups general anesthesia and general/epidural anesthesia at preoperative and postoperative 1st hour and 24th hour after radical cystectomy (56). In another study in degenerative disease of the spine 30 min after incision we observed significant larger concentration of IL-6 in general anesthesia group compared to group of spinal anesthesia (57).

In cesarean section, Jongh *et al.*, measured IL-6, 12 and 24 hours after C/S under either epidural or general anesthesia. In their study, IL-6 levels peaked at 12 hours and remained increased for 24 hours postoperatively with both anesthetic techniques (58). Therefore, it seems that the cytokine response to cesarean section is not influenced by anesthetic technique and is comparable with the changes after elective general surgical procedures. In the same way, Dermitzaki *et al.*, also showed significant increase in IL-6 serum level and no TNF-α in elective C/S. In addition, both groups did not differ in IL-6 or TNF-α serum concentrations at any time point (59).

Blood samples in our study were collected pre-operatively and 30 min after transferring the patient to recovery room after surgery. This could be seen as a limitation to our study. Reikeras *et al.*, reported that IL-6 serum levels peak 6 to 24 hours after surgical procedures (60). Current literature suggests that, after elective surgical procedures, IL-6 remains elevated for 48 to 72 hours (55, 61).

Our results are consistent with those studies, demonstrating a postoperative increase in IL-6 and IL-10 levels, which is influenced by spinal anesthesia, while TNF-α levels were not significantly different between the groups. However, in spinal anesthesia group, there was significant increase in TNF-α while it was not significant in general anesthesia. The results of this study can be substantiated that the level of serum cytokines during surgery and the effect of different anesthetic methods on them can be influenced by the underlying diseases.

The delay of IL-6 increase postoperatively may be related to the synthesis of IL-6 mRNA, which is responsible for its production (62). Lee et al., showed that serum levels peak is 2 h for IL-10 and 2 to 24 hours for TNF-α after surgical procedures (63). Although the results of this study were in line with the results of other studies, it seems that increasing the number of blood samples taken over a longer period can give more conclusive outcomes, regarding the effect of using different anesthetic methods on the level of inflammatory cytokines in the patients. Further studies with higher sample size and also comparing patients with preeclampsia with healthy mothers of cesarean section are required to provide more information about the benefits of using different anesthetic methods on serum levels of inflammatory cytokines in preeclampsia.

Conclusion

Results of the present study demonstrate that spinal anesthesia causes significant difference in post-operation IL-6 and IL-10 serum levels in PE women undergoing cesarean section. But neither general nor spinal anesthesia made such effect on serum levels of TNF-α.

Acknowledgment

This work was done based on the thesis paper on anesthesiology. The authors would like to acknowledge all nurses and physicians of Taleghani Hospital, Shahid Beheshti University of Medical Sciences, Tehran, Iran for their support during the study. The authors also declare that they have no competing interests at all regarding any of the methods or materials or the tests discussed or mentioned in the study.

Conflicts of Interest

The authors declare that they have no conflict of interest.

References

1. Kane SC, Da Silva Costa F, Brennecke SP. New directions in the prediction of pre-eclampsia. Aust N Z J Obstet Gynaecol. 2014;54(2):101-7.
2. Redman CW, Sargent IL. Latest advances in understanding preeclampsia. Science. 2005;308(5728):1592-4..
3. ACOG Committee on Obstetric Practice. ACOG practice bulletin. Diagnosis and management of preeclampsia and eclampsia. Number 33, January 2002. American College of Obstetricians and Gynecologists. Int J Gynaecol Obstet. 2002;77(1):67-75.
4. Saito S, Shiozaki A, Nakashima A, Sakai M, Sasaki Y. The role of the immune system in preeclampsia. Mol Aspects Med. 2007 Apr;28(2):192-209.
5. Raghupathy R. Cytokines as key players in the pathophysiology of preeclampsia. Med Princ Pract. 2013;22 Suppl 1:8-19.
6. Udenze I, Amadi C, Awolola N, Makwe CC. The role of cytokines as inflammatory mediators in preeclampsia. Pan Afr Med J. 2015 10;20:219.
7. Afshari JT, Ghomian N, Shameli A, Shakeri M, Fahmidehkar M, Mahajer E, et al. Determination of Interleukin-6 and Tumor Necrosis Factor-alpha concentrations in Iranian-Khorasanian patients with preeclampsia. BMC Pregnancy Childbirth. 2005;5:14.
8. Romero-Adrian T, Ruiz A, Molina-Vilchez R, Estevez J, Atencio R. Interleukin-2 receptor serum concentrations in normal pregnancy and pre-eclampsia. Invest clín. 2002;43(2):73-8.
9. Hung TH, Charnock-Jones DS, Skepper JN, Burton GJ. Secretion of tumor necrosis factor-alpha from human placental tissues induced by hypoxia-reoxygenation causes endothelial cell activation in vitro: a potential mediator of the inflammatory response in preeclampsia. Am J Pathol. 2004;164(3):1049-61.
10. Laresgoiti-Servitje E, Gomez-Lopez N, Olson DM. An immunological insight into the origins of pre-eclampsia. Hum Reprod Update. 2010;16(5):510-24.
11. Darmochwal-Kolarz D, Leszczynska-Gorzelak B, Rolinski J, Oleszczuk J. T helper 1- and T helper 2-type cytokine imbalance in pregnant women with pre-eclampsia. Eur J Obstet Gynecol Reprod Biol. 1999;86(2):165-70.
12. Daher S, de Arruda Geraldes Denardi K, Blotta MH, Mamoni RL, Reck AP, Camano L, et al. Cytokines in recurrent pregnancy loss. J Reprod Immunol. 2004;62(1-2):151-7.
13. American College of Obstetricians and Gynecologists; Task Force on Hypertension in Pregnancy. Hypertension in pregnancy. Report of the American College of Obstetricians and Gynecologists' Task Force on Hypertension in Pregnancy. Obstet Gynecol. 2013;122(5):1122-31.
14. Leffert LR. What's new in obstetric anesthesia? Focus on preeclampsia. Int J Obstet Anesth. 2015;24(3):264-71.
15. Takacs P, Green KL, Nikaeo A, Kauma SW. Increased vascular endothelial cell production of interleukin-6 in severe preeclampsia. Am J Obstet Gynecol. 2003;188(3):740-4.
16. Ankichetty SP, Chin KJ, Chan VW, Sahajanandan R, Tan H, Grewal A, Perlas A. Regional anesthesia in patients with pregnancy induced hypertension. J Anaesthesiol Clin Pharmacol. 2013;29(4):435-44.
17. Jouppila R, Hollmén A. The effect of segmental epidural analgesia on maternal and foetal acid-base balance, lactate, serum potassium and creatine phosphokinase during labour. Acta Anaesthesiol Scand. 1976;20(3):259-68.
18. Covino BG. Rationale for spinal anesthesia. Int Anesthesiol Clin. 1989;27(1):8-12.
19. Gottumukkala VN, Sharma SK, Philip J. Assessing platelet and fibrinogen contribution to clot strength using modified thromboelastography in pregnant women. Anesth Analg. 1999;89(6):1453-5.
20. Başaran B, Çelebioğlu B, Başaran A, Altınel S, Kutlucan L, Martin JN Jr. Anesthetic practices for patients with preeclampsia or HELLP syndrome: A survey. J Turk Ger Gynecol Assoc. 2016 1;17(3):128-33.
21. Yoo KY, Jeong CW, Park BY, Kim SJ, Jeong ST, Shin MH, et al. Effects of remifentanil on cardiovascular and bispectral index responses to endotracheal intubation in severe pre-eclamptic patients undergoing Caesarean delivery under general anaesthesia. Br J Anaesth. 2009;102(6):812-9.
22. Park BY, Jeong CW, Jang EA, Kim SJ, Jeong ST, Shin MH, et al. Dose-related attenuation of cardiovascular responses to tracheal intubation by intravenous remifentanil bolus in severe pre-eclamptic patients undergoing Caesarean delivery. Br J Anaesth. 2011;106(1):82-7.
23. Yoo KY, Kang DH, Jeong H, Jeong CW, Choi YY, Lee J. A dose-response study of remifentanil for attenuation of the hypertensive response to laryngoscopy and tracheal intubation in severely preeclamptic women undergoing caesarean delivery under general anaesthesia. Int J Obstet Anesth. 2013;22(1):10-8..
24. Bajwa SJS, Kulshrestha A. Anaesthesia for laparoscopic surgery: General vs regional anaesthesia. J Minim Access Surg. 2016;12(1):4-9.
25. Kurosawa S, Kato M. Anesthetics, immune cells, and immune responses. J Anesth. 2008;22(3):263-77.
26. Desborough JP. The stress response to trauma and surgery. BJA: Br J Anaesth. 2000;85(1):109-17.
27. El Azab SR, Rosseel PM, De Lange JJ, van Wijk EM, van Strik R, Scheffer GJ. Effect of VIMA with sevoflurane versus TIVA with propofol or midazolam-sufentanil on the cytokine response during

CABG surgery. Eur J Anaesthesiol. 2002;19(4):276-82.
28. Liu S, Wang B, Li S, Zhou Y, An L, Wang Y, et al. Immune cell populations decrease during craniotomy under general anesthesia. Anesth Analg. 2011;113(3):572-7.
29. Besedovsky H, del Rey A, Sorkin E, Dinarello CA. Immunoregulatory feedback between interleukin-1 and glucocorticoid hormones. Science. 1986;233(4764):652-4.
30. Chrousos GP. The hypothalamic-pituitary-adrenal axis and immune-mediated inflammation. N Engl J Med. 1995;332(20):1351-62.
31. Robertson SA, Bromfield JJ, Tremellen KP. Seminal 'priming' for protection from pre-eclampsia-a unifying hypothesis. J Reprod Immunol. 2003;59(2):253-65.
32. Lai Z, Kalkunte S, Sharma S. A critical role of interleukin-10 in modulating hypoxia-induced preeclampsia-like disease in mice. Hypertension. 2011;57(3):505-14.
33. Taylor BD, Tang G, Ness RB, Olsen J, Hougaard DM, Skogstrand K, et al. Mid-pregnancy circulating immune biomarkers in women with preeclampsia and normotensive controls. Pregnancy Hypertens. 2016;6(4):388-393.
34. Catarino C, Santos-Silva A, Belo L, Rocha-Pereira P, Rocha S, Patrício B, et al. Inflammatory Disturbances in Preeclampsia: Relationship between Maternal and Umbilical Cord Blood. J Pregnancy. 2012;2012:684384.
35. Daneva AM, Hadzi-Lega M, Stefanovic M. Correlation of the system of cytokines in moderate and severe preeclampsia. Clin Exp Obstet Gynecol. 2016;43(2):220-4.
36. Kalinderis M, Papanikolaou A, Kalinderi K, Ioannidou E, Giannoulis C, Karagiannis V, et al. Elevated serum levels of interleukin-6, interleukin-1beta and human chorionic gonadotropin in pre-eclampsia. Am J Reprod Immunol. 2011;66(6):468-75.
37. Pinheiro MB, Martins-Filho OA, Mota AP, Alpoim PN, Godoi LC, Silveira AC, et al. Severe preeclampsia goes along with a cytokine network disturbance towards a systemic inflammatory state. Cytokine. 2013;62(1):165-73.
38. Silva DM, Marreiro Ddo N, Moita Neto JM, Brito JA, Neta EA, Matias JP, et al. Oxidative stress and immunological alteration in women with preeclampsia. Hypertens Pregnancy. 2013;32(3):304-11.
39. Szarka A, Rigo J, Jr ,.Lazar L, Beko G, Molvarec A. Circulating cytokines, chemokines and adhesion molecules in normal pregnancy and preeclampsia determined by multiplex suspension array. BMC Immunol. 2010;11:59.
40. Ferguson KK, McElrath TF, Chen YH, Mukherjee B, Meeker JD. Longitudinal profiling of inflammatory cytokines and C-reactive protein during uncomplicated and preterm pregnancy.Am J Reprod Immunol. 2014;72(3):326-36.
41. Molvarec A, Szarka A, Walentin S, Beko G, Karadi I ,Prohaszka Z, et al. Serum heat shock protein 70 levels in relation to circulating cytokines, chemokines, adhesion molecules and angiogenic factors in women with preeclampsia. Clin Chim Acta. 2011;412(21-22):1957-62.
42. Conrad KP, Miles TM, Benyo DF. Circulating levels of immunoreactive cytokines in women with preeclampsia. Am J Reprod Immunol. 1998;40(2):102-11.
43. Slade MS, Simmons RL, Yunis E, Greenberg LJ. Immunodepression after major surgery in normal patients. Surgery. 1975;78(3):363-72.
44. Walton B. Effects of anaesthesia and surgery on immune status. Br J Anaesth. 1979;51(1):37-43..
45. O'Sullivan ST, Lederer JA, Horgan AF, Chin DH ,Mannick JA, Rodrick ML. Major injury leads to predominance of the T helper-2 lymphocyte phenotype and diminished interleukin-12 production associated with decreased resistance to infection. Ann Surg. 1995;222(4):482-90.
46. Ogawa K, Hirai M, Katsube T, Murayama M, Hamaguchi K, Shimakawa T, et al. Suppression of cellular immunity by surgical stress. Surgery. 2000;127(3):329-36.
47. Yokoyama M, Itano Y, Katayama H, Morimatsu H, Takeda Y, Takahashi T, et al. The effects of continuous epidural anesthesia and analgesia on stress response and immune function in patients undergoing radical esophagectomy. Anesth Analg. 2005;101(5):1521-7.
48. Høgevold HE, Lyberg T, Kahler H, Haug E, Reikeras O. Changes in plasma IL-1beta, TNF-alpha and IL-6 after total hip replacement surgery in general or regional anaesthesia. Cytokine. 2000;12(7):1156-9.
49. Buyukkocak U, Caglayan O, Daphan C, Aydinuraz K, Saygun O, Kaya T, et al. Similar Effects of General and Spinal Anaesthesia on Perioperative Stress Response in Patients Undergoing Haemorrhoidectomy. Mediators Inflamm. 2006;2006(1):97257.
50. Moore CM, Desborough JP, Powell H, Burrin JM, Hall GM. Effects of extradural anaesthesia on interleukin-6 and acute phase response to surgery. Br J Anaesth. 1994;72(3):272-9.
51. Xu Y, Sun Y, Chen H, Wang Y, Wang GN. Effects of two different anesthetic methods on cellular immunity of patients after liver cancer resection. J Biol Regul Homeost Agents. 2016;30(4):1099-1106.
52. Sun H-Z, Song Y-L, Wang X-Y. Effects of Different Anesthetic Methods on Cellular Immune and Neuroendocrine Functions in Patients With Hepatocellular Carcinoma Before and After Surgery. World J Gastroenterol. 2012;18(24):3089-98.
53. Crozier TA, Muller JE, Quittkat D, Sydow M, Wuttke W, Kettler D. Effect of anaesthesia on the cytokine responses to abdominal surgery. Br J Anaesth. 1994;72(3):280-5.
54. Taylor NM, Lacoumenta S, Hall GM. Fentanyl and the interleukin-6 response to surgery. Anaesthesia. 1997;52(2):112-5.
55. Naito Y, Tamai S, Shingu K, Shindo K, Matsui T, Segawa H, et al. Responses of plasma adrenocorticotropic hormone, cortisol, and cytokines during and after upper abdominal surgery. Anesthesiology. 1992;77(3):426-31.
56. Karadeniz MS, Mammadov O, Çiftci HŞ, Usta SA, Pembeci K. Comparing the Effects of Combined General/Epidural Anaesthesia and General Anaesthesia on Serum Cytokine Levels in Radical Cystectomy. Turk J Anaesthesiol Reanim. 2017;45(4):203-9.
57. Risbud MV, Shapiro IM. Role of cytokines in intervertebral disc degeneration: pain and disc content. Nat Rev Rheumatol. 2014;10(1):44-56.
58. De Jongh RF, Bosmans EP, Puylaert MJ, Ombelet WU, Vandeput HJ, Berghmans RA. The influence of anaesthetic techniques and type of delivery on peripartum serum interleukin-6 concentrations. Acta Anaesthesiol Scand. 1997;41(7):853-60.
59. Dermitzaki E, Staikou C, Petropoulos G, Rizos D ,Siafaka I, Fassoulaki A. A randomized study of maternal serum cytokine levels following cesarean section under general or neuraxial anesthesia. Int

J Obstet Anesth. 2009;18(1):33-7.
60. Reikeras O, Borgen P, Reseland JE, Lyngstadaas SP. Changes in serum cytokines in response to musculoskeletal surgical trauma. BMC Res Notes. 2014;7(1):128.
61. Biffl WL, Moore EE, Moore FA, Peterson VM. Interleukin-6 in the injured patient. Marker of injury or mediator of inflammation? Ann Surg. 1996;224(5):647-64.
62. Zhong WW, Burke PA, Hand AT, Walsh MJ, Hughes LA, Forse RA. Regulation of cytokine mRNA expression in lipopolysaccharide-stimulated human macrophages. Arch Surg. 1993;128(2):158-63.
63. Lee TWR, Kowalski S, Falk K, Maguire D, Freed DH, HayGlass KT. High Spinal Anesthesia Enhances Anti-Inflammatory Responses in Patients Undergoing Coronary Artery Bypass Graft Surgery and Aortic Valve Replacement: Randomized Pilot Study .PLoS One. 2016;11(3):e0149942.

26

Thiamine Could Decrease Lactate and Creatinine Level After Coronary Artery Bypass Surgery in Patients with Mild Systolic Dysfunction

Alireza Jahangirifard[1], Shirin Salajegheh[2], Sarvenaz Arab[3], Seyed Bashir Mirtajani[4], Behrooz Farzanegan[1*]

Abstract

Background: During cardiopulmonary bypass, oxidative stress happens in the patient's cells due to blood contact with various levels of synthetic materials. It can activate inflammatory process and release factors such as interleukin 6 (IL-6), C reactive protein (CRP) and neutrophilia, which may hurt different organs. In recent years, many efforts have been made to prevent this type of damage; however, no single treatment has been proposed to reduce this risk. Antioxidant substances such as Thiamine is important in cell defense against free oxygen radicals. Regarding this issue, in this study, effect of Thiamine on lactate levels in patients undergoing coronary artery bypass graft (CABG) surgery has been investigated.

Methods and materials: In this study, 140 patients, 25 to 65 years with mild systolic dysfunction (EF=45-55%) who were candidates for elective CABG surgery in two groups, control and purpose (patients receiving Thiamine), were examined. All of these patients anesthetized in an identical manner, and subjected to a heart-lung pump. Serum lactate levels were measured before, during and six, 12, 18, 24 hours after surgery. All data collected in a questionnaire recorded and evaluated using SPSS statistical software.

Results: Study groups showed no significant differences regarding demographics and underlying diseases. Serum lactate was significantly lower in Thiamine group during the first 24 hours after surgery (except before operation and 2 hours later) ($p < 0.05$). Creatinine level in two groups before surgery was not significantly difference, however, it was significantly lower in case group 24 hours after surgery (1.54±0.14 vs. 1.24±0.19; p: 0.001). In addition, dose of Inotropes in patients who received Thiamine, was significantly lower than the control group (p= 0.001). Extubation was longer in control group (15.4±4.9 vs. 13.15±4.1; p=0.003) while intensive care unit stay was not different.

Conclusion: It seems that Thiamine administration before cardiopulmonary bypass in patients with decreased left ventricular function could decrease serum lactate as tissue perfusion marker and improve kidney function.

Keywords: Thiamine, Coronary artery bypass graft, Systolic dysfunction, Lactate

1. Lung Transplantation Research Center, National Research Institute of Tuberculosis and Lung Diseases (NRITLD), Shahid Beheshti University of Medical Sciences, Tehran, Iran
2. Department of Anesthesiology, Kerman University of Medical Sciences, Kerman, Iran
3. Anesthesiology Research Center, Shahid Beheshti University of Medical Science, Tehran, Iran
4. Mycobacteriology Research Center (MRC), National Research Institute of Tuberculosis and Lung Disease (NRITLD), Shahid Beheshti University of Medical Sciences, Tehran, Iran

Corresponding Author: Behrooz Farzanegan: Tracheal Diseases Research Center, National Research Institute of Tuberculosis and Lung Diseases (NRITLD), Shahid Beheshti University of Medical Sciences, Tehran, Iran;
Email: farzaneganbehrooz@yahoo.com

Introduction

During cardiopulmonary bypass (CPB) surgery, inflammatory responses occur for various reasons (surgical stress, ischemic reperfusion injury, gas micro embolic and particulate) that cause functional impairment in vital organs such as the heart, lungs and kidneys (1). In an accurate statement, it should be noted that stress of surgery leads to inflammatory reactions. However, using CPB exacerbates these inflammatory responses due to increased blood contact with external surfaces (2). These inflammatory responses cause oxidative stress, which is usually associated with the release of inflammatory factors such as C reactive protein (CRP), interleukin 6 (IL-6) and neutrophilia (3). Thus, complications of oxidative stress, by disturbing the balance between free radicals and antioxidants, could exacerbate complications in cardiopulmonary bypass (4). All of these cases indicate that use of antioxidant substances can help to balance effects of increased oxidative stress in patients undergoing cardiopulmonary bypass surgery.

One of the most important markers for improving index of tissue perfusion is serum lactate, which increases during CPB and it is more significant in patients with systolic dysfunction (5). Antioxidant substances such as Thiamine and Glutathione in a form of remission (GSH) have a high degree of cellular defense against oxygen free radicals (6). Thiamine (vitamin B1) have antioxidant effects, and with an unknown mechanism, can improve tissue perfusion and thus improve the index of tissue perfusion, the serum lactate (7). Despite its extracellular function, glutathione plays an important role in purifications of free radicals. High level of GSH reduces loss of oxygen radicals during reperfusion (8). Intracellular GSH is made up of Glycine and Glutamate amino acids and Cysteine containing Thiol (9).

In recent years, many efforts have been made to reduce the damage to organs following cardiopulmonary bypass surgery. Due to spread of different sciences and techniques, there is still no specific method for reducing immunological complications and inflammatory effects of this type of surgery. However, it seems that prescribing antioxidants and drugs during CPB can resolve this problem.

Considering that in patients undergoing cardiopulmonary bypass surgery, serum Thiamine levels are reduced and there has not been any specific research on effects of thiaminc administration on heart function and lactate levels; the research team decided to investigate its effect on serum lactate levels in patients undergoing cardiopulmonary bypass surgery.

Methods

This study designed as a clinical trial and registered in the Iranian clinical trial registry with this code: IRCT2016051412642N24 (dual blinded). Initially, 140 patients with mild heart failure who were selected for coronary artery bypass graft (CABG) surgery (by obtaining consent and the criteria" Aged 25 to 65 years, candidate for elective CABG surgery, mild heart failure (EF between 45% and 55%), thiamine insensitivity, lack of brain problems and lack of post-surgical infections entered the study phase. These patients divided to two groups with 70 participants. At all stage's patients divided between two groups randomly. Two groups including; screening group (300 mg thiamine in 100 ml normal saline 0.9% before CPB) and control group (100 ml normal saline 0.9% before CPB). All patients received a same premedication group (1 mg of lorazepam (P0)) 2 hours and (Morphine 0.1 mg/kg/intramuscular) an hour before surgery. For induction of anesthesia used from Fentanyl, Propofol and Atracurium. Infused Propofol, Fentanyl and Atracurium to maintain anesthesia. Surgery performed using standard on-pump method and patients transferred to the intensive care unit (ICU) intubated and later weaned from ventilator according to standard protocol.

In all patients, serum Lactate levels measured before, during and after surgery (2, 4, 6, 12, 18 and 24 hours after surgery). All data collected in a questionnaire and evaluated using SPSS statistical software (T-test used to compare parametric variables, Mann-Whitney U test, Chi-square tests and Fisher exact test used to compare non-parametric variables in two groups).

Results

The most patients in the study were men and male to female ratio was 63.7% to 36.3% in the control group and 65.5% to 34.5% in the case one. Results of

Table 1: Demographic variables, ASA class, and Ejection fraction of patients in two groups.

	Control (n=70)	Thiamine (n=70)	P-value
Age (year)	56.3±10.2	58.4±9.4	0.25
Height (cm)	167.3±11.4	164.5±12.0	0.33
Weight (Kg)	72.3±15.8	70.1±17.3	0.17
BSA (m2)	1.6±0.16	1.7±0.21	0.39
preoperative EF (%)	45.9±7.3	44.8±6.6	0.48
ASA Class (I/II)	24/46	22/48	0.11
Sex (male/female)	63.7%/36.3	65.5%/34.5%	0.32

EF: Ejection Fraction. ASA: American Society of Anesthesiologists

Table 2: Underlying diseases in two groups of patients.

	Control (n=70)	Thiamine (n=70)	P-value
Diabetes	36(52%)	30(42.5%)	0.22
Hypertension	41 (58.6%)	43 (62.5%)	0.56
Hyperlipidemia	19 (27%)	16 (23%)	0.31
Cigarette smoking	12 (17%)	16 (23%)	0.19
MI	1(1.4%)	1(1.4%)	-
CVA	1(1.4%)	0	-

MI: myocardial Infarction, CVA: Cerebrovascular Accident

this study showed that there was no significant difference between two groups regarding age, sex, height and weight. In addition, according to Table 1, factors such as body surface area (BSA), ejection fraction (EF) and the American society of anesthesiologists (ASA) class had no statistically significant difference (P>0.05).

Table 2 compares underlying diseases in two study groups. Results indicated the meaningless relationship between patients in mentioned groups regarding these issues.

Serum lactate surveyed in patients (before surgery and during 24 hours after surgery) showed a statistically significant difference between two groups (except before and 2 hours after surgery) and this factor was significantly lower in the treatment group than the control group (Table 3).

Results showed that creatinine level in two groups before surgery was not significantly different. However, there was a significant difference in serum creatinine, 24 hours after surgery ($p<0.05$). Table four shows mechanical ventilation time after surgery had a

Table 3: Postoperative serums lactate in two groups of study.

Lactate	Control (n=70)	Thiamine (n=70)	P-value
Before operation (mmol/L)	2.54±0.67	2.63±0.73	0.34
After 2h in ICU	2.25±0.79	2.61±1.7	0.23
After 4h in ICU	3.55±0.64	2.49±0.33	0.001
After 6h in ICU	2.82±0.34	2.28±0.43	0.001
After 12h in ICU	2.29±0.44	2.06±0.41	0.0062
After 18h in ICU	1.96±0.36	1.75±1.25	0.013
After 24h in ICU	1.68±0.61	1.36±0.62	0.032

MV: mechanical ventilation, ICU: Intensive Care Unit

Table 4: Postoperative Base excess (BE) in two groups of study.

	Control (n=70)	Thiamine (n=70)	P-value
Creatinine			
Preoperative (mg/dL)	1.06±0.29	1.01±0.34	0.40
24 h postoperative	1.54±0.14	1.24±0.19	0.001
Duration of MV (hours)	15.4±4.9	13.15±4.1	0.003
Duration of ICU stay (days)	3.73±0.98	3.47±0.93	0.22

MV: mechanical ventilation, ICU: Intensive Care Unit

significant difference in two groups, but duration of ICU stays in two groups did not show any significant difference.

Based on observations made on patients, there

Table 5: Postoperative Base excess (BE) in two groups of study

BE (mEq/L)	Control (n=70)	Thiamine (n=70)	P-value
At entry to ICU	-2.42±2.9	-2.42±2.46	0.99
After 2h in ICU	-3.05±2.2	-3.4±2.65	0.42
After 4h in ICU	-3.8±2.22	-3.41±3.12	0.51
After 6h in ICU	-3.56±2.1	-3.2±2.28	0.50
After 12h in ICU	-2.4±1.99	-1.90±2.20	0.22
After 18h in ICU	-1.21±1.98	-0.78±2.52	0.38
After 24h in ICU	-0.77±2.84	0.45±2.29	0.032

Table 6: Postoperative vasopressor uses in two groups of study

Vasopressor	Control (n=70)	Thiamine (n=70)	P-value
Epinephrine (n)			
After CPB	45	42	0.18
In ICU	45	42	0.18
Epinephrine dose (µ /min)	10.5±1.2	5.46±1.34	0.001
Epinephrine total usage (µg)	36.6±6.8	15.5±4.7	0.001
Dopamine (n)			
After CPB	16	9	0.16
In ICU	19	10	0.075
Dopamine dose (µg/kg/min)	9.7±1.12	4.5±0.98	0.001
Dopamine total usage (µg)	288.5±34.6	112.2±26.6	0.001

were no significant differences in both groups regarding central venous pressure (CVP) during the first 24 hours after ICU admission and the data from these two groups was very close (p>0.05). Although base excess (BE) level was higher in the thiamine recipient group, however, except at 24 hours after surgery, no significant difference observed (Table 5).

Regarding the percentage of patients who received epinephrine and dopamine during and after separation from the CPB and in ICU, there was no significant difference between the two groups ($p > 0.05$). It should be noted that in patients under screening of thiamine, the dose of these two drugs was significantly lower than the control group ($p < 0.005$) (Table 6).

Discussion

Inflammation and accumulation of inflammatory factors, such as cytokines, associated with decreased renal function and increased serum lactate, are common in cardiopulmonary bypass surgery (10). Important factors for starting and continuing inflammation following CPB are not exactly specified. With the onset of inflammation, a large number of inflammatory factors and cells are activated. In the case of CPB, expression of cytokines and inflammatory factors such as endotoxins, tumor necrosis factors (TNFs), Antrodia cinnamomea fruiting bodies (NAKFB) and anaphylatoxins are increased (11). These agents release oxygen-free radicals and proteases by stimulating inflammatory cells, including polymorphonuclear neutrophils (PMN), platelets, and endothelial cells. Inflammation and release of free oxygen radicals followed by tissue damage (12).

Different methods have been proposed to reduce inflammation. Reducing contact time with emergency cardiac care (ECC) (such as off-pump coronary artery bypass (OPCAB) without pump) is one of the ways to reduce inflammation. Of course, along with this method, other methods (such as managing bleeding during surgery, less aortic manipulation in patients with atherosclerosis, using ultrafiltration, reducing prime volume, reducing the CPB duration, using heparin to cover the inner surfaces of tubes and filtering Selection of leukocytes from circulation) are used (13).

About CPB, we could say that cause of increased lactate during cardiac surgery is the reduction of tissue perfusion and low pressure during the pump (11). Mainly, CPB reduces perfusion and reperfusion, however, with the exception of lactate; there are no diagnostic molecular markers for ischemic reperfusion injury. Increased lactate (>3) has proven to be a prognostic factor of mortality in open-heart surgery (14). Results of this study, showed that serum lactate (as a tissue perfusion index) in treatment group in comparison to control group decreased significantly (24 hours after surgery) ($p<0.05$). These results can be important to improvement of patients' condition following the CPB. Reducing free radicals will lead to increased success in surgery outcome and accelerate patient recovery. Thus, based on results, thiamine may play a role in reducing complications and improving the efficiency of patients undergoing cardiopulmonary bypass surgery. However, the effectiveness of thiamine on cardiac factors and its performance has been proven in previous studies. For example, DiNicolantonio and colleagues in 2013 showed that use of thiamine supplements could improve heart function (15). Results of another study, performed by Luger et al. showed that lactate levels were significantly decreased in thiamin-treated patients (48 hours before surgery) (16). Our research results indicate that thiamine reduced creatinine levels. In this case, results are contradictory. For example, in previous studies, it demonstrated that thiamine did not significantly affect acute renal failure (ARF) reduction in patients under CPB (15, 16) and these findings confirmed by Wang et al. (17). However, in the present study only creatinine levels was examined (as a kidney function index). Overall, this decrease in serum levels could be attributed to controlling oxidative and inflammatory factors in the kidneys (18).

In this study, inotropic drug used in thiamine-screened patients was lower than the control group based on Lukienko et al. study. They stated that these results could be linked to the antioxidant properties of thiamine and lower level of lactate in treated group, which can cause better cardiovascular function (19). Meanwhile and based on Maddali and colleagues' observations in 2006, that less inotropic use has provided conditions for reducing the patient's extubating time (20) whereas these results are also observed in our study.

This study has been accompanied by limitations such as inability to measure serum thiamine levels in our country and no assessment of other kidney function markers, which can be addressed more precisely by fixing them.

Conclusion

Use of thiamine before cardiopulmonary bypass can decrease lactate serum level as a marker of reperfusion injury and serum creatinine as a factor for kidney function in patients who have decreased left ventricle function, but the effect of thiamine seems to be limited and higher doses may be needed to further compensate for this damage.

Acknowledgment

None.

Conflicts of Interest

The authors declare that they have no conflict of interest.

References

1. Ruffin Jr RT, Kluger J, Baker WL, Wills SM, Michael White C, Coleman CI. Association between perioperative NSAID use and post-cardiothoracic surgery atrial fibrillation, blood transfusions, and cardiovascular outcomes: a nested cohort study from the AF Suppression Trials (AFIST) I, II and III. Curr Med Res Opin. 2008;24(4):1131-6.

2. Baker WL, Anglade MW, Baker EL, White CM, Kluger J, Coleman CI. Use of N-acetylcysteine to reduce post-cardiothoracic surgery complications: a meta-analysis. Eur J Cardiothorac Surg. 2009;35(3):521-7.

3. Ucar HI1, Tok M, Atalar E, Dogan OF, Oc M, Farsak B, Guvener M, Yilmaz M, Dogan R, Demircin M, Pasaoglu I. Predictive significance of plasma levels of interleukin-6 and high-sensitivity C-reactive protein in atrial fibrillation after coronary artery bypass surgery. Heart Surg Forum. 2007;10(2):E131-5.

4. Wijeysundera DN1, Beattie WS, Rao V, Granton JT, Chan CT. N-acetylcysteine for preventing acute kidney injury in cardiac surgery patients with pre-existing moderate renal insufficiency. Can J Anaesth. 2007;54(11):872-81.

5. Hasanin A, Mukhtar A, Nassar H. Perfusion indices revisited. J Intensive Care. 2017;5:24.

6. Lizard G, Gueldry S, Sordet O, et al. Glutathione is implied in the control of 7-ketocholesterol-induced apoptosis, which is associated with radical oxygen species production. FASEB J. 1998;12(15):1651-63.

7. Manzetti S, Zhang J, van der Spoel D. Thiamin function, metabolism, uptake, and transport. Biochemistry. 2014;53(5):821-35.

8. Eren N, Çakir Ö, Oruc A, Kaya Z, Erdinc L. Effects of N-acetylcysteine on pulmonary function in patients undergoing coronary artery bypass surgery with cardiopulmonary bypass. Perfusion. 2003;18(6):345-50.

9. McBean G. Cysteine, glutathione, and thiol redox balance in astrocytes. Antioxidants (Basel). 2017;6(3): pii: E62.

10. Mao H, Katz N, Ariyanon W, Blanca-Martos L, Adýbelli Z, Giuliani A, Danesi TH, Kim JC, Nayak A, Neri M, Virzi GM, Brocca A, Scalzotto E, Salvador L, Ronco C. Cardiac surgery-associated acute kidney injury. Cardiorenal Med. 2013;3(3):178-99.

11. Koster A, Fischer T, Praus M, Haberzettl H, Kuebler WM, Hetzer R, Kuppe H. Hemostatic activation and inflammatory response during cardiopulmonary bypass: impact of heparin management. Anesthesiology. 2002;97(4):837-41.

12. Ahsan H, Ali A, Ali R. Oxygen free radicals and systemic autoimmunity. Clin Exp Immunol. 2003;131(3):398-404.

13. Laurent T, Markert M, Feihl F, Schaller MD, Perret C. Oxidant-antioxidant balance in granulocytes during ARDS: effect of N-acetylcysteine. Chest. 1996;109(1):163-6.

14. Joudi M, Fathi M, Soltani G, Izanloo A. Factors affecting on serum lactate after cardiac surgery. Anesth Pain Med. 2014;4(4): e18514.

15. DiNicolantonio JJ, Niazi AK, Lavie CJ, O'keefe JH, Ventura HO. Thiamine supplementation for the treatment of heart failure: a review of the literature. Congest Heart Fail. 2013;19(4):214-22.

16. Luger M, Hiesmayr M, Köppel P, et al. Influence of intravenous thiamine supplementation on blood lactate concentration prior to cardiac surgery: a double-blinded, randomised controlled pilot study. Eur J Anaesthesiol. 2015;32(8):543-8.

17. Wang G, Bainbridge D, Martin J, Cheng D. N-acetylcysteine in cardiac surgery: do the benefits outweigh the risks? A meta-analytic reappraisal. J Cardiothorac Vasc Anesth. 2011;25(2):268-75.

18. Nigwekar SU, Kandula P. N-acetylcysteine in cardiovascular-surgery–associated renal failure: a meta-analysis. Ann Thorac Surg. 2009;87(1):139-47.

19. Lukienko PI, Mel'nichenko NG, Zverinskii IV, Zabrodskaya SV. Antioxidant properties of thiamine. Bull Exp Biol Med. 2000;130(9):874-6.

20. Maddali MM, Kurian E, Fahr J. Extubation time, hemodynamic stability, and postoperative pain control in patients undergoing coronary artery bypass surgery: an evaluation of fentanyl, remifentanil, and nonsteroidal antiinflammatory drugs with propofol for perioperative and postoperative management. J Clin Anesth. 2006;18(8):605-10.

Association of Preoperative and Postoperative Brain Natriuretic Peptide Hormone with Morbidity in Adult Patients Undergoing Coronary Artery Bypass Graft Surgery

Mohammad Zia Totonchi[1], Mohammad Forouzeshfard[2], Kamal Fani[3*], Shirin Salajeghe[4], Mehran Ghoreishi[3]

Abstract

Background: Brain natriuretic peptide (BNP) is a cardiac hormone, which its levels as a marker of morbidity in patients undergoing coronary artery bypass grafting (CABG) is still controversial. This study aimed to investigate the relationship between the pre- and postoperative BNP changes and morbidity in adult patients undergoing CABG.

Methods and materials: In this descriptive-analytical study, 50 patients were enrolled underwent elective CABG at the heart center of Rajaei hospital, Tehran, Iran, from September 2016 to May 2017. To determine the serum levels of BNP, blood samples were sent to laboratory at 24 hours before and 24 hours after induction of anesthesia. Duration of intubation, intensive care unit (ICU) stay, and ejection fraction and serum creatinine were considered. Data were analyzed with SPSS Version 22 software and significance level was 5%.

Results: Of patients, 33 (66%) were male and 17 (34%) were female. The mean age ± SD of patients was 61±9 (range 36-82 years). Mean ± SD preoperative BNP level was 919.81±2264.22 pg/ml and postoperative BNP level was 2951.22±4291.27 pg/ml. A significant correlation between pre and postoperative BNP levels and the amount of creatinine, surgical time and length of stay in ICU was not observed. The ejection fraction was correlated with pre and postoperative BNP levels.

Conclusion: Serum levels of BNP at 24 hours before and after cardiac surgery could be a good biomarker for prediction and early diagnosis of heart failure in adults.

Keywords: B- natriuretic peptide, coronary bypass surgery, morbidity

1. Rajaie Cardiovascular center, Medical and Research Center, Tehran, Iran
2. Cancer Research Center, School of Medicine, Semnan University of Medical Sciences, Semnan, Iran
3. Anesthesiology Research Center, School of Medicine, Shahid Beheshti University of Medical Sciences, Tehran, Iran
4. School of Dentistry, Kerman University of Medical Sciences, Kerman, Iran

Corresponding Author: Kamal Fani, MD, Assistant Professor, Anesthesiology Research Center, Velenjak, Chamran Exp Way, Tehran, Iran;
Email: kamalfani@yahoo.com

Introduction

Open heart surgery is a common therapeutic intervention to management and treatment of heart disease that aims to increase the survival and improve the quality of life of these patients (1). Like all other surgeries, this surgery is accompanied by complications that may affect the patient's recovery and health (2). Rate of morbidity in patients undergoing coronary artery bypass grafting (CABG) surgery has not been clearly reported (3-5). Hence, several studies have been conducted to identify prognosis in recovery and to reduce the mortality and morbidity rate after this high risk Surgery (6-9). Study on changes in levels of cardiac biomarkers has been considered in recent years for detecting prognosis of patients after open heart surgery (10, 11). Brain natriuretic peptide (BNP) is a type of heart biomarker or hormone that has been introduced as an indicator of the diagnosis, progression and outcome of treatment in congestive heart failure, acute cerebrovascular accidents and hypertension (12-14). The biomarker is a neuro-hormonal agent that is released by the ventricular myocardium, especially in conditions of increased afterload and ventricular dilation (15). Brain natriuretic peptide, which its bioactive form is N-terminal pro-BNP, has diuretic, natriuretic, vasodilatory, anti-renin-angiotensin-aldosterone characteristics and inhibitory activity on the sympathetic system (14, 16, 17). Concentration of the hormone remains constant after it has increased in the blood, significantly in human plasma, which is easily detectable (14). Normal serum level of N-terminal pro-BNP is less than 300 pg/ml, which increases by aging (15, 18). Level of the hormone affected in several physiological and pathological conditions such as ventricular hypertrophy, left ventricular dysfunction, atrial fibrillation, severe hypertension, aortic stenosis, congestive heart failure, myocardial infarction, pulmonary hypertension, pregnancy hypertension and chronic renal failure (14,19-21). However, BNP as a predictor of cardiovascular events, side effects, and mortality in patients undergoing CABG had been associated with controversial results (22-24). In order that, elevated BNP levels in the early hours after cardiac surgery could be associated with longer hospitalization and higher mortality (25), while Bill et al. (2004) did not report any relationship between BNP levels and ejection fraction, myocardial infarction as an effective factor in morbidity (26). On the other hand, most of these studies examined the relationship between BNP level before and after surgery with patients' morbidity, but relation to determinants of morbidity is less studied.

Regarding the controversial results of previous studies, as well as the evaluation and comparison of BNP levels before and after operation with morbidity, in this study, association of this hormone before and after surgery with factors that can affect the process of recovery and health is examined. Our hypothesis was that preoperative BNP can be like post-operative BNP as a determinative factor in estimating the morbidity of patients after CABG. Therefore, patients with possible post-operative complications can be recognized. The aim of this study was to determine the relationship between pre and post-operative BNP hormone and morbidity in adult patients undergoing CABG surgery.

Methods

In the descriptive-analytic study, patients undergoing elective CABG surgery in the range of 21-89 years who referred to Shahid Rajaie's Heart Center, Tehran, Iran (from September 2016 to May 2017) included the study. Informed consent was obtained from the patients by expressing purpose of the study. All patients who had an emergency or re-operation, as well as simultaneous valve operation, patients with inotrope therapy before surgery and preoperative hematocrit less than 25 were excluded. Sampling was done in convenience method and the sample size was determined according to similar studies. BNP levels were measured in two steps based on samples, which were sent to laboratory at 24 hours before and after surgery. A blood sample (5ml) was collected after that the patient positioned at supine for 15 minutes, and was poured into a tube containing potassium EDTA. Then, serum NT-pro BNP was measured by ELISA with Biomedica Slovakia s.r.o kit (SK-1204) and accurately> 95%.

Demographic and clinical data was collected for pre-operative (24 hours before surgery) and postoperative (24 hours after operation) using a questionnaire. This information includes age, sex, body mass index, underlying illness, history of smoking, ejection fraction (EF), creatinine (Cr), blood urea nitrogen (Bun), glomerular filtration rate before and after surgery, The time of aortic clamp, time of cardiopulmonary bypass, surgical time, number of grafts, duration of intubation and duration of patient's stay in intensive care unit (ICU) were completed.

These patients were considered as morbidity factors:

- low cardiac output (need for inotrope for more than 24 hours or balloon pump placement)
- myocardial infarction (MI: ECG findings and increased cardiac enzymes)
- atrial fibrillation (AF; More than 10 minutes during ICU hospitalization)
- renal failure (Cr>3 or need to dialysis)
- long term intubation (more than 48 hours)
- long term ICU hospitalization (more than 4 days)

SPSS version 20 software using Kolmogrov-Smirnov test (for determination of normality), paired t-test (in parametric data) and dependent Wilcoxon (in nonparametric data) and correlation tests analyzed data. A significant level of 5% was considered.

Results

In this study, 50 patients were evaluated. Of them 33 (66%) were male and 17 (34%) were female. Mean±SD age of patients was 61±9 with a range of 36-82. Most patients (54%, n= 27) were overweight and 21 (42%) people were normal weight and two (4%) were obese. Hypertension had the highest frequency of all comorbidities (60%, n=30). Diabetes mellitus (36%, n=18) and renal failure (4%, n=2) were in the next ranks. Smokers were 19 (38%). Table 1 shows the parameters measured before and after the operation. There was a significant difference between serum creatinine and BNP before and after surgery.

Mean ± SD duration of: surgery was 228.90 ± 43.08, aortic clamp was 48.87 ± 18.17, cardiopulmonary bypass was 90.16 ± 28.21, intubation (hours) was 12.14 ± 4.95 and admission to ICU (day) was 3.28 ± 0.6. Relationship between BNP before and after surgery with sex, smoking and underlying diseases was investigated, which no significant relationship was found (Table 2).

Tables 3 and 4 show correlation between BNP before and after surgery and the variables considered for morbidity (postoperative ejection fraction, postoperative creatinine, duration of intubation, hospitalization in ICU, surgery; aortic clamping and pump times). Among these variables, only ejection fraction had a significant correlation with BNP at both times, before and after the operation.

Discussion

Efforts to identify and assess risks of preoperative and postoperative heart surgery to reduce morbidity and mortality studied. Evaluation of BNP as a criterion in recognition of morbidity in patients undergoing cardiac surgery has been investigated in several studies (18, 20, 26). However, advantage of present study is to examine the level of BNP and its relationship with determinants of morbidity in both

Table 1: Parameters measured before and after the operation.

Variables	Before operation SD± Mean	After operation SD± Mean	P value
Hemoglobin (gr/dl)	1.64 ± 13.73	1.71±13.48	0. 242
Hematocrit (%)	4.79±41.11	4.24±40.81	0.259
Ejection fraction (%)	41.93±11.85	40.81±10.41	0.234
Bun (mg/dl)	6.34±17.51	6.7±17.30	0.421
Creatinine (mg/dl)	0.22 ±0.989	0.31 ± 1.08	0.028
Glomerular filtration rate (ml/min/1.73 m2)	26.05 ±78.84	30.46 ± 76.40	0.448
BNP	919.81± 2364.22	2951.22 ±4291.27	0.000

Table 2: Relationship of mean serum BNP levels before and after surgery with clinical and demographic variables.

Variables		number	BNP1 (pg/ml)	BNP2 (pg/ml)	P value
Gender	female	17	1592.274	5203.411	0.237
	male	33	632.463	1873.939	0.235
Diabetes	+	18	1410.958	4583.611	0.310
	_	32	700.55	2298.93	0.125
Smoking	+	19	461.321	1993.210	0.236
	_	31	1262.96	3816.03	0.237
Hypertension	+	28	1342.623	3213.928	0.237
	_	22	499.67	1667.10	0.236
Kidney disease	+	3	1725.875	2015.25	0.199
	_	47	939.32	3073.00	0.238
Arrhythmia	+	1	85.4	1088	---
	_	49	976.15	3037.75	0.238

before and after cardiac surgery. Open heart surgery is a complex procedure which can lead to morbidity in patients, therefore examining association of BNP in preoperative conditions may be a suitable method to

Table 3: Correlation between preoperative BNP and clinical variables.

Variables		Before surgery	P value
Ejection fraction	50	-0.380	0.006
Creatinine	50	0.114	0.430
Duration of intubation	50	0.108	0.466
Length of ICU hospitalization	50	0.220	0.879
Duration of surgery	50	0.111	0.414
Duration of aortic clamping	50	0.211	0.770
Duration of pump	50	0.151	0.485

predict the complications.

Table 4: Correlation between postoperative BNP and clinical variables

Variables		after surgery	P value
Ejection fraction	50	-0.416	0.003
Creatinine	50	0.068	0.641
Duration of intubation	50	0.044	0.760
Length of ICU hospitalization	50	0.218	0.128
Duration of surgery	50	0.113	0.421
Duration of aortic clamping	50	0.224	0.811
Duration of pump	50	0.131	0.428

In different studies relationship between preoperative BNP serum levels and postoperative morbidity was investigated (22, 27-29), and in some other studies postoperative serum levels of BNP have been considered (30-32). Only in a study, predictive value of BNP serum level before and after operation with morbidity was compared (33). Results of our study showed that postoperative serum BNP levels increased by 3 times in comparison with preoperative CABG after surgery. Increased BNP after surgery has been shown in numerous studies, which can be due to changes in the preload and afterload. In present study, there was a reverse and significant correlation between preoperative and postoperative BNP values and EF after surgery, so that an increased BNP levels was observed in reduced EF. In addition, the relationship between BNP before and after surgery and postoperative creatinine, duration of intubation and duration of ICU stay were observed, however this relationship was not significant. The FDA has approved measuring the NT-proBNP test for the diagnosis of heart failure (14). ProBNP is the most sensitive marker for heart failure or mild cardiac failure (20).

Bosseau et al. showed that although BNP is not a specific hormone for cardiac function, but it can be used as a marker for the diagnosis of congestive heart failure (34). In the study of Hussain et al. BNP levels also had a significant relationship with left ventricular ejection fraction (35). Fox et al concluded that preoperative BNP could be a predictor of post-operative complications, mortality and morbidity (33). In our study, preoperative BNP had a significant correlation with EF after surgery alone. This may be due to the difference in the normal range in the two studies, low sample size in our study and the difference in the factors affecting the BNP level, such as the sex of women and age, which was observed in Fox et al study. Limitations of this study were the low sample size; lack of BNP repeated examination during surgery to determine the rate of BNP increase and the mortality rate of patients.

Conclusion

BNP level can be affected by various factors, but its relationship with EF decreases is significant, which can be used to diagnose the congestive heart failure in patients after open heart surgery. Patients with high levels of BNP before or after surgery may need extra attention due to probable reduced ejection fraction.

Acknowledgment

None.

Conflicts of Interest

The authors declare that they have no conflict of interest.

References

1. Demir A, Aydınlı B, Güçlü ÇY, Yazıcıoğlu H, Saraç A, Elhan AH, Erdemli Ö. Obesity and postoperative early complications in open heart surgery. J Anesth. 2012;26(5):702-10.

2. Murad JA Junior, Machado MN, Fernandes MP, Soares MJF, Grigolo IH, Singulane CC, Godoy MF. B-Type Natriuretic Peptide as a Predictor of Short-Term Mortality in On-Pump Coronary Artery Bypass Grafting. Braz J Cardiovasc Surg. 2017;32(6):462-467.

3. Tully PJ, Baker RA. Depression, anxiety, and cardiac morbidity outcomes after coronary artery bypass surgery: a contemporary and practical review. J Geriatr Cardiol. 2012;9(2):197-208.

4. Pepper J. Nilsson J, Algotsson L, Höglund P, Lührs C, Brandt J. Controversies in off-pump coronary artery surgery. Clin Med Res. 2005;3(1):27-33.

5. Nilsson J, Algotsson L, Höglund P, Lührs C, Brandt J. Comparison of 19 pre-operative risk stratification models in open-heart surgery. Eur Heart J. 2006;27(7):867-74.

6. Faritous ZS, Aghdaie N, Yazdanian F, Azarfarin R, Dabbagh A. Perioperative risk factors for prolonged mechanical ventilation and tracheostomy in women undergoing coronary artery bypass graft with cardiopulmonary bypass. Saudi J Anaesth. 2011;5(2):167-9.

7. Rajaei S, Dabbagh A. Risk factors for postoperative respiratory mortality and morbidity in patients undergoing coronary artery bypass grafting. Anesth Pain Med. 2012;2(2):60-5.

8. Holzmann MJ, Rathsman B, Eliasson B, Kuhl J, Svensson AM, Nyström T, Sartipy U. Long-term prognosis in patients with type 1 and 2 diabetes mellitus after coronary artery bypass grafting. J Am Coll Cardiol. 2015;65(16):1644-1652.

9. Petursson P, Herlitz J, Lindqvist J, Sjöland H, Gudbjörnsdottir S. Prevalence and severity of abnormal glucose regulation and its relation to long-term prognosis after coronary artery bypass grafting. Coron Artery Dis. 2013;24(7):577-82.

10. Shahian DM, Grover FL. Biomarkers and risk models in cardiac surgery. Circulation. 2014;130(12):932-5.

11. Parolari A, Poggio P, Myasoedova V, Songia P, Bonalumi G, Pilozzi A, Pacini D, Alamanni F, Tremoli E. Biomarkers in Coronary Artery Bypass Surgery: Ready for Prime Time and Outcome Prediction? Front Cardiovasc Med. 2016; 2:39.

12. Preeshagul I, Gharbaran R, Jeong KH, Abdel-Razek A, Lee LY, Elman E, Suh KS. Potential biomarkers for predicting outcomes in CABG cardiothoracic surgeries. J Cardiothorac Surg;8:176.

13. van Veldhuisen DJ, Linssen GC, Jaarsma T, van Gilst WH, Hoes AW, Tijssen JG, Paulus WJ, Voors AA, Hillege HL. B-type natriuretic peptide and prognosis in heart failure patients with preserved and reduced ejection fraction. J Am Coll Cardiol. 2013;61(14):1498-506.

14. Macheret F, Heublein D, Costello-Boerrigter LC, Boerrigter G, McKie P, Bellavia D, Mangiafico S, Ikeda Y, Bailey K, Scott CG. Human hypertension is characterized by a lack of activation of the antihypertensive cardiac hormones ANP and BNP. J Am Coll Cardiol. 2012;60(16):1558-65.

15. Daniels LB, Maisel AS. Natriuretic peptides. J Am Coll Cardiol. 2007;50(25):2357-68.

16. Keyzer JM, Hoffmann JJ, Ringoir L, Nabbe KC, Widdershoven JW, Pop VJ. Age-and gender-specific brain natriuretic peptide (BNP) reference ranges in primary care. Clin Chem Lab Med. 2014; 52(9):1341-6.

17. Santhekadur PK, Kumar DP, Seneshaw M, Mirshahi F, Sanyal AJ. The multifaceted role of natriuretic peptides in metabolic syndrome. Biomed Pharmacother. 2017;92:826-35.

18. Potter LR, Yoder AR, Flora DR, Antos LK, Dickey DM. Natriuretic peptides: their structures, receptors, physiologic functions and therapeutic applications. Handb Exp Pharmacol. 2009;(191):341-66.

19. Bansal N, Hyre Anderson A, Yang W, Christenson RH, deFilippi CR, Deo R, Dries DL, Go AS, He J, Kusek JW, Lash JP, Raj D, Rosas S, Wolf M, Zhang X, Shlipak MG, Feldman H. High-sensitivity troponin T and N-terminal pro-B-type natriuretic peptide (NT-proBNP) and risk of incident heart failure in patients with CKD: the Chronic Renal Insufficiency Cohort (CRIC) Study. J Am Soc Nephrol. 2015; 26(4):946-56.

20. Grewal J, McKelvie R, Lonn E, Tait P, Carlsson J, Gianni M, Jarnert C, Persson H. BNP and NT- proBNP predict echocardiographic severity of diastolic dysfunction. Eur J Heart Fail. 2008; 10(3):252-9.

21. Mueller C, Breidthardt T, Laule-Kilian K, Christ M, Perruchoud AP. The integration of BNP and NT-proBNP into clinical medicine. Swiss Med Wkly. 2007; 137(1-2):4-12.

22. Martinez-Rumayor A, Richards AM, Burnett JC, Januzzi JL. Biology of the natriuretic peptides. Am J Cardiol. 2008 Feb 4;101(3A):3-8.

23. Cuthbertson BH, Croal BL, Rae D, Gibson PH, McNeilly JD, Jeffrey RR, Smith WC, Prescott GJ, Buchan KG, El-Shafei H, Gibson GA, Hillis GS. N-terminal pro-B-type natriuretic peptide levels and early outcome after cardiac surgery: a prospective cohort study. Br J Anaesth. 2009; 103(5):647-53.

24. Rodseth RN, Biccard BM, Chu R, Lurati Buse GA, Thabane L, Bakhai A, Bolliger D, Cagini L, Cahill TJ, Cardinale D, Chong CP, Cnotliwy M, Di Somma S, Fahrner R, Lim WK, Mahla E, Le Manach Y, Manikandan R, Pyun WB, Rajagopalan S, Radovic M, Schutt RC, Sessler DI, Suttie S, Vanniyasingam T, Waliszek M, Devereaux PJ. Postoperative B-type natriuretic peptide for prediction of major cardiac events in patients undergoing noncardiac surgery: systematic review and individual patient meta-analysis. Anesthesiology. 2013; 119(2):270-83.

25. Crescenzi G, Landoni G, Monaco F, Bignami E, De Luca M, Frau G, Rosica C, Zangrillo A. Epidural anesthesia in elderly patients undergoing coronary artery bypass graft surgery. J Cardiothorac Vasc Anesth. 2009; 23(6):807-12.

26. Murad Junior JA, Nakazone MA, Machado Mde N, Godoy MF. Predictors of mortality in cardiac surgery: brain natriuretic peptide type B. Rev Bras Cir Cardiovasc. 2015; 30(2):182-7.

27. Fox AA, Nascimben L, Body SC, Collard CD, Mitani AA, Liu KY, Muehlschlegel JD, Shernan SK, Marcantonio ER. Increased

perioperative b-type natriuretic peptide associates with heart failure hospitalization or heart failure death after coronary artery bypass graft surgery. Anesthesiology. 2013; 119(2):284-94.

28. Attaran S, Sherwood R, Desai J, Langworthy R, Mhandu P, John L, El-Gamel A. Brain natriuretic peptide a predictive marker in cardiac surgery. Interact Cardiovasc Thorac Surg. 2009; 9(4):662-6.

29. Eliasdottir S, Klemenzson G, Torfason B, Valsson F. Brain natriuretic peptide is a good predictor for outcome in cardiac surgery. Acta Anaesthesiol Scand. 2008; 52(2):182-7.

30. Berendes E, Schmidt C, Van Aken H, Hartlage MG, Rothenburger M, Wirtz S, Scheld HH, Brodner G, Walter M. A-type and B-type natriuretic peptides in cardiac surgical procedures. Anesth Analg. 2004; 98(1):11-9.

31. Liu H, Wang C, Liu L, Zhuang Y, Yang X, Zhang Y. Perioperative application of N-terminal pro-brain natriuretic peptide in patients undergoing cardiac surgery. J Cardiothorac Surg. 2013; 8:1.

32. Nozohoor S, Nilsson J, Lührs C, Roijer A, Algotsson L, Sjögren J. B-type natriuretic peptide as a predictor of postoperative heart failure after aortic valve replacement. J Cardiothorac Vasc Anesth. 2009; 23(2):161-5.

33. Meersch M, Zarbock A. Prevention of cardiac surgery-associated acute kidney injury. Curr Opin Anaesthesiol. 2017; 30(1):76-83.

34. Fox AA, Shernan SK, Collard CD, Liu K-Y, Aranki SF, DeSantis SM, Jarolim P, Body SC. Preoperative B-type natriuretic peptide is as independent predictor of ventricular dysfunction and mortality after primary coronary artery bypass grafting. J Thorac Cardiovasc Surg. 2008; 136(2):452-61.

35. Kang SH, Park JJ, Choi DJ, Yoon CH, Oh IY, Kang SM, Yoo BS, Jeon ES, Kim JJ, Cho MC, Chae SC, Ryu KH, Oh BH; KorHF Registry. Prognostic value of BNP in heart failure with preserved or reduced EF. Heart. 2015;101(23):1881-8.

36. Maisel AS, Duran JM, Wettersten N. Natriuretic Peptides in Heart Failure: Atrial and B-type Natriuretic Peptides. Heart Fail Clin. 2018; 14(1):13-25.

28

The Balance between Pro-oxidants and Antioxidants in Cardiac Anesthesia

Seyed Mohammad Seyed-Alshohadaei[1*]

1. Anesthesiology Research Center, Shahid Beheshti University of Medical Sciences, Tehran, Iran

Corresponding Author:
Seyed Mohammad Seyed-Alshohadaei, MD, Anesthesiology Research Center, Shahid Beheshti University of Medical Sciences, Tehran, Iran

E-mail: dr.seyed.seyed@gmail.com

Abstract

Due to the development of surgical techniques for controlling the conditions of patients, we are still faced with many conditions and risks in the management of patients' health during and after surgery. Hence, the creation of new methods, access to medicines and things that increase the quality of management and improve patient control conditions are on the agenda of many research teams around the world. Antioxidant substances and their effects on the control of free radicals (as one of the destructive factors on the health of patients undergoing surgery) is one of the research cases that has attracted many researchers in recent years. Cardiac surgery and cardiac anesthesia are among the most challenging types of surgeries. Control and management of patient conditions during this type of surgery is one of the most important challenges of anesthesiology team. This study tries to investigate the importance of antioxidants in controlling conditions and improving the status of patients undergoing cardiac surgery.

Keywords: Antioxidant; Pro-oxidant; Cardiac Anesthesia; Inflammation; Pain

Introduction

Oxidative stress is one of the risk factors for humans. These factors in various organs of the body cause numerous and various injuries, including: asthma in the lung, glomerulonephritis in the kidneys, atherosclerosis in the cardiovascular system, preeclampsia in the fetus, Alzheimer's disease in brain, cataract in the eyes, and even with the application of a multi organ mechanism can cause cancer, diabetes or inflammation. (1)

The source of oxidative stress should be in the balance between oxidative factors (free radicals) and antioxidants. (2)

In this situation, the body's redox system has changed and the consequences of this imbalance appear as stated. Antioxidants as the other pole of this balance are substances that act to protect cells against the harmful effects of free radicals and neutralize them. Antioxidants act their corrective effects in two ways, breaking the cycle or preventing it. In the form of breaking the cycle, when the radical freedom of a single electron is stealing, another free radical is produced, and the cycle continues until it is broken down by an antioxidant, including the antioxidants that act in this way like vitamin E or vitamin C. In the form of prevention, the production of oxidants is prevented by antioxidants, thus reducing the start of cycles. Glutathione peroxidase is an example of antioxidants that act as a preventive method (1)

Pain is considered as a consequence of all surgeries. The cardiovascular surgery as one of the most dangerous types of surgeries is no exception. Control of pain after cardiovascular surgery has a very important role in the success of these types of surgeries, and poor control of postoperative pain have serious complications for patients (3). On the other hand, pain itself causes the oxidative stress in the body (4), while the use of antioxidants in heart surgery has been accompanied by a reduction in oxidative reactions (5). The cardiovascular system is affected by the balance between oxidative stress and antioxidant substances. Therefore, it seems that the control of pain and oxidative damage separately or together can play a significant role in the success and control of the outcome of cardiac surgery.

Pain and oxidants effect:

Pain as an indicator can be a sign of various illnesses. The mechanism of production and the quality of pain vary in each disease; however, the effect of oxidants on pain has been studied and confirmed in several studies. This effect can be achieved by reducing inflammation, reducing the negative effect on nociceptors, cofactors of opioids production or protecting mitochondria (4, 6, 7, 8, and 9). Several studies have shown different results in antioxidant activity for pain relief; however, it is important to control the pain. For example, vitamin C and vitamin E antioxidants in women with pelvic pain and the history of endometriosis have decreased Pain and inflammatory factors in patient's abdominal fluids. Thus, the role of antioxidants in the treatment of these patients is significant (7). Another study has shown that the use of alpha-lipoic acid (as a natural antioxidant) has been effective in reducing peripheral neuropathic pain (10). Combination therapy of antioxidants has also been helpful in treating and relieving pain in patients. For example, the combination of selenium antioxidants, beta-carotene, vitamin C, vitamin E, and methionine shows these results in various studies (4). Melatonin and N-acetylcysteine have similar effects in protecting against oxidative damages and inflammatory markers in cardiac surgery (6).

The combination of antioxidants and analgesics will normalize oxidative stresses. As a result, the use of antioxidants in the treatment of pain can be used to reduce the dose of analgesics and reduce the negative effect of activated oxygen on nociceptors (11). In this case, vitamin C can be mentioned as a cofactor for the production of amide opioids, which high dose administration can reduce the need for opioids in surgery and cancer patients. (8). In another study, an antioxidant effect by Mito Tempo was investigated in neuropathic pain, in which antioxidant activity was assessed with malondialdehyde and reduced glutathione content and overall activity of serum superoxide dismutase in serum and spinal cord. Finally, the results show that antioxidants with mitochondrial effects have reduced neuropathic pain by protecting mitochondria from oxidative damage (9).

Effect of oxidants on CABG surgery:

The inverse relationship between the magnitude of oxidative stress and cardiac performance can be indicative of the effect of oxidative stress. Although this effect has not been seen in patients undergoing cardiac valve surgery, the magnitude of these stresses can be predictive of cardiac function in CABG (12, 13).

Hemodialysis, ischemia and perfusion injuries activate neutrophils during heart surgery and cause stress and activate inflammatory, pre-inflammatory and pre-apoptotic factors. This stress affects various organs in the body. Free radicals are molecules lacking free electrons, which makes them very active. Redox signals are activated in response to changes in the level of ROS (reactive oxygen species), mitochondria and during the cardio pulmonary pump. Blood transfusion from the non-endothelialized cycle is the main source of ROS production during cardiac surgery. The activation of neutrophils in the pulmonary pump is shown by the decrease in L-selectin and the increase of CD11b and CD18. Low level of trisphosphate in damaged area is due to ischemic injury mediated by hypoxanthine. After a period of ischemic injury, reperfusion plays a major role in oxidative stress by initiating a series of events. The pulmonary pump causes mechanical damage to red blood cells, which causes blood cell sensitivity to the membrane complex and, by causing hemoglobin leakage, results in the production of peroxidase. On the other hand, during transfusion, we will encounter oxidative stress. Acute pulmonary and renal damage, two common complications during cardiac surgery, is caused by oxidative damage. The hydroxyl phenol present in propofol is similar to vitamin E. L-arginine plays a role in the immune function and vascular hemostasis, and is a precursor of nitric oxide. Therefore, the addition of L-arginine to the cardioplegia solution decreases myocardial damage and decreases the damage as a result of the activity of superoxide dismutase. The alpha necrosis factor decreases with N-acetylcysteine "administration. Adding N-acetylcysteine" to the cardioplegia solution decreases MDA (Malondialdehyde), glutathione catalase, SOD (Superoxide dismutase), glutathione peroxidase, and glutathione reductase. Mitoquinone mesylate (MitoQ) is an antioxidant by targeting ROS, which is immediately captured by mitochondria and detoxifies ROS (14, 15).

In children, due to the immature heart cells and heart congenital problems, there is more vulnerability to oxidative factors, which leads to poor functioning of heart. Interventions such as glucocorticoids, bypass circuit miniaturization, prime-pump strategies and cardioplegia can reduce the oxidative stress in children's heart surgery (16).

Alpha-lipoic causes the production of other antioxidants, such as glutathione, provided by the block of NRF2 and increase in translation of the enzyme glutathione synthase (17). Glutathione antioxidant systems can stimulate oxidative stress in mitochondria and cause cell toxicity (18). Moreover, intracellular antioxidant systems, such as glutathione and NADPH, can produce ROS (19).

In the cardiovascular system, the antioxidant has a paradoxical ability to simulate oxidative stress (20). The imbalance and increase in the overall serum oxidative state in open-heart surgery can be related to the time of aortic clamp (21). In oxidative stresses in coronary heart disease, antioxidants such as superoxide dismutase 1 and 2, can be measured as biochemical markers for these stresses (22), a new, automated, cheap and easy method is available now to measure the total level of antioxidants versus free radicals (23). The metabolic syndrome is linked to activated protein C, the serum levels of uric acid and the balance of pro oxidants and antioxidants (24).

Conclusion

Control of pain and oxidation factors play an important role in the success of cardiovascular surgery. Pain can cause oxidative damage and also exacerbate the damaging effects of the oxidation of the agent caused by the use of heart pumps, transfusion and other destructive factors. In children, due to their vulnerability, these risks are more severe and the control of these factors seems more necessary. The use of antioxidant agents during cardiac surgery has reduced oxidative damage and decreased pain in patients. However, the use of these agents sometimes paradoxically provokes oxidative stimulation in mitochondria and cellular toxicity, which can be due to the imbalance of the cell oxidant and cell antioxidant factors, which made it vital to measure the balance of oxidant and antioxidant agents.

Future Prospective:

Assessment of the oxidative stress level and antioxidants during coronary heart disease surgeries by measuring stress biomarkers or free radical staining can be useful tool for assessing how antioxidant agents are used preoperatively, during operation and in the post-operative period. Assessing the balance and imbalance of oxidants and antioxidant factors on the course of the diseases by point of care diagnostic systems can determine how to use these vital substances properly.

Acknowledgment

The kind help and assistance received from Anesthesiology Research Center, Shahid Beheshti University of Medical Sciences, Tehran, Iran for this study is highly appreciated.

Conflicts of Interest

The author declares that there is no conflict of interest.

References

1. Pham-Huy LA, He H, Pham-Huy C. Free radicals, antioxidants in disease and health. Int J Biomed Sci. 2008; 4(2): 89–96.

2. Sies H. Oxidative stress: oxidants and antioxidants. Exp Physiol. 1997;82(2):291-5.

3. Zubrzycki M, Liebold A, Skrabal C, Reinelt H, Ziegler M, Perdas E, Zubrzycka M. Assessment and pathophysiology of pain in cardiac surgery. J Pain Res. 2018; 11: 1599–611.
4. Cai GH, Huang J, Zhao Y, Chen J, Wu HH, Dong YL, Smith HS, Li YQ, Wang W, Wu SX. Antioxidant therapy for pain relief in patients with chronic pancreatitis: systematic review and meta-analysis. Pain Physician. 2013;16(6):521-32.
5. Stanger O, Aigner I, Schimetta W, Wonisch W. Antioxidant supplementation attenuates oxidative stress in patients undergoing coronary artery bypass graft surgery. Tohoku J Exp Med. 2014;232(2):145-54.
6. Zakkar M, Guida G, Suleiman M, Angelini GD. Cardiopulmonary bypass and oxidative stress. Oxid Med Cell Longev. 2015;2015:189863.
7. Santanam N, Kavtaradze N, Murphy A, Dominguez C, Parthasarathy S. Antioxidant supplementation reduces endometriosis-related pelvic pain in humans. Transl Res. 2013;161(3):189-95.
8. Carr AC, McCall C. The role of vitamin C in the treatment of pain: new insights. J Transl Med. 2017;15(1):77.
9. Zhan L, Li R, Sun Y, Dou M, Yang W, He S, Zhang Y. Effect of mito-TEMPO, a mitochondria-targeted antioxidant, in rats with neuropathic pain. Neuroreport. 2018;29(15):1275-81.
10. Maglione E, Marrese C, Migliaro E, et al. Increasing bioavailability of (R)-alpha-lipoic acid to boost antioxidant activity in the treatment of neuropathic pain. Acta Biomed. 2015;86(3):226-33.
11. Rokyta R, Holecek V, Pekárková I, et al. Free radicals after painful stimulation are influenced by antioxidants and analgesics. Neuro Endocrinol Lett. 2003;24(5):304-9.
12. Rahsepar AA, Mirzaee A, Moodi F, Moohebati M, Tavallaie S, Khorashadizadeh F, Mottahedi B, Esfehanizadeh J, Azari A, Sajjadian M, Khojasteh R, Paydar R, Mousavi S, Amini M, Ghayour-Mobarhan M, Ferns GA. Prooxidant-antioxidant balance and cardiac function in patients with cardiovascular disease following cardiac surgery. J Heart Valve Dis. 2013;22(3):408-17.
13. Baikoussis NG, Papakonstantinou NA, Verra C, Kakouris G, Chounti M, Hountis P, Dedeilias P, Argiriou M. Mechanisms of oxidative stress and myocardial protection during open-heart surgery. Ann Card Anaesth. 2015;18(4):555-64.
14. Fudulu DP, Gibbison B, Upton T, Stoica SC, Caputo M, Lightman S, Angelini GD. Corticosteroids in Pediatric Heart Surgery: Myth or Reality. Front Pediatr. 2018;6:112.
15. Moris D, Spartalis M, Tzatzaki E, Spartalis E, Karachaliou GS, Triantafyllis AS, Karaolanis GI, Tsilimigras DI, Theocharis S. The role of reactive oxygen species in myocardial redox signaling and regulation. Ann Transl Med. 2017;5(16):324.
16. Fudulu D, Angelini G. Oxidative stress after surgery on the immature heart. Oxid Med Cell Longev. 2016;2016:1971452.
17. Zhang J, Zhou X, Wu W, Wang J, Xie H, Wu Z. Regeneration of glutathione by α-lipoic acid via Nrf2/ARE signaling pathway alleviates cadmium-induced HepG2 cell toxicity. Environ Toxicol Pharmacol. 2017;51:30-7.
18. Zhang H, Limphong P, Pieper J, Liu Q, Rodesch CK, Christians E, Benjamin IJ. Glutathione-dependent reductive stress triggers mitochondrial oxidation and cytotoxicity. The FASEB J. 2012;26(4):1442-51.
19. Korge P, Calmettes G, Weiss JN. Increased reactive oxygen species production during reductive stress: the roles of mitochondrial glutathione and thioredoxin reductases. Biochim Biophys Acta. 2015;1847(6-7):514-25.
20. Handy DE, Loscalzo J. Responses to reductive stress in the cardiovascular system. Free Radic Biol Med. 2017 Aug;109:114-24.
21. Mentese U, Dogan OV, Turan I, Usta S, Dogan E, Mentese SO, Demir S, Ozer T, Aykan AC, Alver A. Oxidant-antioxidant balance during on-pump coronary artery bypass grafting. ScientificWorldJournal. 2014;2014:263058.
22. Peng JR, Lu TT, Chang HT, Ge X, Huang B, Li WM. Elevated levels of plasma superoxide dismutases 1 and 2 in patients with coronary artery disease. Biomed Res Int. 2016;2016:3708905.
23. Erel O. A novel automated method to measure total antioxidant response against potent free radical reactions. Cl Clin Biochem. 2004;37(2):112-9.
24. Ahmadnezhad M, Arefhosseini SR, Parizadeh MR, Tavallaie S, Tayefi M, Darroudi S, Ghazizadeh H, Moohebati M, Ebrahimi M, Heidari-Bakavoli A, Azarpajouh MR, Ferns GA, Mogharebzadeh V, Ghayour-Mobarhan M. Association between serum uric acid, highly sensitive C-reactive protein and pro-oxidant-antioxidant balance in patients with metabolic syndrome. Biofactors. 2018;44(3):263-71.

29

Comparison of retrolaminar paravertebral infiltration of a non-steroid mixture with conventional epidural steroid infiltration in patients suffering from chronic radicular Pain

Sadegh Abdolmohammadi[1]*, Alireza Nekoui[2], Gilbert Blaise[2]

1. Department of Anesthesiology and Pain Medicine, Shahid Beheshti University of Medical Sciences, Loghman Hospital, Tehran, Iran
2. Centre Hospitalier de l'Université de Montréal (CHUM), University of Montreal, Montreal, Quebec, Canada

Corresponding Author: Sadegh Abdolmohammadi, M.D., Assistant Professor, Shahid Beheshti University of Medical Sciences, Loghman Hospital, Department of Anesthesiology, Tehran, Iran.
E-mail: sadegh.abdolmohammadi@smbu.ac.ir

Abstract

Background: Chronic radicular pain is often treated by epidural steroid infiltration (ESI). In 2014, the Food and Drug Administration (FDA) issued a letter warning that ESI may result in rare but serious adverse events, including "loss of vision, stroke, paralysis, and death". In this retrospective study, we compare retrolaminar paravertebral infiltration (PVI) of a non-steroid-mixture with an epidural steroid injection (ESI).

Materials and Methods: We identified 31 patients registered in the Quebec Pain Registry suffering from chronic lumbar or cervical radicular pain referred to the Centre Hospitalier de l'Université de Montréal (CHUM) pain clinic between 2009 to 2014. These patients received ultrasound-guided retrolaminar PVI with a mixture of morphine 1 mg, ketamine 10 mg, neostigmine 0.5 mg, naloxone 2ng, and bupivacaine 10 mg. The control group, matched for gender, age, and DN4 sub-scale score at baseline, consisted of 31 patients with the same pathology; they were treated by fluoroscopic-guided ESI. Principal pathologies in both groups were disc disorders and/or foraminal stenosis. All patients received only one infiltration during the six months following the initial visit. The numerical rating scale (NRS-11) was assessed at the first visit and six months later. The BPI, PCS and SF-12 were compared in both groups. Overall satisfaction with pain relief after six months was assessed with a scale of 1 (very unsatisfied) to 6 (very satisfied).

Results: Average NRS-11 scores for the seven days preceding the first visit and after six months were compared in both groups. The same comparison was made for overall treatment satisfaction. There is no significant difference in the NRS-11 and in the satisfaction scores between the two groups.

Conclusion: Neither of the two methods was shown to be superior to the other in pain relief and overall treatment satisfaction after six months. Considering the possible complications and side effects of ESI, PVI with a non-steroid mixture might be considered as an alternative method. Possibly, multiple PVIs could further decrease pain. Well-designed studies are needed to evaluate this hypothesis.

Keywords: Retrolaminar Paravertebral; Chronic Pain; Epidural Steroid; Morphine; Neostigmine; Ketamine; Naloxone

Introduction

The first therapeutic epidural injection was performed in 1885 by neurologist James Leonard Corning by injecting the local anesthetic cocaine between the lower lumbar spinous processes. The first modern controlled trial evaluating epidural steroid injection (ESI) was performed by Swerdlow et al. in 1970. ESIs are the most widely used pain management procedures in the world. Their use is supported by many placebo-controlled studies and dozens of systematic reviews. Despite the extensive literature on the subject, there continues to be considerable controversy surrounding the safety and efficacy of this procedure (1).

ESI is the most frequently performed procedure in pain clinics throughout the United States, more than doubling between 2000 and 2008 (2). It is estimated that the annual cost to treat back pain alone exceeds $100 billion (3). However, on April 23, 2014, the Food and Drug Administration (FDA) issued a drug safety communication warning that the injection of corticosteroids into the epidural space of the spine may result in rare but serious adverse events and required label changes to warn of rare, but serious neurological problems (4). Specific events reported include, but are not limited to, spinal cord infarction, paraplegia, quadriplegia, cortical blindness, and stroke. This warning resulted from a rapidly expanding body of the literature illustrating the potential for catastrophic neurological complications, including brain and spinal cord infarction following the intra-arterial injection of corticosteroids.

However, all experts did not accept this warning, and there is a debate regarding the risk-benefit of ESI (5). This controversy, along with the lack of sufficient supporting documents showing the ESI as an effective treatment in low back pain syndromes, caused us to consider other possible interventions with different medications. The purpose of this study is to compare the effectiveness of ultrasound-guided retrolaminar PVI with a non-steroid containing mixture versus ESI in patients suffering from chronic cervical or lumbar radicular neuropathic pain.

Methods

We identified two groups of 31 patients registered in Quebec Pain Registry data bank suffering from chronic lumbar or cervical radicular pain who were referred to the pain clinic between 2009 to 2014. Informed consent was obtained from all the patients. All the patients were 18 to 75 years old. The primary cause of the pain was a disc herniation or foraminal stenosis. The neuropathic nature of the pain was diagnosed based on the DN4≥4. All cases with malignancies, congenital anomalies, infection, motor or sensory neurological diseases, cognitive impairment, alcohol, or illicit drug dependence, and past history of lumbar or cervical operations were excluded. All patients were evaluated at the initial visit in the pain clinic and six months later. The patients received only one infiltration during the six months following the initial visit. The data were collected in forms completed by patients and/or a research nurse. Pain intensity was assessed at the first visit and at the six-month follow-up using a numerical rating scale (NRS-11). The BPI, PCS and SF-12 were compared in both groups. Overall satisfaction with pain relief over the six months was assessed with a scale of 1 (very unsatisfied) to 6 (very satisfied) (Statistical analysis software SAS version 9.3).

Using a Broad-spectrum convex transducer (C1-5-D), the case group received an ultrasound-guided (LOGIQ *e*, GE Healthcare, Milwaukee, WI) retrolaminar PVI with a mixture of morphine 1 mg, ketamine 10 mg, neostigmine 0.5 mg, naloxone 2 ng, and bupivacaine 10 mg. The vertebral laminae were identified by ultrasound imaging in a paramedian sagittal plane by sequentially visualizing transverse processes and the corresponding laminae (from lateral to medial). After local anesthesia with lidocaine 2%, the block needle (BD spinal needle Quincke 25 G) was guided to contact the lamina, and the mixture injected was visualized under real-time imaging. The injection was done in the laminae adjacent to the root, which corresponds clinically and radiologically to radicular pain. Radiological images were verified for possible anatomical variations (such as lumbarization of S1 or sacralization of L5). The control group, matched for gender, age, and DN4 sub-scale score at baseline, consisted of 31 patients with the same pathology, pain, and period who were treated by ESI (interlaminar or foraminal) under fluoroscopic control.

Results

Average NRS-11 scores for seven days preceding the first visit were 7.5 (SD=1.7) and 7.2 (SD=1.9) in the case and the control groups, respectively. At the six-month follow-up visit, these scores were 6.9 (SD=1.9) and 6.2 (SD=2.4), respectively (Figure 1). No significant changes were noted in NRS-11 scores at the six-month visit between two groups. Overall satisfaction from pain relief at six months was 3.8 (SD=1.8) and 4.5 (SD=1.5) in the case and the control group, respectively (Figure 2). There was no significant difference in satisfaction score between the two groups.

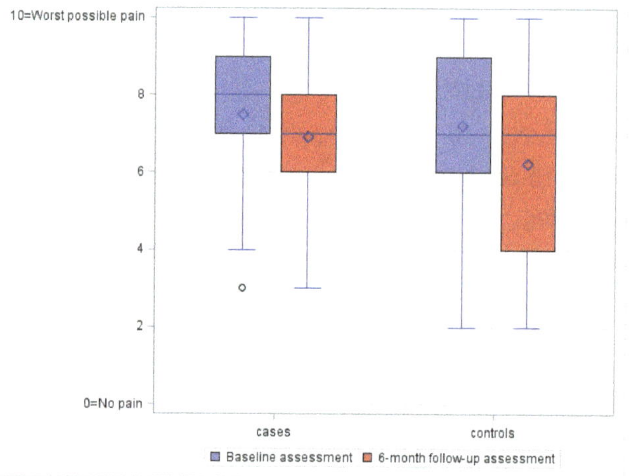

Figure 1. Average NRS-11scores for the seven days preceding the first visit and at the six-month follow-up visit in the case and in the control groups (NRS-11: numerical rating scale).

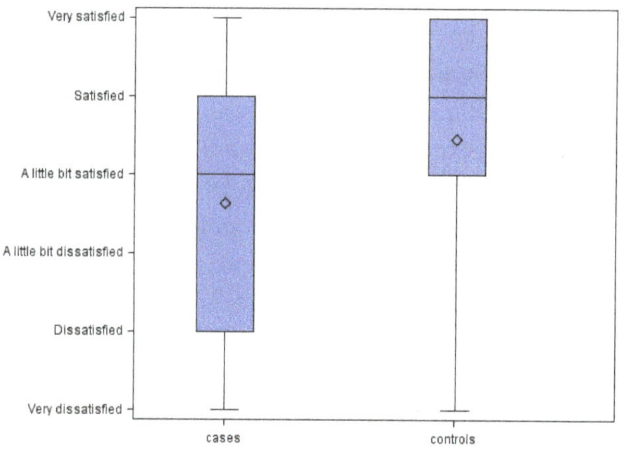

Figure 2. Overall satisfaction from pain relief at the six-month follow-up visit in the case and in the control groups.

Discussion

Based on the Crow W et al. study, it is estimated that the annual cost to treat back pain alone exceeds $100 billion (3). Among those who develop low back pain, approximately 30% will develop either chronic pain or frequent recurrences. Neck pain is less well-publicized, but also exacts a steep socioeconomic toll. Nearly two thirds of patients will experience a significant episode of neck pain over the course of their lives, with the annual prevalence around 30%.

ESI could be considered as the most frequently performed procedures in pain clinics in the United States, and by some estimates, its use has doubled between 2000 and 2008 (2). Although this procedure has historically been utilized for spinal pain of all types, ESI is widely acknowledged to work better for neuropathic pain. However, there continues to be enormous controversy surrounding the short- and long-term effectiveness and, more recently, safety of this treatment (4, 5). The mechanisms by which steroids produce their analgesic effects have been a subject of debate. Inhibition of phospholipase A_2 as an inflammatory mediator by itself (6) and as a rate-limiting factor involved in the production of eicosanoids (prostaglandins, prostacyclins, thromboxanes, and leukotrienes) could be the mechanisms of action. Steroids may inhibit pain via their ability to suppress ectopic discharges from

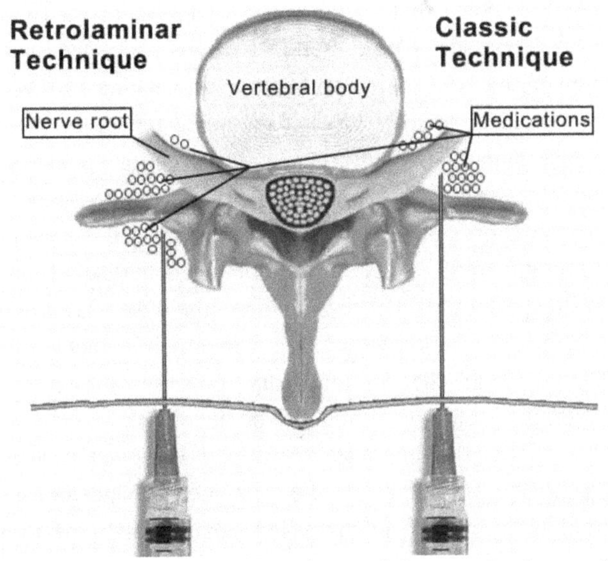

Figure 3. Schematic comparison of the retrolaminar and classic techniques of paravertebral blockade showing a transverse section of the vertebra.

injured nerve fibers (7) and depress conduction in normal unmyelinated C fibers. Other than the steroid effect, local anesthetics act via their increasing the blood flow in the ischemic nerves (8), suppressing ectopic discharges from injured neurons, slowing or halting nociceptive transmission (9), and the washout effect of the injected volume. There is increasing interest in the medical community in finding alternative approaches to treat back pain. First of all, retrolaminar paraspinal space could be considered as an alternative site for injection.

The thoracic paravertebral (TPV) nerve block technique was first described more than one century ago and reintroduced into clinical practice by Eason and Wyatt in 1978. Recently, there have been numerous reports concerning the use of an ultrasound guided paravertebral block. Interestingly, some authors have used ultrasound-guided retrolaminar technique (Figure 3) to infiltrate or to place the catheter (10). The concept that local anesthetic can penetrate the paravertebral space from a laminar injection challenges the classical teaching that the paravertebral space is defined posteriorly as a closed space by the costotransverse ligament. It is possible that the medication trickles through the medial aperture of the superior costotransverse ligament where the dorsal ramus of the spinal nerve exits posteriorly to innervate the paraspinal muscles. It is also possible that the fluid tracks anteriorly through the loose tissues just lateral to the facet joints. The same concept could be considered to explain the diffusion of solution from the retrolaminar space to nerve roots in lumbar and cervical PVI. Moreover, the boundary of the TPV space in the caudal direction is subject to debate. Although some cadaver studies showed that the caudal end of the T12 TPV space is effectively sealed off by the origin of the psoas major muscle, other studies observed communication between thoracic and lumbar paravertebral space (11).

The feasibility of lumbar spine sonography has been reviewed by Darrieutort-Laffite et al. In the cervical spine, Saranteas et al. examined the ultrasound anatomy of the cervical paravertebral space in 20 volunteers (12). They found that there was an excellent visualization of the C3, C4, C5, C6, and C7 transverse processes in all cases. The C5, C6, and C7 nerve roots were excellently identified in all cases. In the present study, all patients with cervical paravertebral infiltration received infiltration between C5 and C7.

The drug mixture we used consisted of morphine, ketamine, neostigmine, naloxone, and bupivacaine. In acute and chronic pain setting, morphine or its related family members are widely used. Its presynaptic and postsynaptic effects are via G-protein-linked opioid mu (mainly), delta, and kappa receptors. Presynaptic interaction inhibits the release of substance-P and calcitonin gene-related peptide by means of interactions with N-type voltage-dependent calcium channels and reduced calcium influx. Postsynaptic activation of opioid receptors leads to inhibition of adenylate-cyclase and also results in the opening of potassium channels, which in turn causes hyperpolarization, rendering the postsynaptic second-order neuron less responsive. Opioid receptors are expressed by central and peripheral neurons as well as by neuroendocrine (pituitary, adrenal), immune, and ectodermal cells (13). So morphine, which is used in the case group, might produce its analgesic effects via penetrating the epidural space and acting centrally and/or peripherally through an anti-inflammatory and analgesic effect on the peripheral nerves in the foraminal area.

Local anesthetics are primarily characterized by their ability to block voltage-gated sodium channels. In addition, to sodium channel blockade, local anesthetics also interact with a wide array of alternative target structures, for example tetrodotoxin-resistant sodium channels, potassium channels, calcium channels, N-methyl-D-aspartate (NMDA) receptors, and G-protein coupled receptors (14). Other than blocking neural transmission, bupivacaine may possibly cause its analgesic effects in chronic pain via the other receptors and mechanisms.

Naloxone is an opioid mu-receptor competitive antagonist. In low doses (in fact, in "ultra-low doses"); it helps control pain and prevents hyperalgesia. A review of the literature suggests that under certain conditions, low-dose opioid antagonists (alone or in combination with opioids) can produce an antinociceptive or analgesic response (15). Furthermore, they have been used successfully in Crohn's disease and irritable bowel syndrome (IBS) to control disease-associated pain. The possible mechanisms of action might be upregulation of opioid receptors, increased levels of endogenous opioids, decreased opioid receptor coupling to stimulatory G-proteins (mediated through filament A), and an inhibition of opioid agonist-induced activation of glial cells (15). In a case report, adding 50 ng/day naloxone to the intrathecal morphine infusion dramatically enhanced the analgesic effect of morphine without apparent side effects for more than three years (16). These mechanisms can explain partly the analgesic role of the naloxone in the mixture. The mechanistic rationale for the naloxone/morphine dose and concentration ratio was based on animal studies and a case report (16) in which an IT naloxone/morphine concentration ratio of $1/10^5$ was efficient in controlling the pain for three years.

Ketamine is an intravenous anesthetic which has an analgesic effect in sub-anesthetic doses. In a review article, De Kock et al. (17) reviewed the effect of ketamine on the inflammatory process. They concluded that ketamine is an immunomodulator that prevents the exacerbation and the extension of local inflammation without blunting the local process and delaying inflammatory resolution. It has an anti-hyperalgesic effect due to its impact on NMDA receptors (18) and an anti-allodynic effect by suppressing toll-like receptor (TLR) mediated signal transduction (19). Ketamine possesses a plethora of other actions that enhance its analgesic properties. These include blocking non-NMDA glutamate and muscarinic cholinergic receptors, facilitating GABA-A signaling, weakly binding to opioid receptors, and possessing local anesthetics as well as possibly neuroregenerative properties (20). Ketamine shows anti-inflammatory (17), antidepressant (21), precognitive (17) effects, as well as a beneficial effect on respiration, which can counter the side effects of morphine. Moreover, the beneficial effects of ketamine in the inflammatory process and post-operative outcome should not be neglected.

Neostigmine was introduced in 1931. It is a reversible inhibitor of the enzyme cholinesterase, which results in an increased concentration of the acetylcholine neurotransmitter. However, due to its hydrophilic nature (presence of a functional quaternary ammonia), it does not cross the dura mater. In 1933, Pellandra reported that intravenous administration of the anticholinesterase drug physostigmine produced analgesia in human beings. Neostigmine has been tested by the intrathecal (22), epidural (23), intra-articular (23), and intravenous (24) approaches to control pain. The analgesia resulting from spinal administration of neostigmine may be due to the increased concentration of acetylcholine and the consequent binding to muscarinic and nicotinic receptors. Epidural neostigmine analgesia seems to be a result of the more central rather than peripheral action. In a study by Laurreti GR et al. (23) in patients undergoing knee surgery, epidural neostigmine resulted in analgesia after the administration of a ten-fold lower dose (1 µg/kg) when compared to knee intra-articular administration, suggesting a central effect. Acetylcholine receptor activation in peripheral nerves is associated with analgesia (25), and intra-articular neostigmine seems to relieve pain after knee arthroscopy. Based on all these mechanisms, it could be hypothesized that neostigmine in the mixture could exert its analgesic effects by spreading on the dorsal root and probably in the epidural space. Due to very low doses of the drugs (especially the ultra-low dose of naloxone), absorption and systemic effects could not be an important factor in the long-term analgesic effect of the mixture.

The pain scores were relatively high in both

groups after six months. The score was only taken once by phone six months after the initial referral to the pain clinic. This score shows the average pain during the seven days before contact, but it does not show the intensity of pain in the days following injection. Overall satisfaction from pain relief is relatively high in both groups. So it can be concluded that the pain management service (including epidural or retrolaminar PVI) after six months had a positive impact on the pain intensity. Interestingly, there is no significant difference between two groups. However, there are the other limitations in this study such as: patient heterogeneity, the multicentric nature of the study, only one infiltration over six months, and missing information concerning pain relief in the days following infiltration.

Conclusion

In order to better understand the outcome of patients treated via retrolaminar PVI using a new mixture, studies need to be undertaken involving a greater number of patients and randomized trials. It would be preferable to study a mixture of two or three drugs instead of five drugs as in the current study; the impact on pain and quality of life should then be evaluated at more frequent intervals. However, based on the FDA warning concerning ESI and the debate surrounding it, finding new approaches and medications for the treatment of spinal radicular pain is an important challenge that needs to be addressed in future studies. This study shows the possibility of using drugs other than steroids in paraspinal interventions.

Acknowledgment

The authors thank Manon Choinière for her assistance in accessing the Quebec Pain Registry, Louis Coupal in extracting data and statistical analysis, and Heather Yampolsky for her editorial assistance.

Conflicts of Interest

The authors declare that they have no conflict of interest.

References

1. Cohen SP, Bicket MC, Jamison D, Wilkinson I, Rathmell JP. Epidural Steroids: A Comprehensive, Evidence-Based Review. Reg Anesth Pain Med. 2013;38:175-200.

2. Manchikanti L, Pampati V, Falco FJ, Hirsch JA. Growth of spinal interventional pain management techniques: analysis of utilization trends and Medicare expenditures 2000 to 2008. Spine. 2013;38:157-68.

3. Crow W, Willis D. Estimating cost of care for patients with acute low back pain: a retrospective review of patient records. J Am Osteopath Assoc. 2009;109:229-33.

4. US Food and Drug Administration. Drug Safety Communications. FDA drug safety communication: FDA requires label changes to warn of rare but serious neurologic problems after epidural corticosteroid injections for pain. www.fda.gov/downloads/Drugs/DrugSafety/UCM394286.pdf.

5. Manchikanti L, Candido KD, Singh V et al. Epidural steroid warning controversy still dogging FDA. Pain Physician. 2014;17:451-74.

6. Saal J. The role of inflammation in lumbar pain. Spine. 1995;20:1821-7.

7. Devor M, Govrin-Lippmann R, Raber P. Corticosteroids suppress ectopic neural discharge originating in experimental neuromas. Pain. 1985;22:127-37.

8. Kobayashi S, Takeno K, Yayama T. Pathomechanisms of sciatica in lumbar disc herniation: effect of periradicular adhesive tissue on electrophysiological values by an intraoperative straight leg raising test. Spine. 2010;35:2004-14.

9. Devor M, Wall P, Catalan N. Systemic lidocaine silences ectopic neuroma and DRG discharge without blocking nerve conduction. Pain. 1992;48:261-8.

10. Jüttner T, Werdehausen R, Hermanns H. The paravertebral lamina technique: a new regional anesthesia approach for breast surgery. J Clin Anesth. 2011;23:443-50.

11. Saito T, Den S, Tanuma K, Tanuma Y, Carney E, Carlsson C. Anatomical bases for paravertebral anesthetic block: fluid communication between the thoracic and lumbar paravertebral regions. Surg Radiol Anat. 1999;21:359-363.

12. Saranteas T, Paraskeuopoulos T, Anagnostopoulou S, Kanellopoulos I, Mastoris M, Kostopanagiotou G. Ultrasound anatomy of the cervical paravertebral space: a preliminary study. Surg Radiol Anat, 2010;32:617-22.

13. Stein C. Opioid Receptors. Annu Rev Med. 2016; 67:433-451.

14. Lirk P, Picardi S, Hollmann MW. Local anaesthetics: 10 essentials. Eur J Anaesthesiol. 2014;31:575-85.

15. Taylor R Jr, Pergolizzi JV Jr, Porreca F, Raffa RB. Opioid antagonists for pain.Expert OpinInvestig Drugs. 2013;22:517-25.

16. Hamann S, Sloan PA, Witt W. Low-dose intrathecal naloxone to enhance intrathecal morphine analgesia: a case report. J Opioid Manag. 2008;4:251-4.

17. De Kock M, Loix S, Lavand'homme P. Ketamine and peripheral inflammation. CNS Neurosci Ther. 2013;19:403-10.

18. Fisher K, Coderre TJ, Hagen NA. Targeting the N-methyl-D-aspartate receptor for chronic pain management. Preclinical animal studies, recent clinical experience and future research directions. J Pain Symptom Manage. 2000;20:358-73.

19. Mei XP, Zhou Y, Wang W et al. Ketamine depresses toll-like receptor 3 signaling in spinal microglia in a rat model of neuropathic pain. Neurosignals. 2011;19:44-53.
20. Cohen SP, Dragovich A. Intrathecal analgesia. Med Clin North Am. 2007;91:251-70.
21. Murrough JW. Ketamine as a novel antidepressant: from synapse to behavior. Clin Pharmacol Ther. 2012;91:303-9.
22. Staikou C, Paraskeva A. The effects of intrathecal and systemic adjuvants on subarachnoid block. Minerva Anestesiol. 2014;80:96-112.
23.Lauretti GR, de Oliveira R, Perez MV, Paccola CA. Postoperative analgesia by intraarticular and epidural neostigmine following knee surgery. J Clin Anesth. 2000;12:444-8.
24.Sethi D, Wason R. Intravenous regional anesthesia using lidocaine and neostigmine for upper limb surgery. J Clin Anesth. 2010;22:324-8.
25. Durate ID, Lorenzetti BB, Ferreira SH. Peripheral analgesia and activation of the nitric oxide-cyclic GMP pathway. Eur J Pharmacol. 1990;186:289-93.

30

Anesthetic considerations in medium-chain acyl-CoA dehydrogenase deficiency

Lisa A. Caplan[1]*, M. Toni Felberg[1]

Abstract

In the 1980's, medium-chain acyl-CoA dehydrogenase deficiency (MCADD) was first described in the literature as three children who presented with coma, hypoglycemia, hyperammonemia, and fatty liver while fasting. These symptoms while similar to Reye's Syndrome, were found to be due to an inability to metabolize medium chain fatty acids during fasting periods. Fatty acids are utilized by the body as essential fuel for skeletal and cardiac muscle, and as an important source of energy during fasting periods. Medium-chain acyl-CoA dehydrogenase is a mitochondrial enzyme required for the beta oxidation of medium chain fatty acids (C4-14), which is deficient in this syndrome. Anesthesiologists may come across these patients in their practice, as MCADD is the most common inhertited disorder of mitochondrial fatty acid oxidation. In addition to determining NPO timing and IV fluid selection, other preoperative issues anesthesiologists must consider are medication management to avoid metabolic decompensation. This manuscript will consider a pediatric patient with MCADD who presented to our pediatric hospital and received a general anesthetic following the guidelines created by our multidisciplinary perioperative team.

Keywords: Medium-chain acyl-CoA dehydrogenase deficiency, Perioperative Guidelines, Anesthetic management of Medium-chain acyl-CoA dehydrogenase deficiency

1. Department of Anesthesiology, Perioperative, and Pain Medicine
Baylor College of Medicine, Texas Children's Hospital, Houston, Texas, United States of America

Corresponding Author:
Lisa A. Caplan M.D. Assistant Professor of Anesthesiology, Baylor College of Medicine, Texas Children's Hospital, Houston, Texas, United States of America. 6621 Fannin Street, Suite W17417, Houston, Texas 77030.

E-mail: lacaplan@texaschildrens.org

Introduction

In 1983, Stanley published a paper in which he described three children who presented with coma, hypoglycemia, hyperammonemia, and fatty liver while fasting (1, 2). These symptoms while similar to Reye's Syndrome, were found to be due to an inability to metabolize medium chain fatty acids during fasting. As such, Stanley may be credited with first publishing medium-chain acyl-CoA dehydrogenase deficiency (MCADD) as a previously unrecognized metabolic disorder of fatty acid oxidation (1, 2). The body utilizes the oxidation of fatty acids not only to provide essential fuel for skeletal and cardiac muscle, but also as an important source of energy during fasting periods (1). While fasting, the brain converts fatty acids to energy in order to conserve glucose levels. The liver will oxidize fatty acids to ketones to servea dual purpose: to provide energy for gluconeogenesis, and generating fat derived substrates to support the brain's metabolic requirements in lieu of glucose (1).

Medium-chain acyl-CoA dehydrogenase is a mitochondrial enzyme required for the beta oxidation of medium chain fatty acids (C4-14) (3, 4). During fasting, adipose tissue will mobilize fatty acids which are then absorbed by the liver and other tissues and converted to acyl-coA esters (3) intracellularily. These esters will then enter the mitochondria as carnitine esters and become re-esterified to acyl co-A esters. The beta oxidation of the esters will liberate electrons as the acyl chain is shortened by an enzymatic process (3). The catalysts are acyl-CoA dehydrogenases, each specific for very-long chain, long-chain, medium-chain, or short chain acyl-co-A esters. Figure 1 is a representation of fatty acid beta-oxidation; medium-chain acyl-CoA dehydrogenase is one of the enzymes responsible for the dehydrogenation of medium-chain fatty acids.

Fatty acids normally undergo β-oxidation during fasting periods to produce ketones. Those with MCADD will accumulate fatty acids during fasting, and not generate ketones. The systemic consequences of MCADD will result in a lack of ketones to meet tissue energy demands manifesting as severe hypoglycemia as well as toxicity of the liver, muscle, and central nervous system as fatty acids and their corresponding acylcarnitines accumulate. Hypoketotic hypoglycemia will develop in times of fasting because of the inability to utilize fat for fuel (2).

MCADD is the most common inherited disorder of mitochondrial fatty acid oxidation (5). It is inherited in an autosomal recessive fashion, occurring primarily in Caucasians with northern European ancestry (2, 3, 5–8). The prevalence has been reported to vary by population studied: 1:4,900 in Germany and 1:17,000 in Taiwan (9). MCADD occurs with a reported incidence of 1 in 12,000- 20,000 births (2, 5, 9).

Diagnosis of MCADD can be accomplished by DNA analysis for mutations or tissue testing of heart, liver, or skeletal muscle for enzyme activity (2, 9). Those affected by MCADD are predominantly homozygous for a single mutation of an A to G nucleotide; the remaining 20% are either carriers of the single gene mutation or compound heterozygotes (2, 10). As of 2009, the United Kingdom performs neonatal screening for MCADD (5). While the Discretionary Advisory Council on Heritable Disorders in Newborns and Children recommends screening for MCADD as a part of the newborn screening panel, conditions tested for in the United States vary by state (11).

Typically those affected with MCADD will exhibit symptoms between 3 months to 2 years of age (mean age 13 months), however neonatal and adult presentations have been reported (5, 9, 10). Roughly 1/3 of affected individuals are asymptomatic throughout life, but will remain at risk for metabolic decompensation in times of fasting (10). Symptoms of MCADD typically manifest after 12-16 hours of fasting when glycogen storesare depleted with no generation of ketones in times of increased energy demands such as: fasting, stress due to surgery, pregnancy, illness, or alcohol binge drinking (5, 8). Although there is no diagnostic stigmata of MCADD, those in acute decompensation may present to physicians with hypoketotic hypoglycemia, encephalopathy, hepatomegaly, vomiting, seizures, coma, or causedeath (5, 9). Table 1 lists the systemic consequences of MCADD. Patients with MCADD are placed at potential risk for aphasia, loss of developmental milestones, and attention deficit disorder attributed to brain damage acquired during metabolic decompensation (8).

There is no specific medical therapy to treat MCADD. Patients are advised to limit exacerbations by limiting nil per os (NPO) times or fasting, which varies by age:

1) 6-12 months: No more than 8 hours
2) 1-2 years: No more than 10 hours
3) 2 years and beyond: No more than 12 hours (8, 9).

During times of stress such as fever, illness, or fasting those with MCADD should ingest additional glucose sources such orange juice or dissolving glucose tablets (9). In a preoperative environment intravenous (IV) fluids with dextrose should be administered until the patient resumes adequate PO intake; point of care glucose testing is not sufficient to assess the energy reserves for those with MCADD (9). The use of carnitine supplementation is controversial though recommended for patients that have a low serum carnitine level (9, 12).

In addition, to determining NPO timing and IV fluid selection, other preoperative issues anesthesiologists must consider are medication management to avoid metabolic decompensation.While inhalational agents, propofol, andneuromuscular blocking agents are not contraindicated in MCADD, they certainly present some controversy (2, 5). Some datasuggests an impairment of fatty acid metabolism associated with anesthetic vapors such as enflurane, thus posing a theoretical increased risk during anesthesia (5, 13).

Cautions in using both depolarizing and non-depolarizing neuromuscular blockers preoperatively have been made. Patients with MCADD may have hypotonia and impaired hepatic metabolism (5, 8); as such may have prolonged effects of certain non-depolarizing agents. Some authors urge caution in the use of succinylcholine in the presence of a potential myopathy (2).

Propofol infusion syndrome (PRIS) is defined by acute bradycardia progressing to asystole during propofol infusion associated with lipoemic plasma, fatty liver enlargement, metabolic acidosis, rhabdomyolysis, and a base excess > -10 mmol (14). PRIS carries an estimated mortality rate of 20%, and is thought to be due to impaired fatty acid metabolism inhibiting the mitochondrial respiratory chain (5). It has been suggested to avoid propofol in patients with MCADD and other mitochondrial disorders, due to the extra fatty acid contents of the soy bean oil and impairment of fatty acid oxidation (4, 5, 15).

Careful multidisciplinary preoperative planning is highly advisable for MCADD patients requiring anesthesia. Ideally they should be the first case of the day, and preoperative dextrose containing IV fluids started to avoid metabolic decompensation. This can be especially challenging in pediatric patients due to cooperation or perhaps difficult IV access. The anesthesiologist should consider risk: benefit of utilizing such anesthetic agents such as volatile anesthetics, neuromuscular blocking agents, and propofol. This manuscript will consider a pediatric patient with MCADD who presented to our pediatric hospital and received a general anesthetic following the guidelines created by a multidisciplinary team consisting of anesthesiology, genetics, and pediatric surgery.

Brief Report

A 19 month old 11.7kg male with a history of MCADD was admitted for possible bilateral orchiopexy for undescended testes. He was diagnosed with MCADD by a newborn screen completed in the state of his birth. He was seen in our pre-operative clinic where a clear note was written in the patient's record including recommendations by the genetics team for management, guided by our institution's metabolic protocol.

The patient was admitted the day before by the genetics service and had an IV placed with D10 ½ normal saline running at 45ml/hr (glucose infusion rate (GIR) of 6.4). He was given 250 mg of levocarnitine intravenously the morning of surgery. Other preoperative considerations for this patient included avoiding muscle relaxants and propofol; the genetics team recommended avoidance of benzodiazepines, barbiturates, and neuromuscular blocking agents. Standard American Society of Anesthesiologists (ASA) monitors (16) were used which included: 3 lead electrocardiogram, noninvasive blood pressure monitor, pulse oximetry, and capnography. Intravenous induction of anesthesia was completed with ketamine 50 mg and fentanyl 20 mcg. He was easily intubated with a 4.0 endotracheal tube without the use of paralytics. Sevoflurane was used for anesthesia maintenance. The patient was extubated deep after no true testes were found, and the procedure was terminated. He was brought to the post anesthesia care unit (PACU) with continued D10 fluid. After an uneventful PACU stay, he was discharged to the floor with D10 fluid until he was able to tolerate solid food. He was discharged by the genetics team later that day with no complications noted in the electronic medical record.

Discussion

In 2013 a multidisciplinary team was assembled at our institution to create preoperative guidelines and best practice recommendations for children with inborn errors of metabolism. The team consisted of pediatric anesthesiologists, geneticists, and pediatric surgeons. They identified best preoperative practices with the dual aim to prevent procedural cancellations or metabolic crises.

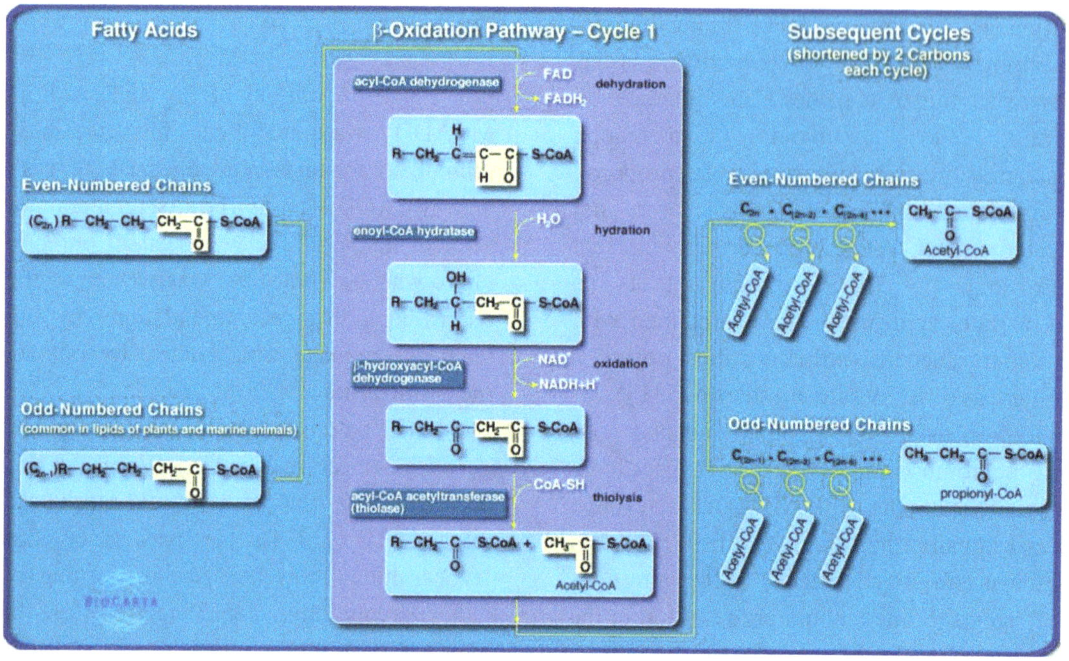

Figure 1. Medium-chain acyl-CoA dehydrogenase (MCAD) is one of the enzymes responsible for dehydrogenation of fatty acids as they cycle through the beta-oxidation spiral. By Modre-Osprian, Robert; Osprian Ingrid; Tilg, Bernhard; Schreier, Gunter; Weinberger, Klaus; and Graner, Armin.

Per our institutional protocol, if a child with MCADD needs a procedure requiring an anesthetic, he/she is referred to our preoperative evaluation clinic for a pre-anesthetic evaluation. Part of this evaluation consists of direct communication with the genetics team for their specific recommendations, i.e. unique preoperative labs, medications and IV fluid management. The day before surgery, if indicated, the patient will be admitted to the hospital and an IV placed prior to becoming NPO. Ideally, to minimize prolonged NPO times due to changes in the schedule, the patient will be the first case in the room.

The NPO policy for our institution follows the ASA NPO guidelines which is 2 hours for clear liquids; 4 hours for breast milk; 6 hours for formula; and 6-8 hours for solid food depending on the fat contents (17). For IV fluids, D10 (or D12.5) ½ NS + 2mEQ/100mL KCl to run with glucose infusion rate (GIR) 8-9 (mg/kg/min). Glucose infusion rate is derived from factors such as the IV fluid infusion rate, the patient's weight, and % of dextrose in the solution. A GIR of 5-8 is considered an average rate to maintain euglycemia (18). If additional fluids are required to replace losses, normal saline or Plasma-Lyte is preferred over Ringer's Lactate since this may theoretically increase acidosis as well as metabolic load on dysfunctional mitochondria.

Our institutional metabolic disorders guidelines also include recommendations for intraoperative anesthetic management. With regards to medications, drugs that are metabolized into odd chain fatty acids should be used cautiously in patients with MCADD which include: succinylcholine, atracurium, mivacurium, and propofol (as it is high in polyunsaturated fats) (19, 20). Some patients may be more sensitive and show prolonged effects to central nervous system depressants, and therefore it is recommended to delay extubation until complete muscle strength as returned. Specific MCADD preoperative fluid recommendations advocate the use of carnitine if it is currently prescribed.

Table 1: Systemic consequences of medium-chain acyl-CoA dehydrogenase deficiency (MCADD).

Organ System	Symptom
Central Nervous System	• Coma • Encephalopathy • Lethargy • Seizures • Sudden death
Cardiac	• Arrhythmia • Cardiovascular arrest
Gastrointestinal	• Abnormal liver function tests • Hepatomegaly • Peripheral lobular fatty liver • Vomiting
Metabolic	• Hyperammonemia • Impaired ketogenesis with hypoketotic hypoglycemia • Metabolic acidosis • Secondary carnitine deficiency

Authors agree that the preoperative management of MCADD requires strategic planning to limit NPO times thus avoid depleting glucose stores with resulting metabolic decompensation (2, 5–7, 12). Table 2 provides a side by side comparison of anesthetic recommendations for MCADD. While these recommendations advocate for glucose containing IV fluids to start preoperatively and continue into the preoperative period, there is no overall consensus of the specific type of fluid nor the GIR (2, 5–7, 12). Our recommendations include guidelines on a specific GIR, as it provides a measure of how quickly a patient receives carbohydrates. While caution has been issued regarding the use of propofol, volatile anesthetics, and muscle relaxants in the context of MCADD, there are case reports of uneventful anesthetics (2, 6, 7).

Our case report considers an uneventful anesthetic utilizing our institution's evidenced based metabolic guidelines which are supported by others in the literature. The British Inherited Metabolic Disease Group provides specific preoperative guidelines for MCADD patients which include recommendations on NPO times and IV/oral glucose replacement (12). Created in 2013, the BIMDG guidelines formalized practices in the United Kingdom which included the preoperative use of 10% glucose solutions (5, 12). Like the BIMDG guidelines, our institutional recommendations share multidisciplinary preoperative planning, limiting NPO times, pre/intra/postoperative use of 10% glucose solutions, and the resumption of a normal diet as soon as feasibly possible.

Allen et al performed a retrospective chart review of 14 patients with MCADD who received a total of 20 general anesthetics over a 17 year period (5). The small number reflects that although MCADD may be the most common inherited form of error in fatty acid oxidation, it is not a disease process that requires multiple procedures for satisfactory quality of life. A majority of these children received glucose containing fluids preoperative hydration per BIMDG recommendations, with 5 reported cases of hyperglycemia (no hypoglycemia or decompensation). Propofol and volatile anesthetics were given, often in combination for these procedures, uneventfully. There was, however, 1 reported case of delayed offset of atracurium; and the authors urge the use of twitch monitoring if neuromuscular blocking agents are used. Allen et al strongly advocate preoperative glucose supplementation following BIMDG, without making specific recommendations on medications to absolutely avoid. Our case report reflects similar results, no incidence of metabolic decompensation when glucose supplementation was given, and the safe use of volatile anesthetics for a brief procedure.

The three decades following Stanley's description of MCADD has greatly expanded the medical communities understanding of this disease.

Table 2: Comparison of anesthetic recommendations for MCADD

	NPO	IV Fluids	Anesthetic Recommendations
Texas Children's Hospital	• Minimum pre-operative fasting interval • Patient admitted the night before surgery to commence IV fluid therapy	• D10 (or D12.5) ½ NS + 2mEQ/100mL KCl to run with GIR 8-9 (weight x GIR x 0.6); • If extra fluids are to be required to replace losses, NS is preferred over Ringer's Lactate	Recommend avoiding benzodiazepines, barbiturates, neuromuscular blocking agents, and propofol.
British Inherited Metabolic Disease Group (BIMDG)	• Minimum pre-operative fasting interval • Feed the child at the time you would feed any other child following an equivalent procedure • Discontinue the intravenous infusion ONLY after the child tolerates food	• IVF to start at time operations starts • 10% glucose 0.45% saline • Fluid/24 hours = 100ml/kg for 1st10kg then 50 ml/kg for next 10kg then 20ml/kg thereafter. Potassium should be added to this solution 10 mmol in 500 ml • Replete carnitine only if deficient	
Allen et al.	Recommends following BIMDG guidelines	Recommends following BIMDG guidelines	• May be safest to avoid propofol; or use 2% formulation to limit fatty acid load • High dose opiate with low dose volatile anesthetic • Recommends antiemetics to control post op nausea vomiting • Cautions use of volatile anesthetics and propofol
Dearlove et al.	Recommend that children for the afternoon operating lists should have a light breakfast and a glucose drink at 1100 h	10% glucose infusion	Reported using thiopental and local anesthetic uneventfully
Justiz et al.	• Limit NPO status to 2–4 h • Close perioperative blood glucose monitoring	• Preoperative intravenous catheter placement • 5% dextrose in lactated Ringer's • Consider adding carnitine	Reported using midazolam, propofol, sevoflurane uneventfully
Wang et al.	• Limit NPO status to 12 hours max	• 10% glucose to start preoperatively • Considering giving carnitine if neurologic status changes	• Preop: assess medical history, neurologic status, coagulations profile, and blood glucose levels • Recommends avoiding succinylcholine • Reported using intrathecal0.25% bupivacaine, fentanyl uneventfully

Apart from dietary management, future treatment may include gene therapy as trials are promising using fiberblast cultures using in vitro studies (21). Anesthetic medications, preoperative guidelines, and glycemic control would benefit from future prospective studies to optimize recommendations (5). Currently, an IRB has been submitted at our institution to prospectively study the impact of these metabolic guidelines and safety with anesthesia.

Conclusion

MCADD is the most common inherited disorder of mitochondrial fatty acid oxidation. Roughly 1/3 of affected individuals are asymptomatic throughout life, but will remain at risk for metabolic decompensation in times of of increased energy demands such as: fasting, stress due to surgery, pregnancy, or illness. Although there is no diagnostic stigmata of MCADD, those in acute decompensation can exhibit hypoketotic hypoglycemia, encephalopathy, hepatomegaly, vomiting, seizures, coma, or cause death. Multidisciplinary preoperative planning is highly advisable for MCADD patients requiring anesthesia. Ideally they should be the first case of the day, and preoperative dextrose containing IV fluids started to avoid metabolic decompensation. This can be especially challenging in pediatric patients due to cooperation or perhaps difficult IV access. The anesthesiologist should consider risk: benefit of utilizing such anesthetic agents such as volatile anesthetics, neuromuscular blocking agents, and propofol.

Acknowledgment

The authors gratefully acknowledge the Texas Children's Hospital physicians who created the "Process for Communicating Special Medical Requirements for Metabolic Patients Undergoing Surgical Procedures". The case report does not contain public health identifiers and an institutional review board (IRB) application was submitted.

Conflicts of Interest

The authors declare that there are no conflicts of interest.

References

1. Stanley CA, Hale DE, Coates PM, et al. Medium-chain acyl-CoA dehydrogenase deficiency in children with non-ketotic hypoglycemia and low carnitine levels. Pediatr Res. 1983;17(11):877-84.

2. Wang SY, Kannan S, Shay D, Segal S, Datta S, Tsen L. Anesthetic considerations for a patient with compound heterozygous medium-chain Acyl-CoA dehydrogenase deficiency. Anesth Analg. 2002;94(6):1595-1597.

3. MD VCB, MPH JEOM. Anesthesia for Genetic, Metabolic, and Dysmorphic Syndromes of Childhood. Second edition. Philadelphia, PA: LWW; 2006.

4. Steiner LA, Studer W, Baumgartner ER, Frei FJ. Preoperative management of a child with very-long-chain acyl-coenzyme A dehydrogenase deficiency. Paediatr Anaesth. 2002;12(2):187-91.

5. Allen C, Perkins R, Schwahn B. A retrospective review of anesthesia and preoperative care in children with medium-chain acyl-CoA dehydrogenase deficiency. Paediatr Anaesth. November 2016.

6. Dearlove OR, Perkins R. MCAD deficiency and anaesthesia. Anaesthesia. 1995;50(3):265.

7. Justiz AC, Mayhew JF. Anesthesia in a child with medium-chain Acyl-CoA dehydrogenase deficiency. Paediatr Anaesth. 2006;16(12):1293-4.

8. Matern D, Rinaldo P. Medium-Chain Acyl-Coenzyme A Dehydrogenase Deficiency. In: Pagon RA, Adam MP, Ardinger HH, et al., eds. GeneReviews(®). Seattle (WA): University of Washington, Seattle; 1993. http://www.ncbi.nlm.nih.gov/books/NBK1424/. Accessed December 8, 2016.

9. Gartner V, McGuire PJ, Lee PR. Child Neurology: medium-chain acyl-coenzyme A dehydrogenase deficiency. Neurology. 2015;85(4):37-40.

10. Loughrey C, Bennett MJ. Screening for MCAD deficiency in newborns. BMJ. 2009;338:b971.

11. Watson RS, Carcillo JA. Scope and epidemiology of pediatric sepsis. Pediatr Crit Care Med J Soc Crit Care Med World Fed Pediatr Intensive Crit Care Soc. 2005;6(3 Suppl):S3-5.

12. British Inherited Metabolic Diseases Group. Management of surgery in children with fat oxidation disorders. 2013. Available at: http://www.bimdg.org.uk/store/guidelines/ Management-of-surgery-in-children-with-fatoxidation- disordersv4-619512-22-05-.

13. Kleemann PP, Jantzen JP, Fenner R, Wiegand UW. [Preoperative increase in the plasma concentration of free fatty acids during minor elective interventions using a conventional anesthesia technic with enflurane]. Anaesthesist. 1986;35(10):604–608.

14. Fudickar A, Bein B. Propofol infusion syndrome: update of clinical manifestation and pathophysiology. Minerva Anestesiol. 2009;75(5):339-44.

15. Farag E, Deboer G, Cohen BH, Niezgoda J. Metabolic acidosis due to propofol infusion. Anesthesiology. 2005;102(3):697-698-699.

16. American Society of Anesthesiology House of Delegates Committee on Standard and Practice. Standards for basic anesthetic monitoring. 2010.

17. American Society of Anesthesiologists Committee. Practice guidelines for preoperative fasting and the use of pharmacologic agents to reduce the risk of pulmonary aspiration: application to healthy patients undergoing elective procedures: an updated report by the American Society of Anesthesiologists Committee on Standards and Practice Parameters. Anesthesiology.

2011;114(3):495-511.
18. Sweet CB, Grayson S, Polak M. Management strategies for neonatal hypoglycemia. J Pediatr Pharmacol Ther JPPT Off J PPAG. 2013;18(3):199-208.
19. Harker HE, Emhardt JD, Hainline BE. Propionic acidemia in a four-month-old male: a case study and anesthetic implications. Anesth Analg. 2000;91(2):309-311.
20. Karagoz AH, Uzümcügil F, Celebi N, Canbay O, Ozgen S. Anesthetic management of a 2-year-old male with propionic acidemia. Paediatr Anaesth. 2006;16(12):1290-1.
21. Schowalter DB, Matern D, Vockley J. In vitro correction of medium chain acyl CoA dehydrogenase deficiency with a recombinant adenoviral vector. Mol Genet Metab. 2005;85(2):88-95.

Perioperative Pain: Molecular Mechanisms and Future Perspectives

Zahra Talebi[1], Ali Dabbagh[1*]

Abstract

Background: Acute perioperative pain is seen in more than 80% of patients undergoing surgery, with almost 75% of them experiencing moderate, severe, or extreme pain; adequate postoperative pain management is not achieved in a satisfactory manner. This styudy was desined ana performed to assess the molecular mechanisms of acute pain management in order to find novel future perspectives.

Materials and Methods: In this narrative review, molecular mechanisms of currently available pain controlling agents were assessed based on 3 steps: preoperative, intraoperative and postoperative phases. Drugs used in each phase and potential novel agents were assessed separately.

Results: many currently available clinical agents were discussed and meanwhile, other potential drugs that could be among the future choices are discussed.

Conclusion: cellular and molecular medicine could open new windows in order to discover novel agents for management of pain; we will have possibly many new agents that will be available in future while they will be different from currently used clinical pain killers.

Keywords: cellular and molecular medicine; pain; perioperative

1. Cardiac Anesthesiology Department, Anesthesiology Research Center, Shahid Beheshti University of Medical Sciences, Tehran, Iran

Corresponding Author:
Ali Dabbagh, MD, Cardiac Anesthesiology Department, Anesthesiology Research Center, Shahid Beheshti University of Medical Sciences, Tehran, Iran.
E-mail: alidabbagh@sbmu.ac.ir

Introduction

The international association for the study of pain, defines pain as "an unpleasant sensory and emotional experience associated with actual or potential tissue damage, or described in terms of such damage" (1). Acute postoperative pain is seen in more than 80% of patients undergoing surgery, with almost 75% of them experiencing moderate, severe, or extreme pain. Based on reports, adequate postoperative pain management is achieved in less than half of surgery patients (2). Effective pain management in surgery patients helps with overall recovery, increases patient satisfaction, and ultimately reduces health care cost. It can also decrease morbidity and improve surgery outcomes (3).

Although several new approaches have been introduced in the past decade as components of a multimodal approach to decrease the side effects and improve quality of analgesia, there hasn't been any major improvement in this field in the past decade. In this article, we reviewed the major mechanisms involved in this process and current clinical strategies in managing this pain in surgical patients (4).

Molecular Mechanisms

Post-operative pain has a biphasic nature,

which makes it more difficult to manage. In the first phase, great nociceptive input is produced in the surgery, where trauma to the tissue results in the production of noxious stimuli. The second phase starts after surgery, when inflammation present at the site, produces more noxious input. These processes initiate pain response in two levels. At peripheral level, the prolonged presence of noxious stimuli results in inflammation and tissue damage. Primary mediators such as prostaglandins, serotonin, leukotrienes, and bradykinins reduce the threshold of high threshold nociceptive afferents and initiate the release of pain mediators such as substance P, CGRP and cholecystokinin in the site of injury, which leads to peripheral sensitization. Hence, weaker stimuli, which normally cannot produce pain, would now be perceived as painful. Histamine, nerve growth factor and norepinephrine are also involved in peripheral sensitization (5). There is also an increased number and proportion of tetrodotoxin-resistant channels in the affected neurons, which leads to the development of spontaneous ectopic activity (6). Reducing the inflammation would be the rational approach in controlling peripheral pain and use of NSAIDs, opioids and local anesthetics is advised.

On the other level, central sensitization occurs as a result of long term potentiation of the central nerves, with NMDA and AMPA glutamate receptors and Wide Dynamic Range (WDR) neurons playing the vital role. WDR neurons receive signals from both innocuous and nociceptive sensory neurons from large areas of the body, but in the case of repeated nociceptive input, their threshold can decrease and their receptive field widen. This is due to NMDA receptor activation that ultimately leads to increased sensitivity of the WDR neurons.

A delta and C fibers bring the Impulses from the peripheral nociceptors to synapse in the lamina II and lamina V; C fibers also synapse in the lamina I of the spinal cord before projecting cranially. In lamina V, neurotransmitters such as glutamate and aspartate, activate amino-3-hydroxyl- 5-methyl-4-proprionic acid (AMPA) and Kainate (KAR) receptors and transmit the pain signal with high speed. These receptors can regulate Na^+ and K^+ ion transfer but are nearly impermeable to Ca^{2+} ions.

NMDA (N-methyl-D-aspartate) glutamate receptor is a membrane protein with an ion channel that works by transferring Na^+ and Ca^{2+} into the cell and simultaneously transferring K^+ to the outside of the cell. Extracellular Mg^{2+} and Zn^{2+} ions can bind to specific sites on the receptor and block the flow of other cations through the open ion channel. Since these receptors are voltage gated, they need a positive change in the cell voltage which is brought upon by an AMPA-induced membrane depolarization, which displaces the magnesium or zinc from the channel passage and clears the way for the calcium ions to enter the neuron. Direct binding of the glutamate can further potentiate this process (5–7).

The accumulation of calcium in cell brings it to a state of excitation without stimulation where spinal neurons are “wind up” and fired rapidly in a transcription independent manner.

The transcription independent central sensitization processes such as wind up and early LTP, are heterosynaptic, and low threshold A Beta input evoke these responses after C fiber conditioning. This kind of central sensitization is reversible and with each repetitive stimulation the pain increases. In the transcription dependent central sensitization, prolonged noxious facilitation, leads to production of modified proteins as a result of activation of certain genes, therefore, Ca^{2+} influx and subsequently production of prostaglandins, nitric oxide, and superoxides increases. This process is believed to be mediated by inflammation and changes in the dorsal root ganglion, the dorsal horn, and irreversible structural modifications in the CNS (5).

This process can ultimately lead to hyperalgesia as a result of central sensitization in spinal cord as well as higher regions of CNS such as anterior cingulate gyrus, amygdale, and rostroventral medulla (5).

The neurokinin receptor (NK1) and cycloxygenase 2 (COX-2) are also involved in central sensitization; however they are not involved in hippocampal LTP. The phosphorylation of synaptic receptors and the insertion of AMPA receptors into the post-synaptic membrane is seen in both hippocampal early phase LTP and central sensitization, but in hippocampal LTP synaptic strengthening is the only mechanism, while other cellular mechanisms and neuronal network changes are involved in central sensitization. These similarities should be noted when treating central sensitization to avoid the disturbance of memory formation and cortical function (8).

Management of pain

In order to effectively manage postoperative pain, appropriate measures should be implemented before, during and after the surgery.

During the operation

Preoperative management:

In the preoperative setting, individual assessment of the patients, patient education, preemptive, and preventive analgesia are the main examples of such measures (2-3, 17).

The analgesic plan, in respect to analgesic efficacy, potential side effects, and effects on recovery should be optimized depending on the surgical procedure. Evidence based recommendations for procedure specific pain management in the common adult surgeries has been developed by the prospect working group, which is a collaboration of surgeons and anesthesiologists, and it can be accessed freely on the website http://www.postoppain.org/.

***Intraoperative* management**

Different neuroendocrine, metabolic, and inflammatory changes are involved in the stress response from the surgery, which can harm organs and ultimately increase postoperative pain. Hypothermia and psychological stress can increase these responses, while deeper levels of anesthesia, neural blockade, and reduced surgical invasiveness can diminish them.

Intravenous Medications

- Lidocaine: Lidocaine is the safest local anesthetic; it can reduce pain and inflammation when administrated as a 100mg IV bolus followed by an infusion of 2 to 3 mg/h in surgeries. Lidocaine has weak analgesic, but potent anti-hyperalgesic effect in humans; it decreases the need for opioids and helps with the early return of bowel function.
- β-blockers: β-blockers can improve surgical stress response and inhibit sympathetic response to tracheal intubation. They also reduce the need for opioid and volatile anesthetic use (3).
- α_2 agonists: clonidine, tizanidine and dexmedetomidine are the most commonly used α_2 agonists in pain management. They can decrease opioid consumption due to their anesthetic and analgesic properties (9). Clonidine is administrated orally and can help with opioid withdrawal pains. Tizanidine acts more rapidly and is more beneficial in patients with spastic disorders. It also has less effects on blood pressure and heart rate (9). Dexmedetomidine is more selective, and it can be administrated IV. It works by hyperpolarization of neurons in locus ceruleus and therefore inhibiting the sympathetic-mediated pain at peripheral nociceptors which inhibits the release of pain mediators such as substance P and glutamate in primary afferent neurons, and the wind up effect in secondary neurons (9–11).
- NMDA inhibitors: In a prospective, randomized, double-blinded study, a 0.5 mg/kg bolus of ketamine followed by continuous intravenous infusion of 0.25 mg/kg/h during the surgery, decreased opioid consumption and reduced areas of hyperalgesia up to 72 h after surgery, compared to placebo or epidural ketamine. IV Ketamine also decreased CPOP for up to 6 months after the surgery (11). Dextromethorphan also works with this mechanism and has shown to be effective in reducing postoperative pain and opioid consumption (effect of preoperative)

Anesthesiology techniques:

Different methods of administration can be used for anesthetic drugs to ensure the optimal analgesia and minimize side effects and use of opioids. The followings are the most commonly used methods used to decrease post-operative pain:

- **Neuraxial techniques of analgesia**, in which epidural or spinal administration of local anesthetic (with a low dose opioid) blocks the nociceptive stimuli and the stress response to surgery. Administration is performed before the surgery and can be continued after the surgery. This technique can also help with postoperative mobilization and reduce the risk of ileus.
- **Transversus Abdominus Plane Blocks,** in which abdominal wall is anesthetized with peripheral nerve block for minor abdominal surgeries.
- **Peripheral Nerve Blocks,** in which afferent nociceptive pathways are blocked.
- **Wound Infiltration Anesthesia,** in which lidocaine or bupivacaine are infiltrated in the wound for local anesthesia. This method is fast acting and

epinephrine can be used to extend the duration of action. A liposomal formulation of bupivacaine has been developed to provide longer durations of action (up to 96 hours), but its clinical use is still limited due to insufficient comparative clinical data.

- **Tumescent Anesthesia,** in which local anesthetic are diluted and administrated subcutaneously in large volumes with epinephrine and other agents.
- **Topical Local Anesthesia,** in which special formulations of local anesthetics with the ability to penetrate the skin (lidocaine and prilocaine, lidocaine-epinephrine-tetracaine and tetracainephenylephrine) are used on intact skin (before surgical incision) or cuts (to facilitate suturing in pediatric patients). Topical oxymetazoline or phenylephrine and lidocaine has also been used for mucosal analgesia (3, 11).

Postoperative Management

Multimodal analgesia, is defined as the use of a combination of different analgesic medication and techniques, with different mechanisms of action in the peripheral and central nervous system to obtain additive or synergistic effects and increase the effectiveness of pain management (2). In this method individual personal and medical needs of patients are considered to obtain the best analgesia plan. Patients' response and side effects are monitored afterwards and required alterations are made depending on patient's needs. Physicians, anesthesiologists and nursing staff should all cooperate to maximize the success of pain management plan (12). Opioids are the key component in multimodal approach and other pharmacological and non-pharmacological interventions are added according to patient's individual needs, to increase their efficacy from other mechanisms, and minimize their side effects. The interventions most commonly used in multimodal analgesia are as follows (3):

- Non-pharmacologic therapies: Transcutaneous electrical nerve stimulation at incision site and cognitive modalities with guided imagery and other relaxation methods, hypnosis, intraoperative suggestions, and music.
- Acetaminophen and NSAIDs, as oral or IV injections to reduce the use of postoperative opioids. A single dose of celecoxib before major surgeries, has shown to reduce post-operative pain and opioid consumption (2).
- Opioids in IV, IM, oral, transdermal, rectal, sublingual, subcutaneous, neuroaxial administration routes, morphine, hydromorphone, fentanyl and tramadol are used more frequently. In patients with severe pain who need more frequent injections, patient controlled IV analgesia with opioids is used (3).
- Gabapentin and pregabalin which can be administrated before or after the surgery (PIIS).
- Corticosteroids (13), dexamethasone (8 mg IV) is the best option, since it can help with nausea and vomiting after the surgery.

Experimental drugs and pain control methods

With the increase in the rate of surgical operations, postoperative pain is gaining more attention in scientific studies, with the aim of finding more effective drugs and procedures with less side effects.

Since various complex mechanisms are involved in the spinal pain amplification caused by surgical insult, numerous therapeutic targets can interfere with this process. Therapies may target neuronal or non-neuronal processes of sensitization. Sensitization is also dependent on calcium influx and inflammation processes. Some therapeutics modulates neuronal activity or by blocking receptor proteins such as NMDA and AMPA receptor, which increase intracellular calcium levels during neuronal activation. Other therapies may target CNS inflammation (11). An overview of the main experimental approaches for management of postoperative pain is presented here.

Acupuncture: auricular acupuncture, in which needles are placed in various parts of the earlobe has been shown to be beneficial in post-operative pain control, but larger studies with improved quality are needed to obtain a definitive conclusion in this matter and justify the routine use of this method (5).

Probiotics: Probiotics has shown beneficial effects on inflammatory pain, by inhibiting pro-inflammatory mediators and increasing the production of anti-inflammatory cytokines in animal models. The adjuvant use of probiotics should be considered in the postoperative period, due to their nonexistent side effects (14).

Magnesium: Administration of IV magnesium

after major GI surgery has shown to reduce postoperative ileus, postoperative severe pain and perioperative analgesic requirements in a randomized clinical trial. Magnesium has no side effects in these doses and its routine administration can be advised for major GI surgeries (15).

Pulsed electromagnetic fields: PEMF improves calmodulin-dependent nitric oxide and/or cyclic guanosine monophosphate signaling, but it can also increase phosphodiesterase activity which inhibits cyclic guanosine monophosphate activity. At certain intervals, this method has demonstrated beneficial effects in postoperative pain in breast reduction patients (16).

Glutamate receptor antagonism: as mentioned before, glutamate plays a key role in central sensitization and pain, and different glutamatergic receptors and pathways have been investigated for their potential in treatment of neuropathic and postoperative pain. Currently ketamine, dextromethorphan, amantadine, and memantine, are clinically available as NMDA receptor antagonists (17). Other drugs such as MK-801 (i.e. dizocilpine), AP5, traxoprodil and norketamine, works with the same mechanism and has been introduced in the literature as treatments for postoperative pain (11). Other than inhibition of the NMDA receptor itself, other molecules involved in the phosphorylation of these receptors can also be considered as therapeutic targets. Examples of such molecules are protein kinase A (PKA) which has a role in phosphorylation of NR1 subunit and the Src. family of protein which are involved in NR2B phosphorylation (11). Although IV administration of ketamine is associated with side effects such as hallucination, combined use of these agents with opioids, while reducing the need for opioids, does not bare any additional side effects when compare to opioids alone (17). AMPA receptors (18) and G protein-coupled metabotropic glutamatenreceptors, mGluR 1 and 5, are other interesting targets in these pathways and several substances has been introduced as antagonists for this receptors (19), but although animal studies were promising, more clinical studies are needed to find the best molecule for human use.

Opioids- New substances and new administrations

Tapentadol is a novel opioid analgesic with potency between tramadol and morphine but with less abuse potential than all other opioid analgesic drugs. It has a unique ability to inhibit norepinephrine reuptake as well as its agonistic effect on μ receptors. Incidence of nausea and vomiting is also lower with this drug compared to oxycodone (5,20,21). It can be used both in preemptive treatment and postoperative period to manage the pain (22). Since the risk for addiction is one of the most important challenges when using opioids, there's an increasing interest focused on development of abuse-deterrent formulations of opioids. Such formulations are based on technologies such as physical or mechanical barriers or the addition of a noxious component (e.g. niacin) or an antagonist (e.g. naloxone, naltrexone) (23). A typical example is slow-release oxycodone formulation that combines a mechanical and a physical barrier effect which prevents crushing or drawing out drug for injection (23). Although these preparations require further evaluation, it has been suggested that they may well become the standard of care in the future (24).

Capsaicin: (8-methyl-N-vanillyl-6-nonenamide) is a TRPV-1 (transient receptor potential vanilloid 1) agonist which can be found in chili pepper seeds, it is non-narcotic and acts peripherally (24). TRPV1 receptors are present on unmyelinated C fiber endings in the periphery, and they tend to be significantly reduced in inflammatory conditions. The activation of the TRPV receptors produces high intensity impulses which lead to the release of substance P, and a burning sensation. C fiber activation is ultimately reduced when substance P is depleted. The A delta and A alpha fibers are not significantly affected by capsaicin. It is available in injection and topical forms. It is thought to have opioid sparing effects and can be used as an adjuvant in a variety of pain disorders, especially in age groups more sensitive to opioid adverse effects. The initial burning sensation with this molecule can be managed with pre-administration of neural blockade before injection of capsaicin. Capsaicin's favorable safety profile makes it an interesting choice in the management of postoperative pain and there are more attempts to identify therapeutically useful agonists and antagonists for the TRPV1 receptor (25, 26).

Immune modulation with glial modulators

According to recent findings astrocytes and microglia, central and peripheral, participate in neuronal hyper excitability and chronic pain (27). These resulted in an increased focus on these cells as targets in pain management. However, although animal studies demonstrate an overall beneficial effect from glial modulators in treatment of pain and central sensitization, and brain glial activation in chronic pain patients has been established, human studies have so far yielded diverse results (28). An example of these modulators is propentofylline, which proved to be beneficial in a variety of rodent pain models in reducing pain hypersensitivity but failed to indicate a beneficial effect in postherpetic neuralgia, in a Phase IIa clinical trial. It seems that different aspects of pain and differences between humans and animal models should be determined carefully to ensure successful translation of use of glia modulators in human (29).

Immune modulation with anti-cytokines agents

Cytokines have also been directly targeted in order to modulate inflammatory processes in pain (30). Intrathecal etanercept as a TNF inhibitor was found effective in preventing phosphorylation of the AMPA-subunit GluR1 in the spinal dorsal horn, and also SNL pain models, with optimal effect achieved when the drug was administrated early after nerve injury (11). Intrathecal IL-1ra was not found beneficial in the SNT model of peripheral nerve injury, but it was found effective in attenuating established mechanical hypersensitivity at 7 days after induction of CCI of the sciatic nerve and reversing mechanical pain hypersensitivity at 96 h after intraplantar CFA injection (31). Interference with IL-1b signaling was also effective in reducing established inflammatory pain. As a biological inhibitor of TNF-a signaling, intraperitoneal injection of Erythropoietin (EPO) and the synthetic peptide ARA290 which mimicks its effects, has demonstrated beneficial effects in SNT nerve injury with reduced SNT-induced inflammation and attenuation of SNT-induced increases in the levels of GFAP, TNF-a, and IL-1b (32). Although these data are highly impressive, the clinical use of these drugs and their risk benefit profile are yet to be determined in larger scale clinical trials.

Antidepressants : Although the efficacy of antidepressants in acute postsurgical pain has been suggested in numerous clinical trials, most of these trials are old and their results are limited by not specifying primary outcomes, disregarding movement-evoked pain, small size and insufficient safety assessment (33,34). Data on use of antidepressants in prevention of chronic postsurgical pain is inclusive with only one of three trials in this indication suggesting any efficacy. Therefore, current evidence does not yet support routine use of any one specific antidepressant for treatment of acute, or prevention of chronic, postsurgical pain and further larger trials are needed to determine optimal dosing and duration of antidepressant treatment, procedure specificity, safety profile, and assessment of movement-evoked pain (35).

Cannabinoids are a group of proteins including endocannabinoids such as anandamide (produced naturally in the body by humans and animal), the phytocannabinoids (found in cannabis and some other plants), and synthetic cannabinoids (manufactured chemically) which act on cannabinoid receptors (36). Since cannabinoid receptors are thought to be involved in analgesic, euphoric and anticonvulsive processes (CB1) and also demonstrate anti-inflammatory and immunosuppressive effects (CB2), cannabinoids represent an interesting target for neuropathic pain management. However the overall clinical data available is still limited and confusing, and suggests limited efficacy from drugs on this category in some neurologic disorders, such as chronic neuropathic pain conditions, in MS and AIDS (24).

Resolvins: A large number of evidence supports the potent anti-inflammatory and pro-resolution actions of omega-3 polyunsaturated fatty acids-derived lipid mediators, such as resolvins, lipoxins, and neuroprotectins in various animal models of inflammation (37). Resolvin E1 (RvE1) is an eicosapentaenoic acid (EPA) derivative that with peripheral spinal, or systemic administration at very low doses, has shown to reduce inflammatory pain, via transient receptor potential ion channel (TRPV1) and modulating microglial signalin (38). Mechanism of RvE1 activates the G-protein-coupled receptor ChemR23, widely expressed in immune cells (macrophages), neurons (primary sensory neurons and spinal cord neurons), and microglia (39).

Calcitonin: Calcitonin is a polypeptide hormone produced naturally in humans by the parafollicular cells of the thyroid gland (40). It is commonly used in treatment of osteoporosis and Paget's disease. Calcitonin's use in acute and chronic pain states has been examined in different studies. A more recent network meta-analysis supports short-term use of calcitonin in later stages of complex regional pain syndrome (24). There is also limited evidence that calcitonin can be used in acute, but not chronic, phantom limb pain after amputation (41).

Vitamin C: Several trials have been conducted on use of vitamin C in postoperative pain. A meta-analysis of the available references in 2016 concluded that there is moderate-level evidence supporting that preoperative dose of 2 g vitamin C can be used as an adjunct for its opioid spring abilities, and high-level evidence is available that supplementation of 1 g/d vitamin C for 50 days is useful in prevention of complex regional pain syndrome type I after extremity surgery (42). Additional studies can be useful in determining overall effectiveness and optimum dosage of vitamin C.

Conclusion

Postoperative pain is a complex phenomenon which depends on several factors, from type of the surgery and the skill of the surgeon to patient's characteristics and background history. Effective management of postoperative pain requires identification of these factors and their underlying molecular mechanisms, and planning an individual approach for each patient accordingly using multimodal analgesia. Pain prevention should be considered in all stages of surgery, preoperative and postoperative period, and each member of the medical team should play their parts optimally to minimize patient's harm and improve surgical outcomes.

Acknowledgment

The authors acknowledge the kind help of Anesthesiology Research Center in administrative issues.

Conflicts of Interest

The authors declare that there are no conflicts of interest.

References

1. Bonica JJ. The need of a taxonomy. Pain. 1979;6(3):247.
2. Chou R, Gordon DB, de Leon-Casasola OA, Rosenberg JM, Bickler S, Brennan T, et al. Management of Postoperative Pain: A Clinical Practice Guideline From the American Pain Society, the American Society of Regional Anesthesia and Pain Medicine, and the American Society of Anesthesiologists' Committee on Regional Anesthesia, Executive Commi. J Pain. 2016;17(2):131–57.
3. Lovich-Sapola J, Smith CE, Brandt CP. Postoperative pain control. Surg Clin North Am. 2015;95(2):301–18.
4. Kang S, Brennan TJ. Mechanisms of postoperative pain. Anesth Pain Med. 2016;11(3):236–48.
5. Vadivelu N, Mitra S, Narayan D. Recent advances in postoperative pain management. Yale J Biol Med. 2010;83(1):11.
6. Neil MJE, Macrae WA. Post surgical pain-the transition from acute to chronic pain. Rev pain. 2009;3(2):6.
7. Paoletti P, Neyton J. NMDA receptor subunits: function and pharmacology. Curr Opin Pharmacol. 2007;7(1):39–47.
8. Ji R-R, Kohno T, Moore KA, Woolf CJ. Central sensitization and LTP: do pain and memory share similar mechanisms? Trends Neurosci. 2003;26(12):696–705.
9. Giovannitti Jr JA, Thoms SM, Crawford JJ. Alpha-2 adrenergic receptor agonists: a review of current clinical applications. Anesth Prog. 2015;62(1):31–8.
10. Kamibayashi T, Maze M. Clinical uses of α2-adrenergic agonists. J Am Soc Anesthesiol. 2000;93(5):1345–9.
11. Deumens R, Steyaert A, Forget P, Schubert M, Lavand'homme P, Hermans E, et al. Prevention of chronic postoperative pain: cellular, molecular, and clinical insights for mechanism-based treatment approaches. Prog Neurobiol. 2013;104:1–37.
12. Elvir-Lazo OL, White PF. Postoperative pain management after ambulatory surgery: role of multimodal analgesia. Anesthesiol Clin. 2010;28(2):217–24.
13. Waldron NH, Jones CA, Gan TJ, Allen TK, Habib AS. Impact of perioperative dexamethasone on postoperative analgesia and side-effects: systematic review and meta-analysis. Br J Anaesth. 2012;aes431.
14. Nazemian V, Shadnoush M, Manaheji H, Zaringhalam J. Probiotics and Inflammatory Pain: A Literature Review Study. Middle East J Rehabil Heal. 2016;3(2).
15. Moharari RS, Motalebi M, Najafi A, Zamani MM, Imani F, Etezadi F, et al. Magnesium can decrease postoperative physiological ileus and postoperative pain in major non laparoscopic gastrointestinal surgeries: a randomized controlled trial. Anesthesiol

pain Med. 2013;4(1).
16. Taylor EM, Hardy KL, Alonso A, Pilla AA, Rohde CH. Pulsed electromagnetic fields dosing impacts postoperative pain in breast reduction patients. J Surg Res. 2015;193(1):504–10.
17. Vorobeychik Y, Willoughby CD, Mao J. NMDA Receptor Antagonists in the Treatment of Pain. In: Treatment of Chronic Pain by Medical Approaches. Springer; 2015. p. 59–65.
18. Gomez-Mancilla B, Brand R, Jürgens TP, Göbel H, Sommer C, Straube A, et al. Randomized, multicenter trial to assess the efficacy, safety and tolerability of a single dose of a novel AMPA receptor antagonist BGG492 for the treatment of acute migraine attacks. Cephalalgia. 2014;34(2):103–13.
19. Vincent K, Cornea VM, Jong Y-JI, Laferrière A, Kumar N, Mickeviciute A, et al. Intracellular mGluR5 plays a critical role in neuropathic pain. Nat Commun. 2016;7.
20. Tzschentke TM, De Vry J, Terlinden R, Hennies H-H, Lange C, Strassburger W, et al. Tapentadol hydrochloride. Drugs Future. 2006;31(12):1053–61.
21. Fidman B, Nogid A. Role of Tapentadol Immediate Release (Nucynta) in the Management Of Moderate-to-Severe Pain. Pharm Ther. 2010;35(6):330.
22. Yadav G, Jain G, Samprathi A, Baghel A, Singh DK. Role of preemptive tapentadol in reduction of postoperative analgesic requirements after laparoscopic cholecystectomy. J Anaesthesiol Clin Pharmacol. 2016;32(4):492.
23. Schaeffer T. Abuse-deterrent formulations, an evolving technology against the abuse and misuse of opioid analgesics. J Med Toxicol. 2012;8(4):400–7.
24. Schug SA, Goddard C. Recent advances in the pharmacological management of acute and chronic pain. Ann Palliat Med. 2014;3(4):263–75.
25. Szallasi A, Sheta M. Targeting TRPV1 for pain relief: limits, losers and laurels. Expert Opin Investig Drugs. 2012;21(9):1351–69.
26. Uchytilova E, Spicarova D, Palecek J. TRPV1 antagonist attenuates postoperative hypersensitivity by central and peripheral mechanisms. Mol Pain. 2014;10(1):67.
27. Ji R-R, Xu Z-Z, Gao Y-J. Emerging targets in neuroinflammation-driven chronic pain. Nat Rev Drug Discov. 2014;13(7):533–48.
28. Loggia ML, Chonde DB, Akeju O, Arabasz G, Catana C, Edwards RR, et al. Evidence for brain glial activation in chronic pain patients. Brain. 2015;138(3):604–15.
29. Gazerani P. Targeting glia in human pain: challenges and opportunities. Future Medicine; 2016.
30. Clark AK, Old EA, Malcangio M. Neuropathic pain and cytokines: current perspectives. J Pain Res. 2013;6:803–14.
31. Mika J, Korostynski M, Kaminska D, Wawrzczak-Bargiela A, Osikowicz M, Makuch W, et al. Interleukin-1alpha has antiallodynic and antihyperalgesic activities in a rat neuropathic pain model. Pain. 2008;138(3):587–97.
32. Jia H, Feng X, Li W, Hu Y, Zeng Q, Liu J, et al. Recombinant human erythropoietin attenuates spinal neuroimmune activation of neuropathic pain in rats. Ann Clin Lab Sci. 2009;39(1):84–91.
33. Fishbain D. Evidence-based data on pain relief with antidepressants. Ann Med. 2000;32(5):305–16.
34. Wong K, Phelan R, Kalso E, Galvin I, Goldstein D, Raja S, et al. Antidepressant Drugs for Prevention of Acute and Chronic Postsurgical PainEarly Evidence and Recommended Future Directions. J Am Soc Anesthesiol. 2014;121(3):591–608.
35. Gilron I. Antidepressant Drugs for Postsurgical Pain: Current Status and Future Directions. Drugs. 2016;76(2):159–67.
36. Russo EB, Hohmann AG. Role of cannabinoids in pain management. In: Treatment of Chronic Pain by Medical Approaches. Springer; 2015. p. 179–95.
37. Serhan CN, Chiang N, Van Dyke TE. Resolving inflammation: dual anti-inflammatory and pro-resolution lipid mediators. Nat Rev Immunol. 2008;8(5):349–61.
38. Xu Z-Z, Berta T, Ji R-R. Resolvin E1 inhibits neuropathic pain and spinal cord microglial activation following peripheral nerve injury. J Neuroimmune Pharmacol. 2013;8(1):37–41.
39. Ji R-R, Xu Z-Z, Strichartz G, Serhan CN. Emerging roles of resolvins in the resolution of inflammation and pain. Trends Neurosci. 2011;34(11):599–609.
40. Visser EJ. A review of calcitonin and its use in the treatment of acute pain. Acute Pain. 2005;7(4):185–9.
41. McCormick Z, Chang-Chien G, Marshall B, Huang M, Harden RN. Phantom Limb Pain: A Systematic Neuroanatomical-Based Review of Pharmacologic Treatment. Pain Med. 2014;15(2):292–305.
42. Chen S, Roffey DM, Dion C-A, Arab A, Wai EK. Effect of perioperative vitamin C supplementation on postoperative pain and the incidence of chronic regional pain syndrome: a systematic review and meta-analysis. Clin J Pain. 2016;32(2):179–85.

Effect of Ketofol instead of Propofol on hemodynamic stabilization for induction of anesthesia in laparatomy

Hamid Kayalha[1], Mohammad Kolahdoozha[2], Siamak Yaghoobi[1], Marzieh Beygom Khezri[1], Seyed Amir Mohajerani[3], Alireza Jahangirifard[4]*

Abstract

Background: Hemodynamic alterations are a common complication during anesthetic induction with intravenous anesthesia. Hypotension due to propofol injection may be very severe in cardiac vascular patients. Ketamine produces increasing significantly, but temporary effect on systematic blood stream, heartbeat, and cardiac output through central sympathetic stimulation. The aim of the study was to determine effect of ketofol and propofol for induction of anesthesia on hemodynamic changes during induction of anesthesia.

Materials and Methods: In the randomized clinical trial study, 96 patients who were candidate for laparotomy enrolled and divided into two random groups of propofol (48 person) and ketofol (48 person). Hemodynamic changes were recorded and examined after induction for 5 and 10 minutes after intubation.

Results: Heart rate was significantly variable in propofol group compared to ketofol group. Systolic, diastolic, and mean arterial blood pressure was not significantly changed during the time period of recording in ketofol group. However, blood pressure was significantly changed during the study in the propofol group.

Conclusion: ketofol is a proper alternative to propofol to stabilize heart rate and blood pressure in laparotomy.

Keywords: Ketofol, Hemodynamic, Anesthesia, Laparatomy

1- Shahid Rajaie Hospital, Qazvin University of Medical Sciences, Qazvin, Iran
2- Kosar Hospital, Qazvin University of Medical Sciences, Qazvin, Iran
3- Anesthesiology Research Center, Shahid Beheshti University of Medical Sciences, Tehran, Iran
4- Lung Transplantation Research Center, National Research Institute of Tuberculosis and Lung Diseases (NRITLD), Shahid Beheshti University of Medical Sciences, Tehran, Iran

Corresponding Author: Alireza Jahangirifard, Assistant Professor, Lung Transplantation Research Center, National Research Institute of Tuberculosis and Lung Diseases (NRITLD), Shahid Beheshti University of Medical Sciences, Tehran, Iran;
E-mail: omidjahangiri_55@yahoo.com

Introduction

Hemodynamic instability is a major complication of anesthesia due to induction, intubation, surgical incision and stress, hypovolemia, anesthesia drugs and volatile anesthetics. Surgical incision and pain cause increase in blood pressure and heart rate.

This challenge is more prominent in patients with ischemic heart diseases, valvular heart diseases, and other cardiovascular diseases. Drugs used for induction of anesthesia decrease blood pressure acutely. Propofol decreases blood pressure by several mechanisms; however, ketamine increases blood pressure vice versa.

Propofol is used at a dose of 1-2.5 mg/kg for induction of anesthesia. Old age, decrease of cardiac reserve and premedication with benzodiazepines and opioids decreases the required dose for induction of anesthesia. Propofol increases the influx of Cl through Cl channels by an effect on GABA receptors.

Ketamine is an antagonist of NMDA receptors could increase systolic and diastolic blood pressure and heart rate by stimulation of sympathetic system. These effects are modified by opioids or volatile anesthetics. Induction of anesthesia is performed by 1-2 mg/kg intravenously or 4-6 mg/kg through intramuscular. Ketamine causes hypnosis and analgesia. Ketamine passes the brain blood barrier and its peak of action is 1 minute by drug redistribution from the brain into the blood stream and then other tissues. The onset of effect of ketamine is 15-30 seconds after intravenous (IV) administration and 3-4 minutes after intramuscular (IM) injection. Duration of effect is 5-10 minutes after IV and 12-25 minutes after IM injection. Propofol rapidly redistribute in blood and other tissues.

Propofol mixed with ketamine (ketofol) is a popular for short procedural sedation and analgesia (1). Ketofol is a combination of the same amount of propofol and ketamine administered for induction of anesthesia. There are a number of recent studies demonstrating the beneficial effects of combination of ketamine and propofol (2); providing cardiovascular stability (3) which could be comparable to etomidate; on the other hand, this combination does not lead to adverse effects of etomidate-associated adrenal insufficiency in critically ill or septic patients (4).

Although in recent studies ketofol has been used for sedation in the emergency department or critically ill patients in ICU (5-7), there are no reports evaluating the use of "ketofol" for induction of anesthesia in elective surgeries. The aim of the study was to determine effect of ketofol and propofol for induction of anesthesia on hemodynamic changes during induction of anesthesia.

Methods

The study was reviewed and approved by the Shahid Beheshti University of Medical Sciences Ethics Committee and been performed in accordance. Information about the study was given comprehensively both orally and in written form to all patients or their accompanying adult. They gave their informed written consent prior to their inclusion in the study.

In a randomized clinical trial, 96 patients candidate for elective laparotomy and ASA class I,II were enrolled and randomly assigned to ketofol and propofol group. Study was performed in a 12 month period from 2014 to 2015.

Exclusion criteria included patients with hypotension or uncontrolled hypertension prior to surgery, heart rate less than 50, pacemaker, bleeding diathesis, difficult intubation or more than 3 attempts for intubation, and required a transfusion prior to surgery.

Groups of study and monitoring

Patients were induced by ketofol in the ketofol group and by propofol in the propofol group. For ketofol group, Ketamine and propofol mixture (ketofol) was prepared 5 mg/mL ketamine and 5 mg/mL propofol, 1:1 mixture in a 20-mL syringe.

Patients were admitted to the operating room and were monitored for pulse oximetry, arterial line, and invasive blood pressure monitoring, electrocardiogram, capnography, bispectral index (BIS) for depth of anesthesia, and cerebral oximetry. Hemodynamic parameters (systolic arterial pressure (SAP), and heart rate (HR) were recorded by an anaesthetist who was blinded to the patient group, at times baseline 0 minutes, and after induction, then after intubation, and the 5 and 10 minutes after intubation.

Induction of anesthesia

Patients were pre-hydrated with 350 ml of normal saline. For pre-medication, Midazolam 0.02 mg/kg and fentanyl 2 μg/kg was administered. After 3 minutes pre-oxygenation, for induction of anesthesia, in Ketofol group, ketofol 1.5 mg/kg and in propofol group 1.5 mg/kg was administered. Then Atracurium 0.5 mg/kg was administered for proper muscle relaxation.

After 3 minutes, patients were intubated with appropriate sized cuffed endotracheal tube. Anesthesia was maintained using propofol 100 μg/kg/min and the mixture of N_2O 50%/O_2 50%. All intubations were performed by the same anesthesiologist.

Blood pressure and heart rate were recorded prior to induction, 3 minutes after induction, after intubation, and 5 and 10 minutes after induction.

Results

In this study, 96 patients candidate for elective

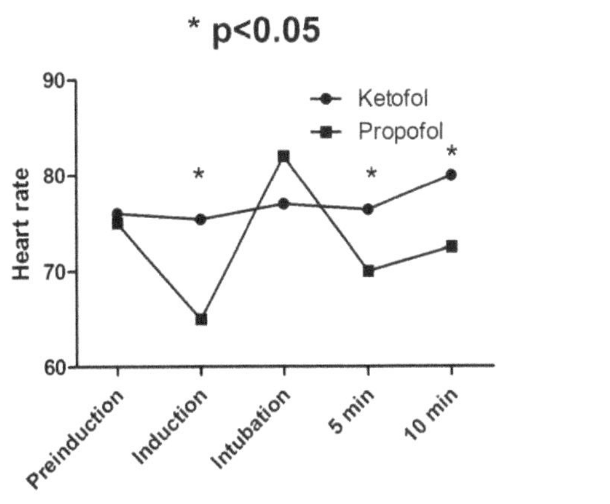

Figure 1. Heart rate in ketofol compare to propofol group.

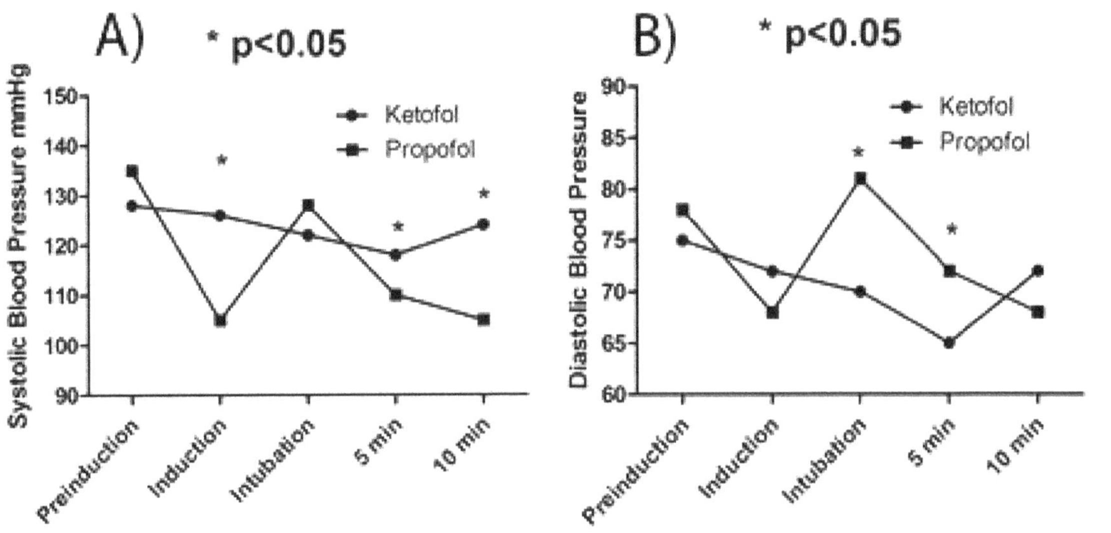

Figure 2. Systolic and diastolic blood pressure in ketofol compare to propofol group.

laparotomy were randomly assigned to one of groups of study. Age, sex, and weight of patients were not significantly different between two groups (Table1).

Heart rate was compared between two groups of study. Heart rate was significantly lower in the propofol group compared to ketofol group at induction (p=0.001) and 5 minutes (p=0.001), and 10 minutes (p=0.001) after intubation. Heart rate was not significantly higher in propofol group compared to ketofol after intubation (p=0.062) (Figure1).

Systolic blood pressure was significantly lower in propofol group compared to ketofol group after induction (p=0.001) and after 5 minutes (p=0.017) and 10 minutes (p=0.002) after intubation. Although systolic BP was higher after intubation in propofol group compare to ketofol but this difference was not significant (p=0.24) (Figure2).

Diastolic blood pressure was lower after induction in propofol group compared to the ketofol group (p=0.054). It was significantly higher in propofol compared to ketofol group at intubation time (p=0.001), 5 minutes after intubation (p=0.001). However, at 10 minutes after intubation, diastolic blood pressure was lower in propofol group compared to ketofol group that was not significant (p=0.10) (Figure 2).

Mean arterial blood pressure (MAP) was significantly lower in propofol group compared to ketofol group at the induction time (p=0.001). At intubation time MAP was significantly higher in propofol group compared to ketofol (p=0.014). MAP was significantly lower in propofol group compared to ketofol at 5 minutes (p=0.015) and 10 minutes (p=0.022) after intubation.

Discussion

In this study, we compared effect of ketofol and propofol on patients underwent elective laparotomy for their hemodynamic changes during induction, intubation and post-intubation time. Our results depicted that ketofol not propofol stabilized hemodynamics during induction, intubation and post-intubation time. Ketofol has a significant effect on the trend of systolic, diastolic, mean blood pressure, and heart rate.

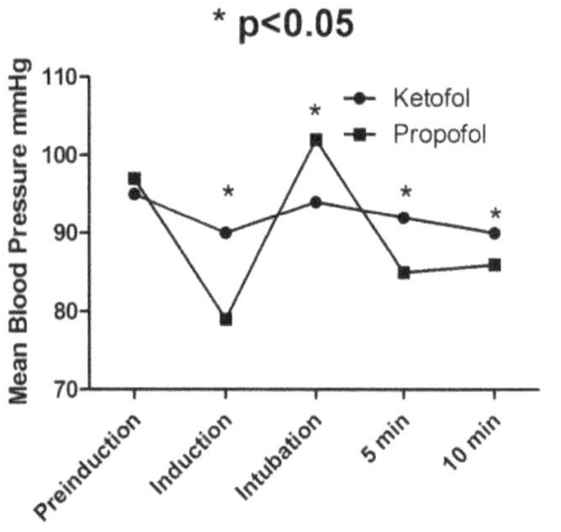

Figure 3. Mean arterial blood pressure in ketofol compare to propofol group.

One of the major challenges in anesthesia is to maintain hemodynamic in a predictable and controlled range during induction and intubation and then the incision of surgery. Ketofol, a combination of ketamin and propofol could maintain hemodynamic during induction, intubation and surgical incision particularly in patients prone to sudden drop or increase in hemodynamic. In a systematic review, ketofol was effective in reducing cardiovascular complications (8). A case series describes the use of the ketofol as an induction agent for intubation in critically ill patients when hemodynamic stability is desired (9). There was no difference between propofol+ketamine versus propofol+etomidate in mean arterial pressure (MAP) and heart rate (HR) during induction of anesthesia in elderly patients (10). Ketofol is a safe and effective induction agent for LMA insertion in children with rapid onset of action and improved hemodynamic stability with less prolonged apnea when compared with propofol (11). Recent reports showed that the number of patients in need of ephedrine was significantly lower and SBP immediately and in 5 min. after PLMA insertion was significantly higher in the ketofol group compared to the propofol group (12). Ketofol improves hemodynamics when compared to addition of fentanyl to propofol, and is associated with better LMA insertion conditions (13).

Mechanism of ketamine by inhibition of afferent pain, sensory inputs and decrease in spinothalamic transmission decrease stimulation of sympathetic responses to pain stimulation including blood pressure and heart rate. Ketamine is rapidly distributed and absorbed into the brain. Ketamine metabolism is in the liver and its elimination half life is 2-3 hours.

Intubation induces disturbances in hemodynamic responses. Propofol decreases hemodynamic variables, including blood pressure and heart rate. Ketofol does not decrease these variables in patients due to blocking severe hemodynamic disturbances and inhibition of sympathetic reactivation in response to pain.

Skin incision appears somewhat in the middle of noxious stimuli, being more stimulating than electrical pain, but much less stimulating than laryngoscopy and intubation (14). The depth of anesthesia is of paramount importance in clinical responses to noxious stimuli. In our study the depth of anesthesia was kept at the BIS:40-60 which is defined as appropriate for depth of anesthesia not-responding to noxious stimuli. Suppressing the most refractory response, hypertension and tachycardia, to the most profound stimulus, intubation, requires yet more opioid and hypnotic. Ketofol seems to suppress pain sensation and decrease the hemodynamic responses better than propofol alone. This potentially could decrease the need for increasing the opioid dose.

Ketofol has its main impact on trend of blood pressure (both systolic and diastolic) and heart rate. This trend follows a stable pattern after induction

Table 1: Demographic characteristics

	Ketofol (n=48)	Propofol (n=48)	p-value
Weight	65.5	67.2	0.3
Age	39.7	36.3	0.4
Sex (Male/Female)	23/22	25/20	0.3

through intubation and in post-intubation time. Such stable trend is probably due to decrease in sympathetic stimulation by somatic pain stimulatory input. This implies the fact that a major barrier to hemodynamic stability is the over-activation of sympathetic nervous system.

Conclusion

Ketofol is a proper alternative to propofol to stabilize heart rate and blood pressure in laparotomy.

Acknowledgment

This study is based on the thesis of Mohammad Kolahdoozha (resident of anesthesiology) and supported by grants from Qazvin University of Medical Sciences, Qazvin,Iran.

Conflicts of Interest

The authors declare that they have no conflict of interest.

References

1. Coulter FL, Hannam JA, Anderson BJ. Ketofol dosing simulations for procedural sedation. Pediatr Emerg Care. 2014;30(9):621-30.
2. Andolfatto G, Willman E. A prospective case series of single-syringe ketamine-propofol (Ketofol) for emergency department procedural sedation and analgesia in adults. Acad Emerg Med. 2011;18(3):237-45.
3. Smischney NJ, Beach ML, Loftus RW, Dodds TM, Koff MD. Ketamine/propofol admixture (ketofol) is associated with improved hemodynamics as an induction agent: a randomized, controlled trial. J Trauma Acute Care Surg. 2012;73(1):94-101.
4. Chan CM, Mitchell AL, Shorr AF. Etomidate is associated with mortality and adrenal insufficiency in sepsis: a meta-analysis. Crit Care Med. 2012;40(11):2945-53
5. Willman EV, Andolfatto G. A prospective evaluation of "ketofol" (ketamine/propofol combination) for procedural sedation and analgesia in the emergency department. Ann Emerg Med. 2007;49(1):23-30.
6. Green SM, Andolfatto G, Krauss BS. Ketofol for procedural sedation revisited: pro and con. Ann Emerg Med. 2015;65(5):489-91.
7. Olson AN, Rao WR, Marienau ME, Smischney NJ. Period Prevalence of Ketamine-Propofol Admixture "Ketofol" in the Operating Room among Anesthesia Providers at an Academic Medical Center. Med Sci Monit. 2015;21:1737-44.
8. Jalili M, Bahreini M, Doosti-Irani A, Masoomi R, Arbab M, Mirfazaelian H. Ketamine-propofol combination (ketofol) vs propofol for procedural sedation and analgesia: systematic review and meta-analysis.Am J Emerg Med. 2015. pii: S0735-6757(15)01130-4.
9. Gallo de Moraes A, Racedo Africano CJ, Hoskote SS, Reddy DR, Tedja R, Thakur L, Pannu JK, Hassebroek EC, Smischney NJ. Ketamine and propofol combination ("ketofol") for endotracheal intubations in critically ill patients: a case series. Am J Case Rep. 2015;16:81-6.
10. Hosseinzadeh H, Eidy M, Golzari SE, Vasebi M.Hemodynamic Stability during Induction of Anesthesia in ElderlyPatients: Propofol + Ketamine versus Propofol + Etomidate. J Cardiovasc Thorac Res. 2013;5(2):51-4.
11. Yousef GT, Elsayed KM.A clinical comparison of ketofol (ketamine and propofol admixture) versus propofol as an induction agent on quality of laryngeal mask airway insertion and hemodynamic stability in children. Anesth Essays Res. 2013;7(2):194-9.
12. Erdogan MA, Begec Z, Aydogan MS, Ozgul U, Yucel A, Colak C, Durmus M. Comparison of effects of propofol and ketamine-propofol mixture (ketofol) on laryngeal mask airway insertion conditions and hemodynamics in elderly patients: a randomized, prospective, double-blind trial. J Anesth. 2013;27(1):12-7.
13. Goh PK, Chiu CL, Wang CY, Chan YK, Loo PL.Randomized double-blind comparison of ketamine-propofol, fentanyl-propofol and propofol-saline on haemodynamics and laryngeal mask airway insertion conditions. Anaesth Intensive Care. 2005;33(2):223-8.
14. Miller RD, Eriksson LI, Fleisher L, Wiener-Kronish JP, Young WL. Millers anesthesia, 8 Ed. Philadelphia: Churchill Livingstone/Elsevier; 2015.

Permissions

All chapters in this book were first published in JCMA, by Shahid Beheshti University of Medical Sciences; hereby published with permission under the Creative Commons Attribution License or equivalent. Every chapter published in this book has been scrutinized by our experts. Their significance has been extensively debated. The topics covered herein carry significant findings which will fuel the growth of the discipline. They may even be implemented as practical applications or may be referred to as a beginning point for another development.

The contributors of this book come from diverse backgrounds, making this book a truly international effort. This book will bring forth new frontiers with its revolutionizing research information and detailed analysis of the nascent developments around the world.

We would like to thank all the contributing authors for lending their expertise to make the book truly unique. They have played a crucial role in the development of this book. Without their invaluable contributions this book wouldn't have been possible. They have made vital efforts to compile up to date information on the varied aspects of this subject to make this book a valuable addition to the collection of many professionals and students.

This book was conceptualized with the vision of imparting up-to-date information and advanced data in this field. To ensure the same, a matchless editorial board was set up. Every individual on the board went through rigorous rounds of assessment to prove their worth. After which they invested a large part of their time researching and compiling the most relevant data for our readers.

The editorial board has been involved in producing this book since its inception. They have spent rigorous hours researching and exploring the diverse topics which have resulted in the successful publishing of this book. They have passed on their knowledge of decades through this book. To expedite this challenging task, the publisher supported the team at every step. A small team of assistant editors was also appointed to further simplify the editing procedure and attain best results for the readers.

Apart from the editorial board, the designing team has also invested a significant amount of their time in understanding the subject and creating the most relevant covers. They scrutinized every image to scout for the most suitable representation of the subject and create an appropriate cover for the book.

The publishing team has been an ardent support to the editorial, designing and production team. Their endless efforts to recruit the best for this project, has resulted in the accomplishment of this book. They are a veteran in the field of academics and their pool of knowledge is as vast as their experience in printing. Their expertise and guidance has proved useful at every step. Their uncompromising quality standards have made this book an exceptional effort. Their encouragement from time to time has been an inspiration for everyone.

The publisher and the editorial board hope that this book will prove to be a valuable piece of knowledge for researchers, students, practitioners and scholars across the globe.

List of Contributors

Samira Rajaei
Immunology Department, School of Medicine, Tehran University of Medical Sciences, Tehran, Iran

Ali Dabbagh
Cardiac Anesthesiology Department, Anesthesiology Research Center, Shahid Beheshti University of Medical Sciences, Tehran, Iran

Kamran Mottaghi, Farhad Safari, Parisa Sezari, Naeime Gholizadeh and Masoud Nashibi
Anesthesiology Research Center, Shahid Beheshti University of Medical Sciences, Tehran, Iran

Masoud Hashemi, Seyed Amir Mohajerani and Peyman Dadkhah
Anesthesiology Research Center, Department of Anesthesiology, Shahid Beheshti University of Medical Sciences, Tehran, Iran

Seyed Mehdi Hoseini Khameneh
Department of Orthopaedics Surgery, Shahid Beheshti University of Medical Sciences, Tehran, Iran

Anahita Hirm anpour, Reihanak Talakoub and Hamed Mansouri
Anesthesia and Critical Care Research Center, Alzahra Hospital, Department of Anesthesiology, School of Medicine, Isfahan University of Medical Sciences, Isfahan, Iran

Nazanin Babaei, Yasaman Aghajani, Noushin Khazaei and Ali Movafegh
Research Development Center, Dr. Ali Shariati Hospital, Tehran University of Medical Sciences, Tehran, Iran

Alireza Saliminia and Omid Azimaraghi
Department of Anesthesiology and Critical Care, Dr. Ali Shariati Hospital, Tehran University of Medical Sciences, Tehran, Iran

Hamid Haji Gholam Saryazdi, Gholamreza khalili, Reihanak Talakoub, Masoud Shahbazi and Saeed Abbasi
Anesthesia and Critical Care Research Center, Alzahra Hospital, Department of Anesthesiology, School of Medicine, Isfahan University of Medical sciences, Isfahan, Iran

Reihanak Talakoub, Gholam Reza Khalili and Babak Haghanifar
Anesthesiology and Critical Care Research Center, Isfahan University of Medical Sciences, Isfahan, Iran

Kamran Mottaghi, Rofeideh Fallahinejadghajari, Parisa Sezari, Mohammadreza Kamranmanesh and Masoud Nashibi
Anesthesiology Research Center, Shahid Beheshti University of Medical Sciences, Tehran, Iran

Seyed Mohammadreza Amouzegar Zavareh and Marzieh Lak
Department of Anesthesiology, School of Medicine, Baqiyatallah University of Medical Sciences, Tehran, Iran

Premal M. Trivedi, Erin A. Gottlieb and Emad B. Mossad
Department of Anesthesiology, Perioperative, and Pain Medicine, Texas Children's Hospital, Division of Pediatric Cardiovascular Anesthesiology, Baylor College of Medicine, Houston, TX, United States of America

Omid Aghadavoudi, Amir Shafa and Zahra Nowrouzi
Anesthesiology and Critical Care Research Center, Isfahan University of Medical Sciences, Isfahan, Iran

Mehrdad Taheri, Alireza Mirkheshti and Yalda Adili
Anesthesiology Research Center, Shahid Beheshti University of Medical Sciences, Tehran, Iran

Alireza Manafi Rasi
Department of Orthopedics, Shahid Beheshti University of Medical Sciences, Tehran, Iran

Reza Taherian
Student Research Committee, School of Medicine, Shahid Beheshti University of Medical Sciences, Tehran, Iran

Mahdi Taherian
Food and Drug Research Institute, Iran Food and Drug Administration, Ministry of Health and Medical Education, Tehran, Iran

Hossein Maghsoudi and Samaneh Haj-alahyar
Biotechnology Research Center, Payamenoor University, Tehran, Iran

Mohammadreza Moshari, Bahman Malek, Maryam Vosoghian, Mastaneh Dahi, Mahshid Ghasemi and Razieh Shekari
Anesthesiology Research Center, Taleghani Hospital, Shahid Beheshti University of Medical Sciences, Tehran, Iran

Mohammadreza Minator-Sajjadi
Taleghani Hospital Clinical Research Development Unit, Shahid Beheshti University of Medical Sciences, Tehran, Iran

Mohammad Reza Moshari, Bahman Malek B, Maryam Vosoughian, Mastaneh Dahi-Taleghani, Mahshid Ghasemi and Seyed Mohammad Seyed-Alshohadaei
Anesthesiology Research Center, Anesthesia Department, Taleghani Hospital, Shahid Beheshti University of Medical Sciences, Tehran, Iran

Siamak Yaghobi and Marzieh-Beigom Khezri
Department of Anesthesiology, School of Medicine, Qazvin University of Medical Sciences, Iran

Amir Hesam Alirezaei
Clinical Research Development Center at Shahid Modarres Hospital, Department of Nephrology, Shahid Beheshti University of Medical Sciences, Tehran, Iran

Mahmood Bakhtiyari
Department of Community Medicine, School of Medicine, Alborz University of Medical Sciences, Karaj, Iran
Department of Epidemiology and Biostatistics, School of Public Health, Tehran University of Medical Sciences, Tehran, Iran

Nilofar Massoudi
Clinical Research Development Center at Shahid Modarres Hospital, Department of Anesthesiology, Shahid Beheshti University of Medical Sciences, Tehran, Iran

Mohammad Fathi
Critical Care Quality Improvement Research Center, Shahid Beheshti University of Medical Sciences, Tehran, Iran

Nilofar Massoudi and Narges-Sadat Ghaemi
Anesthesiology Research Center, Shahid Beheshti University of Medical Sciences, Tehran, Iran

Navid Noraee
Clinical Research and Development Unit at Shahid Modarres Hospital, Department of Anesthesiology, Shahid Beheshti University of Medical Sciences, Tehran, Iran

Dawar Amani and Ali Asadirad
Department of Immunology, School of Medicine, Shahid Beheshti University of Medical Sciences, Tehran, Iran

Shahram Sayyadi, Morteza Jabbari Moghadam, Alireza Mirkheshti, Elham Memary, Dariush Abtahi, Sohrab Salimi and Ardeshir Tajbakhsh
Anesthesiology Research Center, Shahid Beheshti University of Medical Sciences, Tehran, Iran

Kamal Fani, Mona Hashem-Aghaei, Hossein Ali Jelveh-Moghaddam, Golnar Radmand and Ali Dabbagh
Anesthesiology Research Center, Cardiac Anesthesiology Department, Shahid Beheshti University of Medical Sciences, Tehran, Iran

Mahnoosh Foroughi
Cardiovascular Research Center, Shahid Beheshti University of Medical Sciences, Tehran, Iran

Samira Rajaei
Department of Immunology, School of Medicine, Tehran University of Medical Science, Tehran, Islamic Republic of Iran

Kamran Heidari and Masoome Lakestani
Emergency Medicine, Skull Base Research Center, Loghman Hakim Hospital, Shahid Beheshti University of Medical Sciences, Tehran, Iran

Reza Goharani and Mohammadreza Hajiesmaeili
Anesthesiology Research Center, Neurocritical Care Research Center, Loghman Hakim Hospital, Shahid Beheshti University of Medical Sciences, Tehran, Iran

Alireza Jafari, Mohammadreza Kamranmanesh, Homayoun Aghamohammadi, Babak Gharaei and Mehranoosh Noori Khorramabadian
Anesthesiology Research Center, Department of Anesthesia, Shahid Labbafinejad Medical Center, Shahid Beheshti University of Medical Sciences, Tehran, Iran

Behzad Narouie, Payam Sarmadi and Abbas Vali
Urology and Nephrology Research Center; Department of Urology, Shahid Labbafinejad Medical Center, Shahid Beheshti University of Medical Sciences, Tehran, Iran

Reza Valipour
Department of Urology, Tehran Medical Sciences Branch, Islamic Azad University, Tehran, Iran

Mohammadreza Moshari, Ronak Karbalaeifar, Maryam Vosoghian, Bahman Malek and Mastaneh Dahi-Taleghani
Anesthesiology Research Center, Shahid Beheshti University of Medical Sciences, Tehran, Iran

Mohammadreza Moshari, Bahman Malek, Maryam Vosoughian, Mastane Dahi-Taleghani, Ehsan Ghorbani and Seyed Mohammad Seyed-Alshohadaei
Anesthesiology Research Center, Shahid Beheshti University of Medical Sciences, Tehran, Iran

Adel Ebrahimpour
Department of Orthopedic Surgery, Taleghani Hospital, Shahid Beheshti University of Medical Sciences, Tehran, Iran

Abdorasoul Anvaripour and Houshang Shahryari
Anesthesiology department, Bushehr University of Medical sciences, Bushehr, Iran

Sayed Mehran Marashian
Chronic Respiratory Diseases Research Center, National Research Institute of Tuberculosis and Lung Diseases (NRITLD), Shahid Beheshti University of Medical Sciences, Tehran, Iran

Alireza Jahangirifard
Lung Transplantation Research Center, National Research Institute of Tuberculosis and Lung Diseases (NRITLD), Shahid Beheshti University of Medical Sciences, Tehran, Iran

Maryam Vosoughian, Mastaneh Dahi-Taleghani, Mohammadreza Moshari, Shima Rajabi and Farinaz Taheri
Anesthesiology Research Center, Shahid Beheshti University of Medical Sciences, Tehran, Iran

Samira Rajaei
Department of Immunology, School of Medicine, Tehran University of Medical Sciences, Tehran, Iran

Alireza Jahangirifard and Behrooz Farzanegan
Lung Transplantation Research Center, National Research Institute of Tuberculosis and Lung Diseases (NRITLD), Shahid Beheshti University of Medical Sciences, Tehran, Iran

Shirin Salajegheh
Department of Anesthesiology, Kerman University of Medical Sciences, Kerman, Iran

Sarvenaz Arab
Anesthesiology Research Center, Shahid Beheshti University of Medical Science, Tehran, Iran

Seyed Bashir Mirtajani
Mycobacteriology Research Center (MRC), National Research Institute of Tuberculosis and Lung Disease (NRITLD), Shahid Beheshti University of Medical Sciences, Tehran, Iran

Mohammad Zia Totonchi
Rajaie Cardiovascular center, Medical and Research Center, Tehran, Iran

Mohammad Forouzeshfard
Cancer Research Center, School of Medicine, Semnan University of Medical Sciences, Semnan, Iran

Mehran Ghoreishi and Kamal Fani
Anesthesiology Research Center, School of Medicine, Shahid Beheshti University of Medical Sciences, Tehran, Iran

Shirin Salajeghe
School of Dentistry, Kerman University of Medical Sciences, Kerman, Iran

Seyed Mohammad Seyed-Alshohadaei
Anesthesiology Research Center, Shahid Beheshti University of Medical Sciences, Tehran, Iran

Sadegh Abdolmohammadi
Department of Anesthesiology and Pain Medicine, Shahid Beheshti University of Medical Sciences, Loghman Hospital, Tehran, Iran

Alireza Nekoui and Gilbert Blaise
Centre Hospitalier de l'Université de Montréal (CHUM), University of Montreal, Montreal, Quebec, Canada

Lisa A. Caplan and M. Toni Felberg
Department of Anesthesiology, Perioperative, and Pain Medicine Baylor College of Medicine, Texas Children's Hospital, Houston, Texas, United States of America

Zahra Talebi, Ali Dabbagh, Hamid Kayalha, Siamak Yaghoobi and Marzieh Beygom Khezri
Cardiac Anesthesiology Department, Anesthesiology Research Center, Shahid Beheshti University of Medical Sciences, Tehran, Iran1- Shahid Rajaie Hospital, Qazvin University of Medical Sciences, Qazvin, Iran

Mohammad Kolahdoozha
Kosar Hospital, Qazvin University of Medical Sciences, Qazvin, Iran

Seyed Amir Mohajerani
Anesthesiology Research Center, Shahid Beheshti University of Medical Sciences, Tehran, Iran

Alireza Jahangirifard
Lung Transplantation Research Center, National Research Institute of Tuberculosis and Lung Diseases (NRITLD), Shahid Beheshti University of Medical Sciences, Tehran, Iran

Index

www.ingramcontent.com/pod-product-compliance
Lightning Source LLC
LaVergne TN
LVHW080709210926
848485LV00003B/441